T0226487

# Saphenous Vein Graft Lesions and Thrombectomy for Acute Myocardial Infarction

*Editors*

AMAR KRISHNASWAMY
SAMIR R. KAPADIA

# INTERVENTIONAL CARDIOLOGY CLINICS

www.interventional.theclinics.com

*Consulting Editors*
SAMIN K. SHARMA
IGOR F. PALACIOS

April 2013 • Volume 2 • Number 2

**ELSEVIER**

1600 John F. Kennedy Boulevard • Suite 1800 • Philadelphia, Pennsylvania 19103-2899

http://www.theclinics.com

**INTERVENTIONAL CARDIOLOGY CLINICS Volume 2, Number 2**
**April 2013 ISSN 2211-7458, ISBN-13: 978-1-4557-7109-7**

Editor: Barbara Cohen-Kligerman
Developmental Editor: Teia Stone

*Interventional Cardiology Clinics* (ISSN 2211-7458) is published quarterly by Elsevier Inc., 360 Park Avenue South, New York, NY 10010-1710. Months of issue are January, April, July, and October. Subscription prices are USD 188 per year for US individuals, USD 126 per year for US students, USD 281 per year for Canadian individuals, USD 144 per year for Canadian students, USD 281 per year for international individuals, and USD 144 per year for international students. To receive student/resident rate, orders must be accompanied by name of affiliated institution, date of term, and the *signature* of program/residency coordinator on institution letterhead. Orders will be billed at individual rate until proof of status is received. Foreign air speed delivery is included in all *Clinics* subscription prices. All prices are subject to change without notice. **POSTMASTER:** Send address changes to *Interventional Cardiology Clinics*, Elsevier Health Sciences Division, Subscription Customer Service, 3251 Riverport Lane, Maryland Heights, MO 63043. **Customer Service: Telephone: 1-800-654-2452** (U.S. and Canada); **1-314-447-8871** (outside U.S. and Canada). **Fax: 1-314-447-8029. E-mail: journalscustomerservice-usa@elsevier.com** (for print support); **journalsonlinesupport-usa@elsevier.com** (for online support).

*Reprints.* For copies of 100 or more of articles in this publication, please contact the Commercial Reprints Department, Elsevier Inc., 360 Park Avenue South, New York, NY 10010-1710. Tel.: 212-633-3812; Fax: 212-462-1935; E-mail: reprints@elsevier.com.

Printed and bound by CPI Group (UK) Ltd, Croydon, CR0 4YY

Transferred to digital print 2013

# Contributors

## CONSULTING EDITORS

**SAMIN K. SHARMA, MD, FSCAI, FACC**
Director of Clinical Cardiology; Director of Cardiac Catheterization Laboratory, Mount Sinai Medical Center, New York, New York

**IGOR F. PALACIOS, MD, FSCAI**
Director of Interventional Cardiology, Cardiology Division, Heart Center, Massachusetts General Hospital; Associate Professor of Medicine, Harvard Medical School, Boston, Massachusetts

## EDITORS

**AMAR KRISHNASWAMY, MD**
Cleveland Clinic, Cleveland, Ohio

**SAMIR R. KAPADIA, MD**
Cleveland Clinic, Cleveland, Ohio

## AUTHORS

**SAIF ANWARUDDIN, MD**
Assistant Professor of Medicine, Division of Cardiovascular Medicine, Hospital of the University of Pennsylvania, Philadelphia, Pennsylvania

**ANTHONY A. BAVRY, MD, MPH**
Assistant Professor of Medicine, Division of Cardiovascular Medicine, University of Florida, Gainesville, Florida

**DEEPAK L. BHATT, MD, MPH**
Senior Investigator, TIMI Study Group; Professor of Medicine, Harvard Medical School; Chief of Cardiology and Director, VA Boston Healthcare System; Director, Integrated Interventional Cardiovascular Program, Brigham and Women's Hospital, Boston, Massachusetts

**MATTHEWS CHACKO, MD**
Director, Peripheral Vascular Interventions; Co-Director, Cardiology Nurse Practitioner Service; Faculty, Interventional Cardiology, Coronary Care Unit and the Thayer Firm of the Osler Medical Service; Assistant Professor of Medicine, Division of Cardiology, Johns Hopkins Hospital, Johns Hopkins University, Baltimore, Maryland

**CARL A. DRAGSTEDT, DO**
Assistant Professor of Medicine, Division of Cardiovascular Medicine, University of Florida, Gainesville, Florida

**JOSEPH D. FOLEY III, MD**
Interventional Cardiology Fellow, Division of Cardiovascular Medicine, Gill Heart Institute, University of Kentucky, Lexington, Kentucky

**COREY FOSTER, MD**
Fellow, Interventional Cardiology, Cardiovascular Division, Department of Internal Medicine, Washington University School of Medicine, St Louis, Missouri

**SUCHETA GOSAVI, MD**
Department of Internal Medicine, Texas Tech University Health Sciences Center, El Paso, Texas

**HITINDER S. GURM, MD, FACC**
Associate Professor of Internal Medicine, Division of Cardiovascular Disease, Department of Internal Medicine, University of Michigan Cardiovascular Center, University of Michigan, Ann Arbor, Michigan

**AARON HORNE Jr, MD**
Interventional Cardiology Fellow, Division of Cardiology, Johns Hopkins Hospital, Johns Hopkins University, Baltimore, Maryland

**JOHN R. HOYT, MD**
Fellow, Cardiovascular Medicine, Division of Cardiovascular Disease, Department of Internal Medicine, Cardiovascular Center, University of Michigan, Ann Arbor, Michigan

**PEI-HSIU HUANG, MD**
Fellow, Interventional Cardiology, Division of Cardiovascular Medicine, Brigham and Women's Hospital, Harvard Medical School, Boston, Massachusetts

**ELENA LADICH, MD**
Department of Cardiovascular Pathology, CVPath Institute, Inc, Gaithersburg, Maryland

**EVAN LAU, MD**
Interventional Cardiology Fellow, Robert and Suzanne Tomsich Department of Cardiology, Cleveland Clinic Foundation, Cleveland, Ohio

**A. MICHAEL LINCOFF, MD**
Staff Interventional Cardiologist, Vice Chairman and Director, Department of Cardiovascular Medicine, Coordinating Center for Clinical Research, Cleveland Clinic, Cleveland, Ohio

**GABRIEL MALUENDA, MD**
Division of Cardiology, Department of Internal Medicine, Washington Hospital Center, Washington, DC

**DEBABRATA MUKHERJEE, MD, MS, FACC**
Acting Chairman, Department of Internal Medicine, Texas Tech University Health Sciences Center, El Paso, Texas

**MASATAKA NAKANO, MD**
Department of Cardiovascular Pathology, CVPath Institute, Inc, Gaithersburg, Maryland

**FUMIYUKI OTSUKA, MD**
Department of Cardiovascular Pathology, CVPath Institute, Inc, Gaithersburg, Maryland

**AUGUSTO D. PICHARD, MD, FACC**
Division of Cardiology, Department of Internal Medicine, Washington Hospital Center, Washington, DC

**SATYA SHREENIVAS, MD**
Division of Cardiovascular Medicine, Hospital of the University of Pennsylvania, Philadelphia, Pennsylvania

**RENU VIRMANI, MD**
Department of Cardiovascular Pathology, CVPath Institute, Inc, Gaithersburg, Maryland

**PATRICK WHITLOW, MD**
Director of Interventional Cardiology, Robert and Suzanne Tomsich Department of Cardiology, Cleveland Clinic Foundation, Cleveland, Ohio

**WILLIS M. WU, MD**
Interventional Cardiology Fellow, Department of Cardiovascular Medicine, Cleveland Clinic, Cleveland, Ohio

**SAAMI K. YAZDANI, PhD**
Department of Cardiovascular Pathology, CVPath Institute, Inc, Gaithersburg, Maryland

**ALAN ZAJARIAS, MD**
Assistant Professor of Medicine, Cardiovascular Division, Department of Internal Medicine, Washington University School of Medicine, St Louis, Missouri

**KHALED M. ZIADA, MD**
Gill Foundation Professor of Interventional Cardiology, Division of Cardiovascular Medicine, Gill Heart Institute, University of Kentucky, Lexington, Kentucky

# Contents

Saphenous vein grafts (SVGs) are the most used conduits in coronary artery bypass graft (CABG) surgery; however, they are susceptible to accelerated atherosclerosis. Clinical studies have shown 10-year patency rates of SVG can be as low as 50% to 60%. This article highlights changes that are observed following CABG surgery using SVG, including intimal thickening to the development of atherosclerotic changes, and how these changes in vein graft are different from those observed in native atherosclerosis. It also discusses the role of risk factors that contribute to acceleration of SVG atherosclerosis.

Aortocoronary saphenous vein graft is an effective treatment of coronary artery disease and a means of markedly improving long-term prognosis in certain patient subgroups. However, there is a significant failure rate with these conduits. Early failure occurs within the first 1—2 months, most likely from primary thrombosis. Intermediate failure is usually caused by the development of neointimal hyperplasia. Late failure occurs after 3—5 years and results from accelerated atherosclerosis. The impact of saphenous vein graft failure on cardiovascular outcomes is significant, and it is important to implement appropriate therapeutic strategies to prevent or minimize failure rates.

Saphenous vein graft (SVG) percutaneous coronary interventions (PCIs) are associated with adverse clinical events caused by distal embolization in 10% to 20% of cases. Various embolic protection devices (EPDs) have been developed to lower the risk of distal embolization during SVG PCI: distal balloon occlusive devices, distal embolic filters, and proximal balloon occlusive devices. Despite evidence for improved outcomes and cost-effectiveness, rates of national EPD use remain low, the main cause of underutilization being operator preference. With increasing familiarity of operators with EPDs, their use should continue to increase in SVG PCI and lead to better outcomes.

Coronary revascularization using saphenous vein grafts is an important treatment modality for patients with severe coronary artery disease. Percutaneous intervention of these grafts is often the best option for patients who develop severe stenosis of the vein grafts. Use of adjunctive glycoprotein IIb/IIIa inhibitors does not confer added benefit with ischemic endpoints as compared with heparin alone, but it increases the risk of bleeding. Bivalirudin used as the primary anticoagulant lowers the risk of bleeding. No-reflow frequently complicates vein graft interventions but can be treated with vasoactive agents such as calcium channel blockers, adenosine, and nitroprusside.

Percutaneous coronary intervention (PCI) of saphenous vein graft (SVG) is associated with higher adverse event rates, lower procedural success, and inferior long-term patency rates compared with native vessel PCI. The ability to comply with dual antiplatelet therapy, and whether the patient will need an interruption in dual antiplatelet therapy, should be considered when deciding whether to implant a drug-eluting stent (DES) or bare metal stent (BMS) in an SVG. DES should be used for SVG PCI because they seem to reduce target vessel revascularization. This article reviews the evolution and contemporary evidence regarding use of DES versus BMS in SVG PCI.

Percutaneous interventions of (usually degenerated) saphenous vein grafts (SVG) are associated with higher risk of distal embolization and worse clinical outcomes, including target vessel revascularization, myocardial infarction, and death, as compared with percutaneous coronary intervention of native coronary arteries. Embolic protection devices have demonstrated value in reducing the risk of embolization and postprocedural enzyme elevation after SVG interventions. Frequently, however, such devices are not used or cannot be used. As a result, novel stenting strategies intended to decrease the risk of periprocedural myocardial infarction seem to play a major role in enhancing the results following SVG interventions.

Interventions on vein graft occlusions are technically feasible procedures but carry significant risk for periprocedural complications and demonstrate questionable long-term patency. For those circumstances in which recanalization of a graft occlusion is warranted, the authors have highlighted some of the procedural considerations and available techniques that may help maximize chances for success. This should not be mistaken for a wholesale endorsement of vein graft chronic total occlusion interventions. Before undertaking a procedure of this complexity, the operator must put strong consideration into the risks, benefits, and alternatives for a given patient.

Coronary interventions of degenerated saphenous vein grafts (SVGs) continue to present a management challenge. Although repeat coronary artery bypass grafting

(CABG) remains a significant risk factor for operative mortality, percutaneous coronary intervention (PCI) is still associated with a high risk for periprocedural events. There is a lack of consensus on the optimal treatment strategy for patients with severe stenosis of SVGs. It is imperative to review the characteristics of native versus SVG disease, risk factors for complications after SVG intervention, procedural treatment strategies important to the decision on which therapeutic strategy to follow, and measures to mitigate the risks of periprocedural complications.

Because of greater patient comorbidities, more diffusely diseased vessels, and the greater possibility of mechanical complications, saphenous vein graft interventions are fraught with complications. The greatest risk is a higher risk of periprocedural myocardial infarction due to distal embolization of microemboli. The risk for no-reflow in a patient with concomitant native critical vessel disease can have grave consequences. Minimizing the risk of periprocedural myocardial infarction with the use of distal embolic protection, understanding the role of adjunctive pharmacotherapy, and learning how to manage less common but serious mechanical complications during saphenous vein graft interventions are important to ensure optimal patient outcomes.

Primary percutaneous coronary intervention is the favored mode of reperfusion therapy for ST-elevation myocardial infarction (STEMI) when able to be performed in a timely fashion in appropriately selected patients. However, controversy about the role of coronary thrombectomy in the management of STEMI persists because of a paucity of favorable historical data. After the TAPAS trial thrombectomy has gained favor in recent years. The results of the TOTAL, TASTE, and SMART percutaneous coronary intervention trials will provide further insight into the use of thrombectomy in STEMI. This article examines the relevant trial evidence regarding how to best manage and apply thrombectomy in clinical practice.

Thrombectomy in the setting of primary percutaneous coronary intervention allows for improved macrovascular and microvascular perfusion, possible limitation of infarct size, and the preservation of left ventricular function and myocardial viability. The beneficial tissue level effects of thrombectomy have translated into an improvement in cardiovascular mortality. A variety of thrombectomy devices are currently available, including aspiration thrombectomy catheters and rheolytic catheters. A review of the various types of thrombectomy devices available, clinical evidence for their use, clinical pearls for use, and device troubleshooting are presented.

Patients with unstable coronary syndromes are often found to have intracoronary thrombus on angiography. Despite advancements in catheter-based treatments for coronary disease, these lesions remain challenging, as percutaneous coronary intervention of thrombus-containing lesions may be associated with worse outcomes. This article reviews the literature on adjunctive pharmacotherapy in the treatment of thrombotic coronary lesions with special focus on ST-segment elevation myocardial infarction, lesions with high thrombus burden, and saphenous vein graft intervention.

# INTERVENTIONAL CARDIOLOGY CLINICS

**NOW AVAILABLE FOR YOUR iPhone and iPad**

# Preface

# Saphenous Vein Graft Stenosis and Thrombotic Lesions in Acute Myocardial Infarction

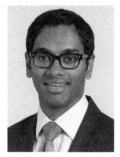 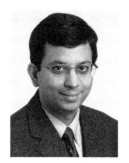

Amar Krishnaswamy, MD    Samir R. Kapadia, MD

*Editors*

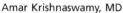

This issue of *Interventional Cardiology Clinics* provides a comprehensive review of two important clinical scenarios faced by interventional cardiologists: saphenous vein graft (SVG) stenosis and thrombotic lesions in acute myocardial infarction.

The use of SVGs is a mainstay in the surgical revascularization of coronary artery disease. Unfortunately, these conduits possess a limited lifespan, and patients often require repeat revascularization using percutaneous coronary intervention (PCI). Dr Mukherjee and colleagues and Dr Virmani and colleagues provide a comprehensive analysis of the natural history and histopathologic mechanisms of SVG failure and an understanding of the reasons for the high-risk nature of these interventions. Drs Ziada, Pichard, and Gurm and colleagues discuss the use of specific methods and devices to optimize the short-term and long-term results of SVG PCI, including embolic protection devices, intravascular imaging, and stent choice. Drs Lincoff and Wu provide a guide to the

appropriate use of adjunctive pharmacotherapies for SVG PCI, including antithrombotic treatments and strategies to combat the no-reflow phenomenon, while Drs Anwarrudin and Shreenivas provide a toolkit for operators when they encounter any of the myriad complications of SVG intervention. Drs Zajarias and Foster and Drs Whitlow and Lau address two important concepts: whether it is preferable to intervene on the native coronary artery in the setting of SVG disease and strategies for successful intervention on vein graft chronic total occlusion, respectively.

Acute myocardial infarction and thrombus-laden lesions present another difficult treatment setting for the practicing interventionalist. Dr Bavry and Dr Dragstedt provide a comprehensive analysis of the literature pertaining to both mechanical and aspiration thrombectomy, and Drs Chacko and Horne discuss the devices available for thrombectomy and their use. Finally, Dr Bhatt provides an understanding of the adjunctive intravenous,

Intervent Cardiol Clin 2 (2013) xi–xii
http://dx.doi.org/10.1016/j.iccl.2013.01.001
2211-7458/13/$ – see front matter © 2013 Published by Elsevier Inc.

intracoronary, and oral pharmacotherapy that is necessary for the successful treatment of patients with thrombotic coronary occlusion.

Each of these articles is meant to fit together to provide a comprehensive review of these topics, but they are written in such a way that even as stand-alone articles they provide the reader with a suitable understanding of the issues at hand. Our job as editors was made easy by the considerable effort put forth by these internationally recognized authors and their fellows, as well as the tireless labors of Ms Barbara Cohen-Kligerman to bring this publication to fruition. We give each and every one of them our sincerest thanks and hope that you find this publication a helpful and practical resource in your interventional cardiology practice.

Amar Krishnaswamy, MD
Cleveland Clinic
9500 Euclid Avenue, J2-3
Cleveland, OH 44195, USA

Samir R. Kapadia, MD
Cleveland Clinic
9500 Euclid Avenue, J2-3
Cleveland, OH 44195, USA

E-mail addresses:
KRISHNA2@ccf.org (A. Krishnaswamy)
kapadis@ccf.org (S.R. Kapadia)

# Pathology of Saphenous Vein Grafts

Saami K. Yazdani, PhD, Fumiyuki Otsuka, MD,
Masataka Nakano, MD, Elena Ladich, MD,
Renu Virmani, MD*

## KEYWORDS

• Saphenous vein grafts • Coronary artery bypass graft • Pathology • Anastomosis

## KEY POINTS

- Saphenous vein grafts (SVGs) are susceptible to accelerated atherosclerosis as compared with native coronary arteries, thus limiting the long-term benefits of coronary artery bypass graft surgery.
- As early as the first year after surgery, thickening of the wall by neointimal growth and infiltration of foamy macrophages is observed.
- SVG stenosis is associated with the development and expansion of necrotic cores and the occurrence of hemorrhage, leading to expansion and eventually rupture of the plaque.
- A better understanding of the mechanisms leading to SVG stenosis will facilitate the findings of more robust therapeutic strategies to reduce the need for percutaneous or surgical intervention.

## INTRODUCTION

Coronary artery bypass graft (CABG) surgery remains a cornerstone for the treatment of severe coronary artery atherosclerosis.[1,2] CABG surgery has been shown to prolong life, especially in patients with multivessel coronary artery (3-vessel disease) and left main disease in patients with arterial anatomy in whom percutaneous approaches are unlikely to afford long-term lumen patency (eg, heavily calcified lesions and diffused atherosclerotic disease). Although arterial grafts have been shown to be superior for CABG, they are not always available, which has led to the use of the more plentiful and more easily harvestable saphenous vein grafts (SVGs).[3,4] SVGs, unlike their arterial counterparts, are susceptible to the rapid development of atherosclerosis; therefore interventional procedures are common after 5 to 10 years.[5,6] The reported rates of vein bypass graft occlusion are 8% early after the operation, 13% at 1 year, 20% at 5 years, 41% at 10 years, and 45% at more than 11.5 years.[7,8] This article discusses the pathologic stages of the disease and other factors leading to the failure of saphenous vein bypass grafts.

## EARLY CHANGES

Within the first 72 hours after placement, a thin layer of platelets and fibrin is deposited along the vein graft intimal surface. During this period, acute inflammatory cells are often present in the walls of the grafts. Diffused intimal hyperplasia consisting of smooth muscle cells in a proteoglycan and collagen matrix is always observed in vein grafts in place for over 1 month.[9–12] The mechanism of this remodeling process[11] is believed to involve responses to endothelial injury and hemodynamic stress as the vein wall is subjected to the increased distending pressure of the arterial circulation. These hemodynamic changes lead

Dr Virmani is a consultant for Medtronic AVE, Abbott Vascular, W.L. Gore, Atrium Medical, Arsenal Medical, and Lutonix.
Department of Cardiovascular Pathology, CVPath Institute, Inc. 19 Firstfield Road, Gaithersburg, MD 20878, USA
* Corresponding author.
E-mail address: rvirmani@cvpath.org

to increased levels of intracellular adhesion molecule-1 (ICAM-1), vascular adhesion molecule-1 (VCAM-1), and monocyte chemotactic protein-1 (MCP-1).[13] The initial extent of intimal thickening is inversely proportional to flow though the graft,[14] suggesting that the differences in flow rates between arterial and venous beds play an important role in the progression of vein graft disease.[15] Alteration in flow may also diminish nitric oxide production and trigger smooth muscle cell proliferation.[16] In vein grafts that demonstrate long-term patency, the vein lumen diameter approximates the lumen diameter of the native coronary artery to which it is anastomosed.[17] Over the course of a year after bypass surgery, medical smooth muscle cell loss with focal medial fibrosis and adventitial thickening is commonly seen.[6]

## VEIN GRAFT THROMBOSIS

Early graft failure due to thrombotic complications may occur secondary to damage to the vein itself during harvest and insertion, leading to excessive endothelial injury; poor run-off due to plaque present at the anastomosis and/or severe distal native coronary atherosclerosis; or technical factors (eg, graft twisting or kinking or distal arterial dissection during creation of the anastomosis).[8,11,18–20] Vein graft occlusion rates within the first postoperative month range from 3% to 12%, and occlusion is secondary to graft thrombosis in most cases.[7,8,21] Pathologically, the vein graft is obstructed and distended with thrombus in its entire course in patients who do not survive the early postoperative period. Additionally, acute myocardial infarction is seen in the territory supplied by the thrombosed grafts. In patients who survive at least several months following CABG surgery in which acute vein graft thrombosis occurred, the graft appears as a thin fibrous cord throughout its length. Histologically, the vein wall is markedly contracted, and the small lumen is occluded by organized thrombus characterized by a collagen and proteoglycan matrix containing smooth muscle cells and small recanalization channels.

## CHRONIC VEIN GRAFT VASCULOPATHY: FIBROINTIMAL HYPERPLASIA AND ATHEROSCLEROSIS

For most vein grafts, vasculopathy develops as an insidious lesion that is a major cause of morbidity and mortality. With the continued high volume of patients treated with CABG surgery and the aging of the population, the rates of repeat revascularization procedures (catheter-based and repeat CABG surgery) are increasing. During the first 6 years after CABG surgery, the rate of vein graft occlusion is 1% to 2% per year; from 6 to 10 years postoperatively, the occlusion rate increases to 4% per year.[22,23] By 10 years after CABG surgery, only 60% of vein grafts are patent, and only 50% of vein grafts are free of significant lumen stenosis.[7,21,24,25]

The basic lesions of chronic vein graft vasculopathy are intimal hyperplasia, atherosclerosis, and combined atherosclerosis and fibrointimal proliferation. In an autopsy study of 177 SVGs in place 1 to 14 years antemortem, 25 demonstrated atherosclerosis; 66 demonstrated fibrointimal hyperplasia without atherosclerosis, and 26 were fibrous cords (chronic total occlusion).[26] While the accumulation of fibrointimal hyperplasia did not cause severe graft narrowing in most cases, it was associated with greater than 50% lumen area narrowing in 30% of grafts. Of grafts with atherosclerosis, 84% had greater than 50% lumen area narrowing (of which 64% had >75% lumen area stenosis).[26]

## SVG DISEASE—RISK FACTORS

Risk factors for native coronary artery atherosclerosis, particularly abnormal serum lipids, have also been correlated with atherosclerosis of bypass vein grafts.[17,25–28] From clinical studies of the known atherosclerotic risk factors, elevated serum total cholesterol, low-density lipoprotein (LDL) cholesterol and triglycerides, and low serum high-density lipoprotein (HDL) cholesterol levels appear to be important in the development of chronic vein graft atherosclerosis.[29–31] Reducing LDL cholesterol levels to less than 100 mg/dL with the lipid-lowering agent lovastatin (40 to 80 mg/day) with or without cholestyramine (8g/day) is associated with an increased frequency of vein graft patency.[32]

Morphologic studies from autopsy hearts have been generally supportive of the association of abnormal lipid levels and vein graft disease, and have provided histologic confirmation of the presence of atherosclerotic lesions (in contrast to fibrointimal hyperplasia).[26–28] In the previously noted morphologic autopsy study of vein grafts, 68% of atherosclerotic vein grafts were associated with hypercholesterolemia, compared with only 15% with fibrointimal hyperplasia.[26]

Morphological and angiography studies have also shown that cigarette smoking is a risk factor for vein graft atherosclerosis.[28,33] Studies of the relationship between diabetes mellitus and vein graft atherosclerosis have yielded inconsistent results.[8] There was a trend toward a higher mean serum glucose level in patients with vein graft atherosclerosis studied at autopsy versus those with fibrointimal hyperplasia.[26] In contrast to abnormal lipid levels and vein graft atherosclerosis, systemic hypertension appears to be associated with fibrointimal hyperplasia. Among autopsy vein grafts, 75% of grafts exhibiting fibroinitmal hyperplasia (without atherosclerosis) were from patients with hypertension versus 25% of vein grafts with atherosclerosis,[26] although ruptured plaques may be seen more often in patients with hypertension.[8,22,28,34]

## SVG ATHEROSCLEROSIS: PROGRESSION

To examine the progression of vein graft atherosclerotic lesions, the authors recently performed serial sectioning of morphological assessment of 31 SVGs from 16 patients in whom vein grafts were in place at least 2 years (mean age of vein graft 8.5 ± 5.9 years, range 2–22 years).[35] There were 589 vein graft sections examined, of which 333 demonstrated fibrointimal thickening (FIT), and the remaining 256 showed atherosclerotic changes. Atherosclerotic lesions were classified as: intimal xanthoma (IX) or superficial foam cell lesions, characterized by surface foam cell

accumulation without a fibrous cap or lipid core (**Fig. 1**); fibroatheroma with necrotic core (FA), which had well-developed necrotic cores (**Fig. 2**); lesions with hemorrhagic necrotic cores (HNCs); and plaque ruptures (PRs) (**Fig. 3**).

In IX lesions (fatty streak), there was accumulation of macrophages along the intimal surface; the vein graft intima consisted of proteoglycan and collagen (see **Fig. 1**). In a previous study, vein graft intimal smooth muscle cell apoptosis was observed at sites of foam cell accumulation, raising the possibility that a foam cell-derived factor can induce smooth muscle cell death.[36] In the authors' study, there was a continuous significant progression of lumen area percent stenosis from IX lesion (37% ± 9% stenosis) to fibroatheroma (46% ± 17%) to hemorrhagic lipid core lesions (52% ± 19%) (**Table 1**). Once a lipid core forms in an atherosclerotic vein graft, the risk of core hemorrhage increases as the lipid core size increases (see **Table 1**). Therefore, vein graft atherosclerotic stenosis progression likely passes though phases of macrophage deposition on the vein graft intima followed by development of a lipid core; lipid core hemorrhage results in greater lumen stenosis progression. These data suggest

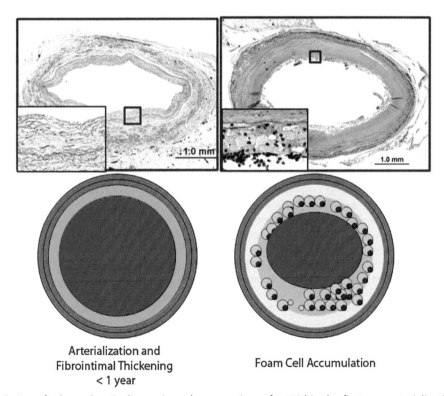

Arterialization and
Fibrointimal Thickening
< 1 year

Foam Cell Accumulation

**Fig. 1.** Initiation of atherosclerotic disease in saphenous vein grafts. Within the first year, arterialization and fibroinitmal thickening (higher magnification) of the vein graft are observed. This is followed by foam cell accumulation (higher magnification) within the neointima.

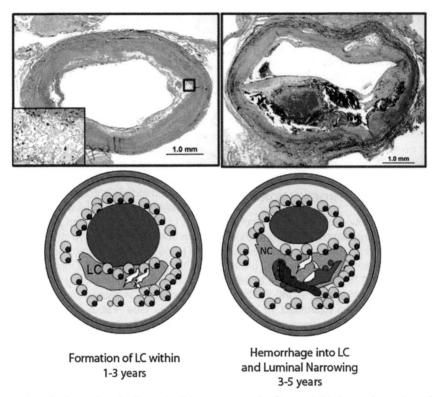

**Fig. 2.** Progression of atherosclerotic disease in SVGs. Between the first and third year, formation of a lipid core (LC) (higher magnification) is observed. After 4 to 5 years, hemorrhage into the lipid core and moderate-to-severe lumen narrowing are observed.

that inhibition of foam cell adherence is a potential therapeutic target for preventing SVG atherosclerosis and may be the mechanism for enhanced vein graft patency as has been demonstrated in lipid-lowering trials.[32]

In patients with vein graft atherosclerosis, acute plaque rupture and lumen thrombosis are important mechanisms of morbidity and mortality.[29,37] In the authors' study of vein graft atherosclerosis progression, plaque rupture and acute thrombosis were identified in 23% of sections with lipid core present. The mean lumen area stenosis in ruptured plaques was 75% plus or minus 24%, which corresponds to a diameter stenosis of 55% plus or minus 23% (95% confidence interval 42%–67%). Similar to lipid core hemorrhage, the risk of plaque rupture increased as the total lipid core size increased and as the percentage of the entire atherosclerotic plaque area. In vein graft atherosclerosis, a diameter stenosis of at least 55% with lipid core area of at least 5.1 mm$^2$ that occupies at least 44% of the total plaque area were morphologic predictors of plaque rupture and lumen thrombosis. Fibrous caps were 2.6-fold thinner in plaques with cap rupture compared with nonrupture plaques. Further, vein

graft plaque rupture sites were frequently long (mean length 6.6 mm) and multifocal (3.2 rupture sites per vein graft); they additionally were associated with long segments of plaque (2.1 cm) containing large, nonruptured lipid cores. This finding underscores the diffuse nature of vein graft atherosclerosis and the limited therapeutic benefit of percutaneous treatment that only addresses short focal lesion stenosis. Currently, there is an expanding use of interventional strategies (eg, embolic protection devices) in which multiple areas are treated to reduce the incidence of necrotic core prolapse and embolization during stenting.[18]

## SVG DISEASE: COMPARISON TO CORONARY ATHEROSCLEROSIS

The histology of SVG atherosclerosis differs somewhat from native coronary atherosclerosis and may reflect the relatively rapid development of atherosclerotic disease in vein grafts less than 10 years. Typically, advanced atherosclerosis in vein grafts consists of a friable foam cell-rich lesion containing a large lipid (necrotic) core or several cores and a thin fibrous cap.[6,38,39] Intraplaque

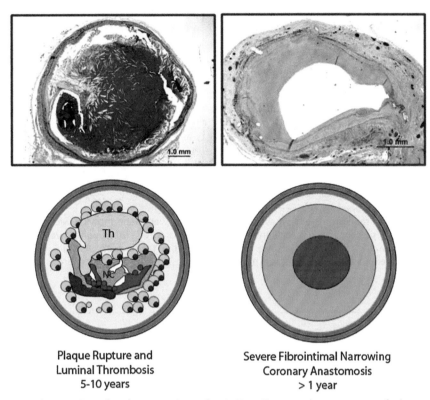

**Fig. 3.** Rupture and narrowing of saphenous vein grafts. At 5 to 10 years, plaque rupture of a large necrotic core accompanied with hemorrhage often leads to luminal thrombus. At the coronary anastomosis, fibroinitmal growth is commonly observed, whereas atherosclerosis is uncommon. NC, necrotic core; Th, thrombus.

hemorrhage within the large core is common (see **Fig. 3**), even in small plaques, but fibrocalcific lesions in vein grafts are rare and the significance debated (**Fig. 4**).[39–42] Just as in native coronary arteries, rupture of the fibrous cap can precipitate acute thrombus formation leading to acute myocardial infarction (**Fig. 5**).[29,37] The friable, necrotic features of vein graft atherosclerotic plaques are probably responsible for the high incidence of distal emobolization (resulting in non-Q wave myocardial infarction and elevation of serum levels of cardiac enzymes) when these vessels are treated with catheter-based therapies (balloon angioplasty and stents).

On the other hand, native vessel coronary artery disease takes at least 4 to 5 decades and is a slow-growing process with many more stages of plaque progression. The fatty streak lesion is observed in the first and second decades, especially in thoracic and abdominal aorta and midright

**Table 1**
**Lesion morphology, stenosis, and lipid core size of SVBG (>2 years)**

| Changes in SVBG | Incidence Per Lesion (%) | Number of Sections (%) | IEL Area (mm²) | Stenosis (%) | Lipid Core Area (mm²) | % Lipid Core |
|---|---|---|---|---|---|---|
| Fibrointimal thickening (FIT) | 28 (90.3) | 333 (56.5) | 10.97 ± 2.28 | 34 ± 15 | - | - |
| IX | 23 (74.2) | 111 (18.8) | 12.36 ± 3.02 | 37 ± 9 | - | - |
| FA | 20 (64.5) | 70 (11.9) | 14.08 ± 2.59 | 46 ± 17 | 1.5 ± 1.9 | 18 ± 19 |
| HNC | 17 (54.8) | 44 (7.5) | 14.62 ± 2.72 | 52 ± 19 | 2.8 ± 3.3 | 28 ± 31 |
| PR | 10 (32.3) | 31 (6.3) | 15.35 ± 3.56 | 75 ± 24 | 9.3 ± 7.9 | 57 ± 51 |

*Abbreviations:* IEL, internal elastic lamina; SVBG, saphenous vein bypass graft.
   *Reproduced from* Yazdani SK, Farb A, Nakano M, et al. Pathology of drug-eluting versus bare-metal stents in saphenous vein bypass graft lesions. JACC Cardiovasc Interv 2012;5:668; with permission.

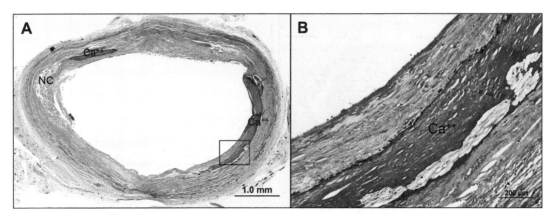

**Fig. 4.** Calcification of a saphenous vein bypass graft. (*A*) A low-power image showing wide open vein graft with calcified sheets ($Ca^{++}$) present in the intima and small necrotic core (NC). (*B*) A high-power image showing thin sheet calcification close to the luminal surface. (*Reproduced from* Yazdani SK, Otsuka F, Nakano M, et al. Do animal models of vein graft atherosclerosis predict outcomes in man? Atherosclerosis 2012;223:104; with permission.)

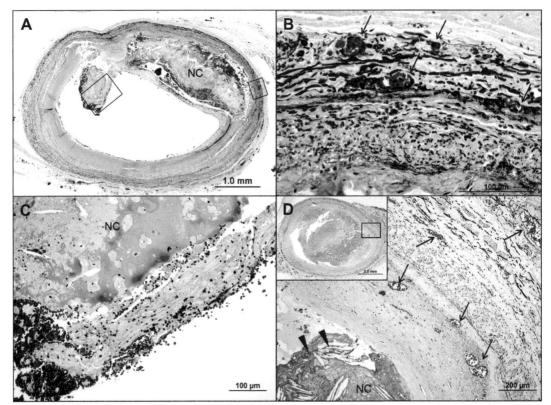

**Fig. 5.** Plaque rupture with intraplaque hemorrhage and angiogenesis. (*A*) A low-power image showing a moderately narrowed bypass vein graft of 5 years in duration with plaque hemorrhage within a large necrotic core (NC). Boxed areas highlight the angiogenesis (*B*) and rupture sites (*C*). (*B*) A high-power view showing angiogenesis (*arrows*), which are mostly located in the vein wall with few present in the neointima. (*C*) A high-power image showing the rupture of the thin fibrous cap with underlying necrotic core filled with fibrin and red cells. (*D*) A low-power image showing an occluded vein graft with plaque rupture and overlying thrombus. A high-power image represents remarkable angiogenesis (*arrows*) within the plaque and adventitia as well as intraplaque hemorrhage within the necrotic core (*arrow heads*). (*Reproduced from* Yazdani SK, Otsuka F, Nakano M, et al. Do animal models of vein graft atherosclerosis predict outcomes in man? Atherosclerosis 2012;223:103; with permission.)

coronary arteries; however, with age, these lesions tend to regress.

In advanced atherosclerotic lesions, true vein graft aneurysms may form; these lesions may be multiple and are most often seen in grafts present over 5 years.[43–45] Vein graft aneurysms contain large poorly formed thrombi that occupy a large portion of the lumen. Another feature of degenerated atherosclerotic vein grafts is medial atrophy or complete disruption; in the latter instance, there may be extrusion of plaque contents into the adventitia associated with an adventitial inflammatory reaction (forming a psedoaneurysm).

## SVG FAILURE: ANASTOMOSIS

The proximal and distal sites of anastomosis (junction between graft and host vessel) are frequent sites of late graft failure, an effect that is partly related to adaptive responses to hemodynamic factors including wall shear stress.[46,47] Within the authors' study at the aortic anastomosis, approximately 67% of sites showed only fibrointimal proliferation, and 33% of sites had atherosclerotic plaque (with or without lipid core formation). At the distal anastomosis of the SVG to the native coronary artery, only 4% of sites demonstrated atherosclerotic plaque, and 96% of sites showed fibrointimal thickening (see **Fig. 3**).

## SUMMARY

Compared with native coronary arteries, SVGs undergo more rapid atherosclerotic lesion development, thus limiting the long-term benefits of CABG surgery. As early as the first year after surgery, thickening of the wall by neointimal growth and infiltration of foamy macrophages are observed. SVG stenosis is associated with the development and expansion of necrotic cores and the occurrence of hemorrhage, leading to expansion and eventually rupture of the plaque. A thorough understanding of the mechanisms leading to SVG stenosis will facilitate the development of more robust therapeutic strategies to reduce the need for percutaneous or surgical intervention.

## REFERENCES

1. Yusuf S, Zucker D, Peduzzi P, et al. Effect of coronary artery bypass graft surgery on survival: overview of 10-year results from randomised trials by the Coronary Artery Bypass Graft Surgery Trialists Collaboration. Lancet 1994;344:563–70.
2. Davis KB, Chaitman B, Ryan T, et al. Comparison of 15-year survival for men and women after initial medical or surgical treatment for coronary artery disease: a CASS registry study. Coronary Artery Surgery Study. J Am Coll Cardiol 1995;25:1000–9.
3. Tsui JC, Dashwood MR. Recent strategies to reduce vein graft occlusion: a need to limit the effect of vascular damage. Eur J Vasc Endovasc Surg 2002; 23:202–8.
4. Nwasokwa ON. Coronary artery bypass graft disease. Ann Intern Med 1995;123:528–45.
5. Hamby RI, Aintablian A, Handler M, et al. Aortocoronary saphenous vein bypass grafts. Long-term patency, morphology and blood flow in patients with patent grafts early after surgery. Circulation 1979;60:901–9.
6. Virmani R, Atkinson JB, Forman MB. Aortocoronary saphenous vein bypass grafts. Cardiovasc Clin 1988;18:41–62.
7. Fitzgibbon GM, Kafka HP, Leach AJ, et al. Coronary bypass graft fate and patient outcome: angiographic follow-up of 5,065 grafts related to survival and reoperation in 1,388 patients during 25 years. J Am Coll Cardiol 1996;28:616–26.
8. Motwani JG, Topol EJ. Aortocoronary saphenous vein graft disease: pathogenesis, predisposition, and prevention. Circulation 1998;97:916–31.
9. Bulkley BH, Hutchins GM. Accelerated "atherosclerosis". A morphologic study of 97 saphenous vein coronary artery bypass grafts. Circulation 1977;55: 163–9.
10. Kern WH, Dermer GB, Lindesmith GG. The intimal proliferation in aortic-coronary saphenous vein grafts. Light and electron microscopic studies. Am Heart J 1972;84:771–7.
11. Vlodaver Z, Edwards JE. Pathologic changes in aortic-coronary arterial saphenous vein grafts. Circulation 1971;44:719–28.
12. Ip JH, Fuster V, Badimon L, et al. Syndromes of accelerated atherosclerosis: role of vascular injury and smooth muscle cell proliferation. J Am Coll Cardiol 1990;15:1667–87.
13. Zou Y, Dietrich H, Hu Y, et al. Mouse model of venous bypass graft arteriosclerosis. Am J Pathol 1998;153:1301–10.
14. Morinaga K, Eguchi H, Miyazaki T, et al. Development and regression of intimal thickening of arterially transplanted autologous vein grafts in dogs. J Vasc Surg 1987;5:719–30.
15. Meyerson SL, Skelly CL, Curi MA, et al. The effects of extremely low shear stress on cellular proliferation and neointimal thickening in the failing bypass graft. J Vasc Surg 2001;34:90–7.
16. Rao GN, Berk BC. Active oxygen species stimulate vascular smooth muscle cell growth and proto-oncogene expression. Circ Res 1992;70: 593–9.
17. Barboriak JJ, Batayias GE, Pintar K, et al. Pathological changes in surgically removed aortocoronary vein grafts. Ann Thorac Surg 1976;21:524–7.

18. Virmani R, Atkinson JB, Forman MB. Aortocoronary bypass grafts and extracardiac conduits. New York: Churchill Livingstone; 1991.

19. Waller BF, Roberts WC. Remnant saphenous veins after aortocoronary bypass grafting: analysis of 3,394 centimeters of unused vein from 402 patients. Am J Cardiol 1985;55:65–71.

20. Barboriak JJ, Pintar K, Van Horn DL, et al. Pathologic findings in the aortocoronary vein grafts. A scanning electron microscope study. Atherosclerosis 1978;29:69–80.

21. Bourassa MG. Fate of venous grafts: the past, the present and the future. J Am Coll Cardiol 1991;17: 1081–3.

22. Domanski MJ, Borkowf CB, Campeau L, et al. Prognostic factors for atherosclerosis progression in saphenous vein grafts: the postcoronary artery bypass graft (Post-CABG) trial. Post-CABG Trial Investigators. J Am Coll Cardiol 2000;36:1877–83.

23. Mehta D, Izzat MB, Bryan AJ, et al. Towards the prevention of vein graft failure. Int J Cardiol 1997; 62(Suppl 1):S55–63.

24. Acinapura AJ, Rose DM, Jacobowitz IJ, et al. Internal mammary artery bypass grafting: influence on recurrent angina and survival in 2,100 patients. Ann Thorac Surg 1989;48:186–91.

25. Campeau L, Enjalbert M, Lesperance J, et al. The relation of risk factors to the development of atherosclerosis in saphenous-vein bypass grafts and the progression of disease in the native circulation. A study 10 years after aortocoronary bypass surgery. N Engl J Med 1984;311:1329–32.

26. Atkinson JB, Forman MB, Vaughn WK, et al. Morphologic changes in long-term saphenous vein bypass grafts. Chest 1985;88:341–8.

27. Lie JT, Lawrie GM, Morris GC Jr. Aortocoronary bypass saphenous vein graft atherosclerosis. Anatomic study of 99 vein grafts from normal and hyperlipoproteinemic patients up to 75 months postoperatively. Am J Cardiol 1977;40:906–14.

28. Neitzel GF, Barboriak JJ, Pintar K, et al. Atherosclerosis in aortocoronary bypass grafts. Morphologic study and risk factor analysis 6 to 12 years after surgery. Arteriosclerosis 1986;6:594–600.

29. Solymoss BC, Nadeau P, Millette D, et al. Late thrombosis of saphenous vein coronary bypass grafts related to risk factors. Circulation 1988;78:I140–3.

30. Linden T, Bondjers G, Karlsson T, et al. Serum triglycerides and HDL cholesterol—major predictors of long-term survival after coronary surgery. Eur Heart J 1994;15:747–52.

31. Daida H, Yokoi H, Miyano H, et al. Relation of saphenous vein graft obstruction to serum cholesterol levels. J Am Coll Cardiol 1995;25:193–7.

32. The effect of aggressive lowering of low-density lipoprotein cholesterol levels and low-dose anticoagulation on obstructive changes in saphenous-vein coronary-artery bypass grafts. The Post Coronary Artery Bypass Graft Trial Investigators. N Engl J Med 1997;336:153–62.

33. FitzGibbon GM, Leach AJ, Kafka HP. Atherosclerosis of coronary artery bypass grafts and smoking. CMAJ 1987;136:45–7.

34. Pregowski J, Tyczynski P, Mintz GS, et al. Incidence and clinical correlates of ruptured plaques in saphenous vein grafts: an intravascular ultrasound study. J Am Coll Cardiol 2005;45:1974–9.

35. Yazdani SK, Farb A, Nakano M, et al. Pathology of drug-eluting versus bare-metal stents in saphenous vein bypass graft lesions. JACC Cardiovasc Interv 2012;5:666–74.

36. Kockx MM, De Meyer GR, Bortier H, et al. Luminal foam cell accumulation is associated with smooth muscle cell death in the intimal thickening of human saphenous vein grafts. Circulation 1996;94: 1255–62.

37. Walts AE, Fishbein MC, Matloff JM. Thrombosed, ruptured atheromatous plaques in saphenous vein coronary artery bypass grafts: ten years' experience. Am Heart J 1987;114:718–23.

38. Sisto T, Yla-Herttuala S, Luoma J, et al. Biochemical composition of human internal mammary artery and saphenous vein. J Vasc Surg 1990;11: 418–22.

39. Mautner SL, Mautner GC, Hunsberger SA, et al. Comparison of composition of atherosclerotic plaques in saphenous veins used as aortocoronary bypass conduits with plaques in native coronary arteries in the same men. Am J Cardiol 1992;70: 1380–7.

40. Walts AE, Fishbein MC, Sustaita H, et al. Ruptured atheromatous plaques in saphenous vein coronary artery bypass grafts: a mechanism of acute, thrombotic, late graft occlusion. Circulation 1982; 65:197–201.

41. Castagna MT, Mintz GS, Ohlmann P, et al. Incidence, location, magnitude, and clinical correlates of saphenous vein graft calcification: an intravascular ultrasound and angiographic study. Circulation 2005;111:1148–52.

42. Lardenoye JH, de Vries MR, Lowik CW, et al. Accelerated atherosclerosis and calcification in vein grafts: a study in apoe*3 leiden transgenic mice. Circ Res 2002;91:577–84.

43. Pintar K, Barboriak JJ, Johnson WD, et al. Atherosclerotic aneurysm in aortocoronary vein graft. Arch Pathol Lab Med 1978;102:287–8.

44. Taliercio CP, Smith HC, Pluth JR, et al. Coronary artery venous bypass graft aneurysm with symptomatic coronary artery emboli. J Am Coll Cardiol 1986; 7:435–7.

45. Liang BT, Antman EM, Taus R, et al. Atherosclerotic aneurysms of aortocoronary vein grafts. Am J Cardiol 1988;61:185–8.

46. Leask RL, Butany J, Johnston KW, et al. Human saphenous vein coronary artery bypass graft morphology, geometry and hemodynamics. Ann Biomed Eng 2005;33:301–9.

47. Butany JW, David TE, Ojha M. Histological and morphometric analyses of early and late aortocoronary vein grafts and distal anastomoses. Can J Cardiol 1998;14:671–7.

# Natural History of Saphenous Vein Grafts

Sucheta Gosavi, MD, Debabrata Mukherjee, MD, MS*

## KEYWORDS

• Saphenous vein grafts • Bypass surgery • Graft failure

## KEY POINTS

- The natural history of saphenous vein graft suggests significant failure rate with only 80% of saphenous vein grafts remaining patent 5 years after surgery and about 60% remaining patent at 7–10 years.
- Saphenous vein graft failure is related to 3 distinct but interrelated pathologic processes: thrombosis, intimal hyperplasia, and atherosclerosis.
- Early thrombosis is a major cause of vein graft loss during the first month after bypass surgery, whereas during the remainder of the first year, intimal hyperplasia forms a template for subsequent atherogenesis, which thereafter predominates.
- The spectrum of risk factors predisposing to vein graft atherosclerosis and its clinical sequelae is broadly similar to that recognized for native coronary disease.
- The clinical impact of saphenous vein graft failure is significant, and concerted multifaceted strategies are needed to prevent graft failure.
- Important elements of this preventive strategy include continued improvements in surgical technique and the optimal use of the most effective antithrombotic agents and more intensive risk factor modification (in particular early and aggressive lipid-lowering drug therapy and complete smoking cessation).

## INTRODUCTION

Aortocoronary saphenous vein graft (SVG) implantation in humans was first performed by Garrett and colleagues[1] in May 1967, and later the technique was further refined by Favaloro.[2] This advance in surgical practice led to an effective treatment of coronary artery disease and a means of markedly improving long-term prognosis in certain patient subgroups. However, with demonstration of the dramatic benefits obtained by saphenous vein grafting came the recognition of significant failure rate with these conduits (**Fig. 1**). Here we review the natural history of vein grafts, compare SVGs with other conduits, and describe strategies to favorably modify the failure rate and improve long-term patency.

## PATHOGENESIS OF SVG FAILURE

SVG failure has a trimodal distribution.[3] Early failure occurs within the first 1–2 months, most likely from primary thrombosis caused by technical factors, poor runoff into small or severely diseased distal coronary arteries, or unrecognized intrinsic saphenous vein disease at the time of implantation.[4,5] Intermediate failure of saphenous vein grafts is usually caused by the development of neointimal hyperplasia, which is most prominent in the first year after bypass surgery but may occur

Department of Internal Medicine, Texas Tech University Health Sciences Center, 4800 Alberta Avenue, El Paso, TX 79905, USA
* Corresponding author.
E-mail address: debabrata.mukherjee@ttuhsc.edu

Intervent Cardiol Clin 2 (2013) 251–258
http://dx.doi.org/10.1016/j.iccl.2012.11.001
2211-7458/13/$ – see front matter © 2013 Elsevier Inc. All rights reserved

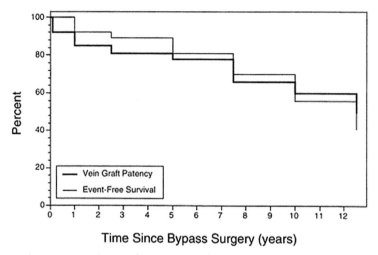

**Fig. 1.** Long-term graft patency and event-free survival after saphenous vein bypass surgery. (*Adapted from Motwani JG, Topol EJ. Aortocoronary saphenous vein graft disease: pathogenesis, predisposition, and prevention. Circulation 1998;97(9):916–31; with permission.*)

up to 3 years after implantation.[6] Late failure occurs after 3–5 years and results from accelerated atherosclerosis.[7]

### Primary Thrombosis

The harvesting of venous conduits itself is associated with focal endothelial disruption.[8] The high-pressure distension used to overcome venospasm during harvesting may also cause endothelial cell loss and medial damage.[8] Loss of the endothelial monolayer results in the accumulation of fibrin on the luminal surface, the adherence of platelets and neutrophils, and a reduction in tissue plasminogen activator production.[9–11] Endothelial loss may also activate the extrinsic coagulation cascade by tissue factor that is constitutively expressed in the exposed subendothelium. Thrombomodulin is an important membrane-bound antithrombotic regulatory protein that forms a 1:1 complex with thrombin, leading to activation of the circulating anticoagulant molecule, protein C. The process of vein harvesting attenuates the activity of thrombomodulin by up to 30%, which has an additional procoagulant effect.[12]

In addition, the inherent antithrombotic properties of veins are weaker compared with those of arteries. Heparan sulfate, a proteoglycan molecule with anticoagulant properties mediated by potentiation of antithrombin III, is less prominent in the media and in the poorly developed internal elastic lamina of veins compared with arteries.[13] Production of nitric oxide (NO) and prostacyclin, both potent inhibitors of platelet activation, is lower in veins than in arteries, and NO production is further reduced by bypass grafting.[14] Bypass surgery not only affects the local production of factors influencing hemostasis but also alters their circulating levels, with a particularly marked perioperative elevation of plasma fibrinogen, and these changes also favor a prothrombotic response.[15]

The tendency for early graft occlusion resulting from these prothrombotic effects may be amplified by technical factors that reduce graft flow, including intact venous valves, anastomotic stricture, or graft implantation proximal to an atheromatous segment. In addition, saphenous veins, particularly when denuded, are highly sensitive to circulating vasoconstrictors, including the most potent endogenous vasoconstrictor, endothelin-1. The circulating concentration of endothelin-1 shows a marked initial increase followed by an additional slower increment, after the onset of cardiopulmonary bypass,[16] and the resulting venoconstrictor response may further attenuate flow and promote stasis. In SVGs, the predominant vasomotor response to thrombin is a constrictor one, in contrast to the thrombin-mediated vasorelaxation that occurs via endothelial receptors in internal mammary arteries, further promoting thrombosis in SVGs.[17]

### Neointimal Hyperplasia

Neointimal hyperplasia, defined as the accumulation of smooth muscle cells and extracellular matrix in the intimal compartment, is the major pathology responsible for graft failure between 1 month and 1 year after implantation. Many veins may exhibit mild intimal or medial fibrosis before grafting.[18] However, nearly all veins implanted into the arterial circulation develop further intimal thickening within

4–6 weeks, which may reduce the lumen by up to 25%, but this process, in itself, rarely produces significant stenosis.[19] Exaggerated neointimal hyperplasia may, however, lead to significant obstruction and graft failure.

Initially, medial smooth muscle cells proliferate in response to several growth factors and cytokines released from platelets and from activated endothelial cells and macrophages. This is followed by migration of smooth muscle cells into the intima, with subsequent further proliferation. Later, synthesis and deposition of extracellular matrix by activated smooth muscle cells leads to a progressive increase in intimal fibrosis and a reduction in cellularity.[20]

The endothelial cell plays a key role in regulating intimal growth through several tonic growth-inhibitory mechanisms. Endothelial loss markedly attenuates these growth-modulating effects. Furthermore, as neoendothelium forms, it does so over a layer of platelets and fibrin that has been deposited on the thrombogenic basement membrane. This nonocclusive thrombus is progressively organized into fibrotic tissue as the abundant platelet component releases growth factors, which promote ingress and proliferation of smooth muscle cells.[9]

In contrast to the arterial injury model, in the venous graft, the major component of intimal hyperplasia occurs after endothelial regeneration. Thus, additional mechanisms operate in the grafted vein.[10] One such mechanism relates to the transient ischemia that happens on explantation, with reperfusion after grafting. This ischemia-reperfusion cycle not only reduces endothelial production of antiproliferative mediators such as prostacyclin, NO, and adenosine[21] but also markedly increases superoxide radical formation that directly promotes smooth muscle cell proliferation.[22] Loss of the vasa vasorum blood supply, on which veins are relatively more dependent than are arteries, may also promote a continuing cycle of ischemia and fibrosis. In vitro evidence also indicates that thrombin may cause much more pronounced proliferation of smooth muscle cells in saphenous veins compared with internal mammary arteries.[17]

An additional mechanism for graft neointima formation may involve perivascular fibroblasts, which translocate through the media of newly placed vein grafts and differentiate into myofibroblasts, acquiring α-smooth muscle actin. The intima of human saphenous vein grafts retrieved during repeat bypass surgery exhibits a profile of cytoskeletal proteins similar to that of myofibroblasts in porcine vein grafts, suggesting a role for these cells in graft intimal hyperplasia in the clinical setting.[23]

The hemodynamic conditions inside blood vessels lead to the development of superficial stresses near the vessel walls, which can broadly be divided into 2 categories: (1) circumferential wall stress caused by pulse pressure variation inside the vessel and (2) shear stress caused by blood flow. Normal wall stresses caused by blood pressure are transferred to all vessel wall layers (intima, media, and adventitia). On the other hand, shear stress is applied mainly to the inner layer of the arterial wall in contact with the blood, the vascular endothelium.[24] The acute, pronounced increase in wall stress incurred by saphenous veins on exposure to arterial pressures is a potential factor promoting intimal fibrosis. This increased wall stress, significantly upregulates vein graft intimal receptors for basic fibroblast growth factor, a potent vascular smooth muscle cell mitogen released from damaged endothelial and smooth muscle cells.[25]

On the other hand, distension of veins under arterial pressure increases vein diameter and reduces mean blood velocity, both favoring decrease in shear stress.[20] The reduction in shear stress increases the shear-regulated production of several potent mitogens, including platelet-derived growth factor, basic fibroblast growth factor, and endothelin 1, and attenuates the production of growth inhibitors such as transforming growth factor-β and NO, thus, shifting the balance toward smooth muscle cell proliferation and intimal hyperplasia. The switch from high to normal shear stress is associated with an increase in intimal thickening because of increased smooth muscle cell proliferation and extracellular matrix deposition.

## Accelerated Atherosclerosis

After the first year of bypass surgery, atherosclerosis is the dominant process responsible for SVG failure. Although the progression of native vessel coronary disease is also important in symptom recurrence, angiographic studies indicate that among patients who present with unstable angina, non–ST-elevation myocardial infarction, or ST-segment-elevation myocardial infarction after previous bypass surgery, the culprit lesion in 70%–85% of cases is an atherosclerotic vein graft stenosis, often with superimposed thrombus.[26,27] Necropsy studies have found evidence of atheromatous plaques as early as 1 year after bypass surgery, but hemodynamically important stenoses resulting in recurrent symptoms rarely occur before 3 years after grafting, and the clinical impact of vein graft atheroma increases markedly after 5–7 years.[7,28–30]

The histologic types and stages of atherosclerotic lesion development in native coronary arteries have been comprehensively reviewed by the

American Heart Association Council on Arteriosclerosis.[31] Although the fundamental process of atheroma development and the predisposing factors are similar in vein grafts, certain histologic differences are present compared with native vessel disease. A major difference is the rapidly progressive nature of the atherosclerotic process in saphenous vein grafts. As in other situations in which accelerated forms of atherosclerosis occur, a pivotal factor in the rapidity of progression of vein graft atheroma is chronic endothelial cell injury and dysfunction.[9,32]

On histopathology, vein graft atheroma has more foam cells and inflammatory cells, including multinucleate giant cells, than native coronary atheroma with appearances similar to experimental models of immune-mediated atherosclerosis.[30] Morphologically, vein graft atherosclerosis tends to be diffuse, concentric, and friable with a poorly developed or absent fibrous cap and little evidence of calcification, whereas native vessel atheroma is proximal, focal, eccentric, and nonfriable with a well-developed fibrous cap and frequent calcification. Intravascular ultrasound evidence suggests that the focal compensatory enlargement observed in atherosclerotic-native coronary arteries (Glagov's law) does not appear to occur in stenotic saphenous vein grafts.[33] The lipid handling of saphenous veins is also relatively proatherogenic, with slower lipolysis, more active lipid synthesis, and higher lipid uptake than in native coronary arteries.[34]

## STRATEGIES TO MODIFY THE NATURAL HISTORY OF SVG FAILURE
### Smoking Cessation

In the Coronary Artery Surgery Study (CASS), among smokers randomly assigned to bypass surgery, survival rate at 10 years was 68% for persistent smokers and 84% for those who stopped smoking within 6 months of surgery (relative risk of death, nonquitter/quitter = 1.73; $P$ = .018).[35] The benefit of smoking cessation in the surgically treated patients points to the specific impact of smoking in reducing survival in this group through its effects in promoting vein graft disease.

The CASS data are complemented by a 15-year prospective follow-up study of 415 patients after SVG grafting.[36] In this study, compared with patients who stopped smoking since surgery, persistent smokers at 1 year after surgery had 2.3 times the risk of myocardial infarction and 2.5 times greater need for reoperation. Even greater elevations of risk for myocardial infarction, reoperation, and angina pectoris were observed in patients still smoking 5 years after surgery. No statistically significant differences in outcome at 1 or 5 years were observed in this study between patients who had stopped smoking after surgery and nonsmokers, further indicating the marked reduction in risk afforded by complete cessation of smoking.[36]

### Lipid-Lowering Drug Therapy

Two angiographic trials of lipid-lowering therapy, the Cholesterol-Lowering Atherosclerosis Study (CLAS I and II)[37,38] and the Post-Coronary Artery Bypass Grafting (Post-CABG) Trial,[39] included exclusively patients who had previously undergone bypass surgery. Another clinical trial of secondary prevention with pravastatin, the Cholesterol and Recurrent Events (CARE) Trial, included a substantial proportion of patients (1091 of 4159 patients; 26.2%) with a history of bypass surgery.[40] The 2 lipid-lowering trials (CARE and Post-CABG) both underscore the need for an increasingly aggressive approach to cholesterol lowering in patients with established ischemic heart disease, including those with prior surgical revascularization. In the CARE trial, patients with average levels of total and low-density lipoprotein (LDL) cholesterol treated with pravastatin for 5 years showed a marked (24%) reduction in risk of the composite end point of fatal and nonfatal coronary events and the need for myocardial revascularization ($P$ = .003).[40]

In the Post-CABG trial,[39] follow-up angiography, performed in 1192 patients at a mean of 4.3 years after recruitment, showed that aggressive lowering of LDL cholesterol with lovastatin reduced the progression of vein graft disease (defined as per-patient percentage of grafts with a decrease of 0.6 mm or more in lumen diameter), the rate of vein graft occlusion, and the number of new vein graft lesions, compared with moderate lowering of LDL cholesterol with lovastatin. Additional data from this trial indicated that the aggressive cholesterol-lowering regimen (but not the moderate regimen) afforded equivalent benefits in reducing disease progression irrespective of graft age at initiation of drug therapy.[41] Although the primary end points in the Post-CABG Trial were angiographic, the observed reduction in angiographic disease progression was reflected in a reduction in need for further revascularization in the aggressively treated compared with the moderately treated group.

In a study using serial intravascular ultrasound, lumen loss was associated with an increase in plaque area and a decrease in SVG area (plaque growth and negative remodeling) with a linear relationship between follow-up LDL cholesterol and plaque growth leading to lumen loss during follow-up.[42] Based on current national guidelines, all CABG surgery patients should receive statin therapy unless otherwise contraindicated.[43]

## Antithrombotic Agents

Aspirin in the Veterans Administration (VA) Cooperative Studies increased vein graft patency at 60 days[44] and at 1 year[45] after coronary bypass surgery compared with placebo. The effect of aspirin in improving 1-year vein graft patency in the VA study population was markedly dependent on grafted native vessel diameter: if the grafted vessel diameter was ≤2 mm, aspirin significantly reduced vein graft occlusion over placebo (20.1% vs 32.3%; $P = .008$); for vein grafts placed to vessels greater than 2 mm in diameter, aspirin did not appear to improve patency. Available data indicate that aspirin is effective in improving vein graft patency only if commenced no later than 1 day after surgery.[44–46]

In a meta-analysis from the Antiplatelet Trialists' Collaboration, low-dose aspirin was associated with improved graft patency, as assessed by coronary angiography, at an average of 1 year after surgery.[47] The pooled odds reduction for SVG closure was 41% (8% absolute risk reduction) with low-dose aspirin (75–325 mg/d) compared with placebo. Current guidelines state that aspirin is the drug of choice for prophylaxis against early SVG closure. It is the standard of care and should be continued indefinitely given its benefit in preventing subsequent clinical events.[43]

The Clopidogrel After Surgery for Coronary Artery DiseasE (CASCADE)[48] trial indicated that compared with aspirin monotherapy, the combination of aspirin plus clopidogrel did not significantly reduce SVG intimal hyperplasia 1 year after CABG. A registry analysis suggested that among patients with myocardial infarction revascularized by CABG, clopidogrel-treated patients had a lower risk of the combined end point of death or recurrent myocardial infarction.[49] Given the negative results of the CASCADE study and other data available to date, there is not enough evidence to support the routine use of clopidogrel after CABG.[50]

## COMPARISON WITH OTHER CONDUITS

The internal thoracic artery, with its excellent long-term patency (especially when used to the left anterior descending vessel), remains the preferred primary conduit in most patients undergoing CABG. Among patients undergoing first-time elective CABG, the use of a radial artery graft compared with SVG did not result in greater 1-year patency in a multicenter, randomized VA Cooperative Studies Program controlled trial.[51] Another study suggested that radial artery grafts may have lower patency rates than left internal mammary artery and saphenous vein grafts.[52] Overall, the internal thoracic artery should be used as the preferred conduit whenever feasible (**Fig. 2**).

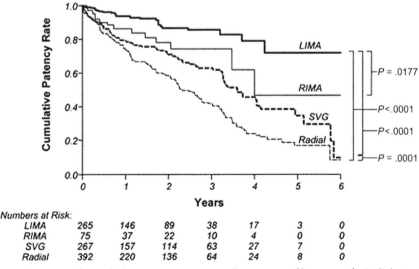

**Fig. 2.** Kaplan-Meier curves of cumulative patency rates according to type of bypass graft. Radial artery grafts were associated with worst patency rate of all graft types. LIMA, Left internal mammary artery; RIMA, Right internal mammary artery; SVG, Saphenous vein graft. (*Adapted from* Khot UN, Friedman DT, Pettersson G, et al. Radial artery bypass grafts have an increased occurrence of angiographically severe stenosis and occlusion compared with left internal mammary arteries and saphenous vein grafts. Circulation 2004;109(17):2086–91; with permission.)

## SUMMARY

The natural history of SVG suggests significant failure rate with only 80% of SVGs remaining patent 5 years after surgery and about 60% remaining patent at 7–10 years.[53] SVG failure is related to 3 distinct but interrelated pathologic processes: thrombosis, intimal hyperplasia, and atherosclerosis. Early thrombosis is a major cause of vein graft loss during the first month after bypass surgery, whereas during the remainder of the first year, intimal hyperplasia forms a template for subsequent atherogenesis, which thereafter predominates. The spectrum of risk factors predisposing to vein graft atherosclerosis and its clinical sequelae is broadly similar to that recognized for native coronary disease. However, the pathogenic effects of these risk factors are amplified by loss of the anatomic and functional integrity of the endothelium during and after grafting, by inherent deficiencies of the vein as a conduit, and by transposition of the vein into the high-pressure arterial circulation. The clinical impact of saphenous vein graft failure is significant, and concerted multifaceted strategies are needed to prevent graft failure. Important elements of this preventive strategy include continued improvements in surgical technique and the optimal use of the most effective antithrombotic agents; more intensive risk factor modification, in particular, early and aggressive lipid-lowering drug therapy; and complete smoking cessation.

## REFERENCES

1. Garrett HE, Dennis EW, DeBakey ME. Aortocoronary bypass with saphenous vein graft. Seven-year follow-up. JAMA 1973;223(7):792–4.

2. Favaloro RG. Saphenous vein graft in the surgical treatment of coronary artery disease. Operative technique. J Thorac Cardiovasc Surg 1969;58(2): 178–85.

3. Conti VR, Hunter GC. Gene therapy and vein graft patency in coronary artery bypass graft surgery. JAMA 2005;294(19):2495–7.

4. Cataldo G, Braga M, Pirotta N, et al. Factors influencing 1-year patency of coronary artery saphenous vein grafts. Studio Indobufene nel Bypass Aortocoronarico (SINBA). Circulation 1993;88(5 Pt 2):II93–8.

5. Lesperance J, Bourassa MG, Biron P, et al. Aorta to coronary artery saphenous vein grafts. Preoperative angiographic criteria for successful surgery. Am J Cardiol 1972;30(5):459–65.

6. Barboriak JJ, Pintar K, Van Horn DL, et al. Pathologic findings in the aortocoronary vein grafts. A scanning electron microscope study. Atherosclerosis 1978;29(1):69–80.

7. Lie JT, Lawrie GM, Morris GC Jr. Aortocoronary bypass saphenous vein graft atherosclerosis. Anatomic study of 99 vein grafts from normal and hyperlipoproteinemic patients up to 75 months postoperatively. Am J Cardiol 1977;40(6):906–14.

8. Roubos N, Rosenfeldt FL, Richards SM, et al. Improved preservation of saphenous vein grafts by the use of glyceryl trinitrate-verapamil solution during harvesting. Circulation 1995;92(Suppl 9): II31–6.

9. Verrier ED, Boyle EM Jr. Endothelial cell injury in cardiovascular surgery. Ann Thorac Surg 1996; 62(3):915–22.

10. Dilley RJ, McGeachie JK, Tennant M. Vein to artery grafts: a morphological and histochemical study of the histogenesis of intimal hyperplasia. Aust N Z J Surg 1992;62(4):297–303.

11. Nachman RL, Silverstein R. Hypercoagulable states. Ann Intern Med 1993;119(8):819–27.

12. Cook JM, Cook CD, Marlar R, et al. Thrombomodulin activity on human saphenous vein grafts prepared for coronary artery bypass. J Vasc Surg 1991; 14(2):147–51.

13. Cox JL, Chiasson DA, Gotlieb AI. Stranger in a strange land: the pathogenesis of saphenous vein graft stenosis with emphasis on structural and functional differences between veins and arteries. Prog Cardiovasc Dis 1991;34(1):45–68.

14. Angelini GD, Christie MI, Bryan AJ, et al. Surgical preparation impairs release of endothelium-derived relaxing factor from human saphenous vein. Ann Thorac Surg 1989;48(3):417–20.

15. Moor E, Hamsten A, Blomback M, et al. Haemostatic factors and inhibitors and coronary artery bypass grafting: preoperative alterations and relations to graft occlusion. Thromb Haemost 1994;72(3):335–42.

16. te Velthuis H, Jansen PG, Oudemans-van Straaten HM, et al. Circulating endothelin in cardiac operations: influence of blood pressure and endotoxin. Ann Thorac Surg 1996;61(3):904–8.

17. Yang Z, Ruschitzka F, Rabelink TJ, et al. Different effects of thrombin receptor activation on endothelium and smooth muscle cells of human coronary bypass vessels. Implications for venous bypass graft failure. Circulation 1997;95(7):1870–6.

18. Thiene G, Miazzi P, Valsecchi M, et al. Histological survey of the saphenous vein before its use as autologous aortocoronary bypass graft. Thorax 1980; 35(7):519–22.

19. Chesebro JH, Fuster V. Platelet-inhibitor drugs before and after coronary artery bypass surgery and coronary angioplasty: the basis of their use, data from animal studies, clinical trial data, and current recommendations. Cardiology 1986;73(4–5):292–305.

20. Allaire E, Clowes AW. Endothelial cell injury in cardiovascular surgery: the intimal hyperplastic response. Ann Thorac Surg 1997;63(2):582–91.

21. Holt CM, Francis SE, Newby AC, et al. Comparison of response to injury in organ culture of human saphenous vein and internal mammary artery. Ann Thorac Surg 1993;55(6):1522–8.

22. Rao GN, Berk BC. Active oxygen species stimulate vascular smooth muscle cell growth and proto-oncogene expression. Circ Res 1992;70(3):593–9.

23. Shi Y, O'Brien JE Jr, Mannion JD, et al. Remodeling of autologous saphenous vein grafts. The role of perivascular myofibroblasts. Circulation 1997; 95(12):2684–93.

24. Papaioannou TG, Stefanadis C. Vascular wall shear stress: basic principles and methods. Hellenic J Cardiol 2005;46(1):9–15.

25. Nguyen HC, Grossi EA, LeBoutillier M 3rd, et al. Mammary artery versus saphenous vein grafts: assessment of basic fibroblast growth factor receptors. Ann Thorac Surg 1994;58(2):308–10 [discussion: 310–1].

26. Chen L, Theroux P, Lesperance J, et al. Angiographic features of vein grafts versus ungrafted coronary arteries in patients with unstable angina and previous bypass surgery. J Am Coll Cardiol 1996;28(6):1493–9.

27. Douglas JS Jr. Percutaneous approaches to recurrent myocardial ischemia in patients with prior surgical revascularization. Semin Thorac Cardiovasc Surg 1994;6(2):98–108.

28. Kalan JM, Roberts WC. Morphologic findings in saphenous veins used as coronary arterial bypass conduits for longer than 1 year: necropsy analysis of 53 patients, 123 saphenous veins, and 1865 five-millimeter segments of veins. Am Heart J 1990;119(5):1164–84.

29. Neitzel GF, Barboriak JJ, Pintar K, et al. Atherosclerosis in aortocoronary bypass grafts. Morphologic study and risk factor analysis 6 to 12 years after surgery. Arteriosclerosis 1986;6(6):594–600.

30. Ratliff NB, Myles JL. Rapidly progressive atherosclerosis in aortocoronary saphenous vein grafts. Possible immune-mediated disease. Arch Pathol Lab Med 1989;113(7):772–6.

31. Stary HC, Chandler AB, Dinsmore RE, et al. A definition of advanced types of atherosclerotic lesions and a histological classification of atherosclerosis. A report from the Committee on Vascular Lesions of the Council on Arteriosclerosis, American Heart Association. Circulation 1995;92(5): 1355–74.

32. Boyle EM Jr, Lille ST, Allaire E, et al. Endothelial cell injury in cardiovascular surgery: atherosclerosis. Ann Thorac Surg 1997;63(3):885–94.

33. Nishioka T, Luo H, Berglund H, et al. Absence of focal compensatory enlargement or constriction in diseased human coronary saphenous vein bypass grafts. An intravascular ultrasound study. Circulation 1996;93(4):683–90.

34. Shafi S, Palinski W, Born GV. Comparison of uptake and degradation of low density lipoproteins by arteries and veins of rabbits. Atherosclerosis 1987; 66(1–2):131–8.

35. Cavender JB, Rogers WJ, Fisher LD, et al. Effects of smoking on survival and morbidity in patients randomized to medical or surgical therapy in the Coronary Artery Surgery Study (CASS): 10-year follow-up. CASS Investigators. J Am Coll Cardiol 1992;20(2):287–94.

36. Voors AA, van Brussel BL, Plokker HW, et al. Smoking and cardiac events after venous coronary bypass surgery. A 15-year follow-up study. Circulation 1996;93(1):42–7.

37. Blankenhorn DH, Nessim SA, Johnson RL, et al. Beneficial effects of combined colestipol-niacin therapy on coronary atherosclerosis and coronary venous bypass grafts. JAMA 1987;257(23): 3233–40.

38. Cashin-Hemphill L, Mack WJ, Pogoda JM, et al. Beneficial effects of colestipol-niacin on coronary atherosclerosis. A 4-year follow-up. JAMA 1990; 264(23):3013–7.

39. The effect of aggressive lowering of low-density lipoprotein cholesterol levels and low-dose anticoagulation on obstructive changes in saphenous-vein coronary-artery bypass grafts. The Post Coronary Artery Bypass Graft Trial Investigators. N Engl J Med 1997;336(3):153–62.

40. Sacks FM, Pfeffer MA, Moye LA, et al. The effect of pravastatin on coronary events after myocardial infarction in patients with average cholesterol levels. Cholesterol and Recurrent Events Trial investigators. N Engl J Med 1996;335(14):1001–9.

41. Campeau L, Hunninghake DB, Knatterud GL, et al. Aggressive cholesterol lowering delays saphenous vein graft atherosclerosis in women, the elderly, and patients with associated risk factors. NHLBI post coronary artery bypass graft clinical trial. Post CABG Trial Investigators. Circulation 1999;99(25): 3241–7.

42. Hong YJ, Mintz GS, Kim SW, et al. Disease progression in nonintervened saphenous vein graft segments a serial intravascular ultrasound analysis. J Am Coll Cardiol 2009;53(15):1257–64.

43. Eagle KA, Guyton RA, Davidoff R, et al. ACC/AHA 2004 guideline update for coronary artery bypass graft surgery: summary article: a report of the American College of Cardiology/American Heart Association Task Force on Practice Guidelines (Committee to Update the 1999 Guidelines for Coronary Artery Bypass Graft Surgery). Circulation 2004;110(9): 1168–76.

44. Goldman S, Copeland J, Moritz T, et al. Improvement in early saphenous vein graft patency after coronary artery bypass surgery with antiplatelet therapy: results of a Veterans

Administration Cooperative Study. Circulation 1988;77(6):1324–32.

45. Goldman S, Copeland J, Moritz T, et al. Saphenous vein graft patency 1 year after coronary artery bypass surgery and effects of antiplatelet therapy. Results of a Veterans Administration Cooperative Study. Circulation 1989;80(5):1190–7.

46. Stein PD, Dalen JE, Goldman S, et al. Antithrombotic therapy in patients with saphenous vein and internal mammary artery bypass grafts. Chest 1995; 108(Suppl 4):424S–30S.

47. Collaborative overview of randomised trials of anti-platelet therapy–II: maintenance of vascular graft or arterial patency by antiplatelet therapy. Antipla-telet Trialists' Collaboration. BMJ 1994;308(6922): 159–68.

48. Kulik A, Le May MR, Voisine P, et al. Aspirin plus clo-pidogrel versus aspirin alone after coronary artery bypass grafting: the clopidogrel after surgery for coronary artery disease (CASCADE) Trial. Circula-tion 2010;122(25):2680–7.

49. Sorensen R, Abildstrom SZ, Hansen PR, et al. Effi-cacy of post-operative clopidogrel treatment in patients revascularized with coronary artery by-pass grafting after myocardial infarction. J Am Coll Cardiol 2011;57(10):1202–9.

50. Kulik A, Ruel M. Clopidogrel after coronary artery bypass graft surgery insufficient evidence. J Am Coll Cardiol 2011;58(10):1084–5.

51. Goldman S, Sethi GK, Holman W, et al. Radial artery grafts vs saphenous vein grafts in coronary artery bypass surgery: a randomized trial. JAMA 2011; 305(2):167–74.

52. Khot UN, Friedman DT, Pettersson G, et al. Radial artery bypass grafts have an increased occurrence of angiographically severe stenosis and occlusion compared with left internal mammary arteries and saphenous vein grafts. Circulation 2004;109(17): 2086–91.

53. Motwani JG, Topol EJ. Aortocoronary saphenous vein graft disease: pathogenesis, predisposition, and prevention. Circulation 1998;97(9):916–31.

# Embolic Protection Devices for Saphenous Vein Graft Percutaneous Coronary Interventions

Joseph D. Foley III, MD, Khaled M. Ziada, MD*

## KEYWORDS

- Percutaneous coronary intervention • Saphenous vein graft • Embolic protection devices
- Embolization • Periprocedural complications

## KEY POINTS

- Percutaneous coronary interventions (PCI) of saphenous vein grafts (SVGs) are complicated by distal embolization, which results in periprocedural myocardial infarction (MI) in 10% to 20% of cases.
- Embolic protection devices (EPDs) consistently lower the rates of major adverse cardiac events associated with these procedures to 5% to 10%.
- Although EPDs add to the cost of the SVG PCI procedure, they are considered cost-effective because of their favorable impact on adverse outcomes and length of stay in hospital.
- According to the American College of Cardiology/American Heart Association (ACC/AHA) PCI guideline update of 2011, use of an EPD during SVG PCI when technically feasible has a class 1b recommendation.
- National registry data indicate considerable underutilization of embolic protection devices during SVG PCI, with use ranging from 20% to 50%, mainly because of operator preference.
- With the strong recommendation of ACC/AHA PCI guideline updates and with improved training and familiarity with the devices, EPD usage should continue to increase.

## INTRODUCTION

### Scope and Mechanisms of Saphenous Vein Graft Disease

Although saphenous vein grafts (SVGs) have been and are currently used in almost every coronary artery bypass grafting (CABG) surgery, long-term patency of these conduits remains suboptimal. Up to 15% fail within the first year and an additional 1% to 2% fail every year between years 1 and 6. Beyond the sixth year after CABG, SVG failure rate approaches 4% per year. At 10 years the overall failure rate is roughly 40%, and nearly half of all surviving vein grafts demonstrate significant degenerative atherosclerotic changes.[1–4]

Mechanisms of SVG failure vary and can be classified according to the time since implantation. Early failure is generally defined as graft failure within the first 30 days after CABG and is typically associated with thrombosis, spasm, or a technical problem related to the surgical anastomosis of the

Sources of support: None.
Conflict of interest: None.
Division of Cardiovascular Medicine, Gill Heart Institute, University of Kentucky, 900 South Limestone Street, 326 Charles T. Wethington Building, Lexington, KY 40536-0200, USA
* Corresponding author.
E-mail address: khaled.ziada@uky.edu

Intervent Cardiol Clin 2 (2013) 259–271
http://dx.doi.org/10.1016/j.iccl.2012.11.008

SVG. Graft failure between 1 and 12 months following implantation is most likely associated with perianastomotic intimal hyperplasia leading to stenosis and, possibly, occlusion. Late failure beyond 12 months is usually related to a novel stenosis within the graft or native coronaries, and is commonly associated with advanced atherosclerotic degenerative changes within the SVG conduits.[5]

## High-Risk Nature of SVG Disease

Repeat revascularization is undertaken in close to 20% of all patients within 10 years after CABG surgery.[6] Because of the higher morbidity and mortality with repeat CABG surgery, percutaneous interventional approaches have become standard for obstructive lesions affecting SVGs.[7] These procedures represent some of the highest-risk subgroups of patients undergoing percutaneous coronary intervention (PCI), primarily owing to the risk of periprocedural complications. Reduced antegrade flow (slow-flow or no-reflow phenomena) and major adverse cardiac events (MACE) (predominantly periprocedural myocardial infarction [MI]) occur in approximately 5% to 20% of SVG PCI in comparison with less than 1% with native coronary PCI.[8] In a registry of 1056 patients who underwent SVG intervention, 15% suffered a periprocedural MI, defined by a creatine kinase MB (CK-MB) fraction greater than 5 times the upper limit of normal (ULN).[9]

Periprocedural MIs carry significant prognostic implications. The 1-year mortality in those who develop larger periprocedural MI (CK-MB >5× ULN) exceeds 11%, compared with 6.5% in those with minor CK-MB elevations and 4.8% in patients who had no CK-MB elevation after the procedure.[9]

## Pathophysiology of Periprocedural MIs

The primary mechanism leading to periprocedural MI in SVG PCI is related to distal embolization from the site of angioplasty in the body of the graft to the distal microvasculature, eventually leading to myonecrosis and elevation of serum enzymes.[10] The embolized material consists of debris (atherosclerotic plaque and thrombotic elements) with particles ranging in size from approximately 50 to greater than 600 μm. Neutrophils and macrophages are also identified.[11] There is evidence to suggest that larger plaque volumes measured by intravascular ultrasonography and the degree of change in plaque size from before to after stenting increase the risk of distal embolization.[12] Platelets play a significant role in the development of periprocedural MIs, although this factor may be more important in native coronaries than in SVG PCI.

At the time of PCI, exposed intraplaque contents stimulate platelet activation and aggregation at the site of PCI, but probably in the downstream microvasculature as well. Thus, platelet aggregates not only cause mechanical plugging of the microcirculation but also lead to biochemical responses caused by their interaction with the injured endothelium, the neutrophils, and with more platelets. The release of vasoactive substances such as serotonin and endothelin-1 from the activated platelets and the injured endothelium lead to intense microvascular vasoconstriction, which perpetuates myonecrosis.[10,13]

The phenomenon of distal embolization and periprocedural MI can be mitigated by a combination of pharmacologic and mechanical interventions.[10] Pharmacologic intervention is discussed in "Pharmacotherapy During Saphenous Vein Graft Intervention" by Willis M. Wu and A. Michael Lincoff elsewhere in this issue. The focus of this article will be on distal embolic protection devices (EPDs) during SVG PCI.

## EMBOLIC PROTECTION DEVICES

The 3 general categories for EPD are: (1) distal balloon occlusive devices; (2) distal filters; and (3) proximal balloon occlusive devices. Each of the categories has specific characteristics that affect their efficacy, utility, and suitability for each individual case. **Table 1** summarizes the general differences between the 3 categories of EPD.[14] **Table 2** describes the technical specifications of each of the available EPDs, which may affect the feasibility of using them in different lesion subsets.

## Distal Balloon Occlusive Devices

### GuardWire

The protypical EPD in this category is the PercuSurge GuardWire (Medtronic, Sunnyvale, CA). The GuardWire consists of a 0.014-inch (0.356-mm) hollow guide wire with a soft occlusion balloon toward the distal end, and a 2.5-cm steerable tip beyond the balloon. The GuardWire is used to cross the lesion, and the balloon is positioned distal to the lesion in a relatively disease-free segment. A low-pressure inflation of the balloon then occludes the graft and prevents downstream flow. Angioplasty, stenting, and postdilation are all performed as necessary. An aspiration catheter is then advanced over the wire and any debris is removed with a slow distal-to-proximal pullback within the column of stagnant blood between the guide catheter and the site of distal balloon occlusion. After aspiration, the balloon is deflated and the GuardWire is withdrawn to restore forward flow (**Fig. 1**).[15]

**Table 1**
**Characteristics of different categories of embolism protection devices**

|  | Distal Filter | Distal Balloon Occlusion | Proximal Occlusion |
|---|---|---|---|
| Antegrade perfusion | Uninterrupted | Temporarily interrupted | Temporarily interrupted |
| Distal-vessel visualization | Unhindered | Not possible during inflation | Possible via inner sheath |
| Efficacy of embolic protection | May allow passage of emboli smaller than pore size (~100 μm) | Once inflated, traps all emboli | All particles can be aspirated |
| Vasoactive substances | Pass unimpeded | Can be aspirated completely | Can be aspirated completely |
| Crossing profile | 0.04–0.05″ (1.01–1.27 mm) | 0.026–0.033″ (0.660–0.838 mm) | No crossing, deployed proximal to lesion |
| Embolization during device positioning | Likely to occur | Less likely to occur | None, because device does not cross lesion |
| Retrieval profile | Occasionally difficult if filter full of debris | Not a problem after balloon deflation | Not a problem, device is proximal to lesion |
| Flexibility of guide-wire use | None, because filter is attached to wire (except Spider RX) | None, because balloon is attached to wire | Excellent, device can be used with any wire |
| Effect of distal disease on device | May not be feasible if no disease-free segment | May not be feasible if no disease-free segment | Device is proximal, distal disease irrelevant |

*Data from* Ziada KM, Mukherjee D. Peri-procedural myocardial infarction and embolism protection devices. In: Topol E, Tierstein P, editors. Textbook of interventional cardiology. 6th edition. Philadelphia: Saunders Elsevier; 2011. p. 372–87.

**Table 2**
**Technical specifications of various embolic protection devices**

| Device Name, Manufacturer | Material | Guide Wire (Inches) | Pore Size (μm) | Guide Catheter (French) | Length (cm) | Vessel Size (mm) | Crossing Profile (French) |
|---|---|---|---|---|---|---|---|
| Distal Balloon Occlusive Devices | | | | | | | |
| GuardWire, Medtronic | Hollow hypotube | 0.014, 0.018 | n/a | 6 | 200, 300 | 2.5–5.0, 3.0–6.0 | 2.1–2.7 |
| TriActiv, Kensey-Nash | Hollow Hypotube | 0.014 | n/a | 7, 8 | 190, 340 | 3.0–5.0 | |
| Distal Embolic Filters | | | | | | | |
| FilterWire EZ/EX, Boston Scientific | Polyurethane filter | 0.014 | 110 | 6 | 190, 300 | 2.25–3.5, 3.5–5.5 | 3.2 |
| SpiderFx, Ev3 Inc | Nitinol filter | 0.014, 0.018 | 167–209 | 6 | 190, 320 | 3.0–7.0 | 3.2 |
| Cardioshield, Abbott Vascular | Nitinol filter | 0.014, 0.018 | 100 | 6 | | | |
| Interceptor PLUS, Medtronic | Nitinol & platinum filter | 0.014 | Inflow: 1400; distal: 100 | 6 | 180 | 2.5–6.0 | 2.7 |
| Proximal Balloon Occlusive Devices | | | | | | | |
| Proxis, St. Jude Medical | | 0.014 | n/a | 7 | 126 | 2.5–5.0 | n/a |

0.014 inch = 0.356 mm; 0.018 inch = 0.457 mm.
*Abbreviation:* n/a, no data available.

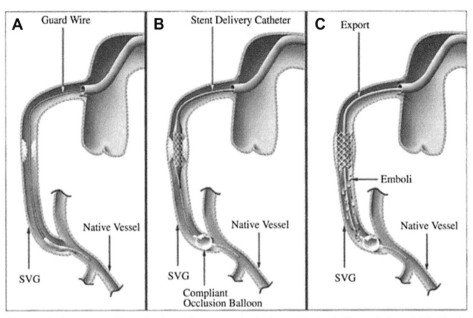

**Fig. 1.** The GuardWire system. The wire is used to cross the lesion with the balloon deflated (*A*). The balloon is then inflated to occlude the graft distal to the site of the lesion (*B*). After PCI is completed, debris is aspirated using the Export catheter (*C*). (*From* Gorog DA, Foale RA, Malik I. Distal myocardial protection during percutaneous coronary intervention: when and where? J Am Coll Cardiol 2005;46:1437; with permission.)

The seminal clinical trial that established the efficacy of the GuardWire system was the SAFER (Saphenous Vein Graft Angioplasty Free of Emboli Randomized) Trial, completed in 2002.[16] This trial randomized 800 patients with stable clinical presentation who had an SVG culprit lesion to either the GuardWire system or placebo during SVG PCI. Patients were included only if their SVG was considered suitable for EPD use. The primary efficacy end point was freedom from MACE (death, MI, or revascularization) at 30 days postprocedure, The GuardWire was associated with a significant reduction in MACE (9.6% vs 16.5% with placebo, *P*<.004). The reduction in MACE was primarily driven by the reduction in periprocedural MIs with GuardWire use (8.6% vs 14.7%, *P* = .008) and fewer no-reflow phenomena (3% vs 9%, *P* = .02) (**Fig. 2**).[16] In the subgroup of patients who received glycoprotein IIb/IIIa inhibitors during the procedure, clinical benefit of the GuardWire was still evident (MACE in 10.7% vs 19.4% in the placebo group, *P* = .008). These findings led to approval of this device by the Food and Drug Administration (FDA) in August 2001. With the development of more EPD systems, this device is no longer produced by its manufacturer.

## TriActiv

The TriActiv system (Kensey-Nash, Exton, PA) was the second distal balloon occlusive EPD that received FDA approval for use in the United States. Similar to the GuardWire, this system uses a distal balloon that is inflated with a prefilled $CO_2$ inflator before PCI. After completing the PCI, stagnant debris and blood proximal to the occlusive balloon are actively extracted using a microflush catheter that is advanced into the vein graft and attached to an automated pump, which in turn flushes and extracts all debris in the stagnant column of blood. The occlusive balloon is deflated only after adequate extraction is performed, and downstream flow is then restored (**Fig. 3**).[17]

The TriActiv system was approved by the FDA for use in SVG PCI based on the results from 2 randomized trials. The first included 113 patients who were randomized to the TriActiv system or any other EPD. The final results demonstrated the noninferiority of the TriActiv system at 30 days.[18] A larger study of more than 600 patients further established the efficacy of this system in the protection of distal embolism. Patients were randomized to TriActiv versus distal balloon occlusion or a distal-filter device. The TriActiv system resulted in a noninferior outcome compared with other devices. There was an increased risk of bleeding with TriActiv use, which was attributed to the need for a larger guiding catheter. This device is no longer produced by its manufacturer, so there are no distal balloon occlusion devices now available on the United States market.

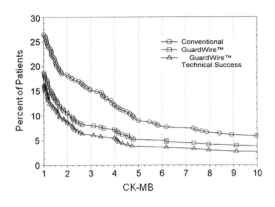

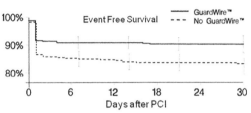

**Fig. 2.** The SAFER trial. (*Top*) Cumulative distribution-function curve of peak cardiac enzyme values after assignment to placebo (395 patients), GuardWire (406 patients), and the per-protocol subgroup with technically successful GuardWire use (366 patients). Each curve shows the percentage of patients whose creatine kinase MB (CK-MB) elevation (expressed as a multiple of institutional upper limit of normal) exceeded the value on the x-axis. (*Bottom*) Kaplan-Meier curves for survival free of major adverse cardiac events during 30 days of follow-up after percutaneous coronary intervention (PCI). (*From* Baim DS, Wahr D, George B, et al. Randomized trial of a distal embolic protection device during percutaneous intervention of saphenous vein aorto-coronary bypass grafts. Circulation 2002;105:1285–90; with permission.)

## Distal Embolic Filters

Several distal filters were developed over the last decade, and are available for use in adjunction with interventional procedures in various arterial beds. Those discussed here include the FilterWire EZ, SpiderFX, Cardioshield, and Interceptor PLUS. Filters specific to carotid embolic protection, such as Angioguard, Accunet, and Emboshield, are beyond the scope of this article and are not discussed.

### FilterWire EZ

The FilterWire EZ (Boston Scientific Corp, Natick, MA) is one of the most popular EPDs in the United States today. The FilterWire consists of a 0.014-inch wire that has a polyurethane filter basket near its distal end. The filter basket has a radiopaque nitinol loop at its base. Distal to the filter basket protrudes a radiopaque shapeable

spring coil tip of the guide wire (**Fig. 4**).[19] The currently used version has pores that are 100 to 110 μm in diameter. The FilterWire can be used in SVGs ranging between 3.5 and 5.5 mm in diameter. Before introducing the device into the guiding catheter, the filter is retracted into an introducing sheath under heparinized saline to collapse the filter basket and dispel the air bubbles. The collapsed filter and its introducing sheath are then used to cross the lesion, with the shapeable tip of the wire leading through the body of the graft. The filter basket is then deployed in a distal relatively disease-free portion of the graft by retracting the introducing sheath. The wire then serves as a standard angioplasty wire. During PCI, blood flow through the pores of the filter is preserved, and injecting contrast for visualization is not affected by the deployed filter. When the PCI is complete, a retrieval sheath is advanced over the wire and used to collapse the filter basket securely. The retrieval sheath and the collapsed filter trapping the embolic debris inside it are then removed as one unit.

The pivotal clinical trial that led to FilterWire approval by the FDA in August 2004 was The FilterWire EX Randomized Evaluation (FIRE) trial.[20] In this multicenter trial, 650 patients were randomized to either a PercuSurge GuardWire or a FilterWire EX for distal EPD during SVG PCI. Patients were excluded if they had an acute or recent MI, SVG age less than 6 months, true aorto-ostial lesions 10 mm or less from ostium, reference diameter less than 3.5 mm or greater than 5.5 mm, Thrombolysis In Myocardial Infarction flow grade 0, lesion within 25 mm of the distal anastomosis, unprotected Y-limb branch vessel proximal to the study device, planned use of atherectomy devices, or left ventricular ejection fraction of less than 25%. All patients received aspirin before the procedure and dual antiplatelet therapy afterward. Use of glycoprotein IIb/IIIa inhibitors was left to the operator's discretion. The primary end point was the 30-day composite occurrence of MACE, including death, MI (as defined by postprocedural CK-MB elevation ≥3 times normal), or target-vessel revascularization (TVR). The primary composite end point occurred in 9.9% of FilterWire EX patients and 11.6% of GuardWire patients (*P* = .53). Most MACE events consisted of non–Q-wave MIs. The rates of periprocedural MIs were almost identical between the two devices (7.8% with FilterWire vs 8.4% with GuardWire) (**Fig. 5**). A 1-sided test for noninferiority was satisfied at the *P* = .0008 level, thus proving that the FilterWire EX is noninferior to the GuardWire in patients undergoing SVG PCI.

As the design of the wire was modified to the FilterWire EZ, 2 small, prospective nonrandomized

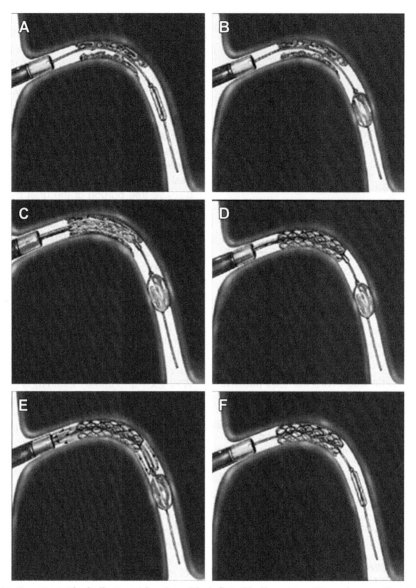

**Fig. 3.** The TriActiv system. The balloon guide wire with deflated balloon is positioned across the stenosis (*A*) and the occlusion balloon is inflated (*B*). A stent is delivered over the balloon guide wire (*C*) and deployed at the lesion (*D*). The flush catheter is advanced over the balloon guide wire and saline is infused via holes in the distal end. Extraction of fluid and debris is through the guiding catheter (*E*). The occlusion balloon is deflated and flow is restored (*F*). (*From* Carrozza JP Jr, Caussin C, Braden G, et al. Embolic protection during saphenous vein graft intervention using a second-generation balloon protection device: results from the combined US and European pilot study of the TriActiv Balloon Protected Flush Extraction System. Am Heart J 2005;149:1136; with permission.)

registries were used to demonstrate its safety and similarity in performance to the EX design. Inclusion and exclusion criteria were similar to those of the FIRE trial. The MACE rates were not different from those of the FIRE trial, and the EZ design is thus the one that is currently available for use in the United States.[21] The FilterWire EZ is the most commonly used EPD for SVG PCI, probably because of its ease of use and the reasonable crossing profile (**Fig. 6**).

### SpiderFX

The SpiderFX (ev3 Endovascular Inc, Plymouth, MN) is another distal embolic filter made of a nitinol braid. Unlike the FilterWire EZ, the SpiderFX filter is separate from the angioplasty wire, which allows operators to use the wire of their choice to cross the lesion, then deliver the filter distal to the lesion over the wire. The SpiderFX also comes in different sizes (3–7 mm) (**Fig. 7**). The pore size is 167 to 209 μm, which is significantly larger than the

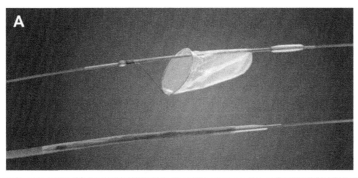

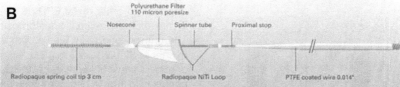

**Fig. 4.** The FilterWire system. (*A*) The FilterWire is composed of a polyurethane filter basket premounted on a 0.014-inch guide wire and preloaded on a delivery sheath. The pore size is 100 to 110 μm. (*B*) The FilterWire is compatible with a 6F guiding catheter, has a crossing profile of 3.2F, and can protect saphenous vein grafts 3.5 to 5.5 mm in diameter. A landing zone distal to the lesion of greater than 25 to 30 mm is required. After PCI is completed, a retrieval sheath is used to capture and remove the filter. NiTi, nitinol; PTFE, polytetrafluoroethylene. (*From* Lee MS, Park SJ, Kandzari DE, et al. Saphenous vein graft intervention. JACC Cardiovasc Interv 2011;4:839; with permission.)

FilterWire (110 μm). Data from the SPIDER (Saphenous Vein Graft Protection In a Distal Embolic Protection Randomized) trial was presented in 2005.[22] This study was performed to evaluate the safety and efficacy of the SPIDER/SpideRX EPD during SVG PCI. A total of 747 patients were randomized to either the SPIDER/SpideRX system or a control EPD group (which included both the GuardWire and FilterWire distal EPDs). Inclusion and exclusion criteria were similar to FIRE and SAFER, as previously described. The primary end point was 30-day MACE (death, MI, TVR, and urgent CABG). The primary end point was reached in 9.2% in the SPIDER group versus 8.7% with other devices (*P* not significant). The results were statistically significant for noninferiority (*P* = .012) with this device when compared with other EPDs evaluated in this study (mostly FilterWire).

## Cardioshield

The Cardioshield is another distal-filter device that is mainly of historical interest, as it is no longer available for clinical use. The main clinical trial that ultimately led to its demise was CAPTIVE.[23] CAPTIVE was a randomized trial comparing the Cardioshield with the PercuSurge GuardWire. A total of 650 patients were enrolled and followed for the 30-day primary composite end point of death, MI, emergent CABG, or TVR. Originally designed as a superiority study, the statistical design was changed during the trial to a noninferiority design. The

primary end point was reached in 11.4% with Cardioshield versus 9.1% with GuardWire (*P* = .37). However, this did not satisfy the statistical threshold for noninferiority (*P* = .057). No further trials have been published on this device.

## Interceptor PLUS

The Interceptor PLUS Coronary Filter System (Medtronic AVE, Sunnyvale, CA) is a novel catheter-based filter EPD. It consists of a steerable vascular filter, an actuator handle, a torque handle, a peel-away introducer, and a guide-wire introducer. Using the actuator handle, the filter is deployed and collapsed. Once the filter is expanded, blood and embolic material first pass proximally through 4 large inflow openings proximally and then distally through numerous distal-filter 100-μm pores that allow for perfusion while trapping embolic debris (**Fig. 8**).

This EPD was evaluated in the AMEthyst (Assessment of the Medtronic AVE Interceptor Saphenous Vein Graft Filter System) trial in 2008.[24] This trial randomized nearly 800 patients undergoing SVG PCI to the Interceptor PLUS or to either the GuardWire or FilterWire. The primary end point was 30-day MACE, which consisted of death, MI, or TVR. The end point was reached in 8% in the Interceptor group versus 7.3% in the control group (*P* = .77; *P* = .025 for noninferiority). No further trials have been published on this device.

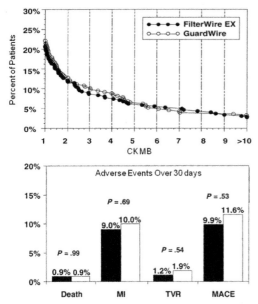

**Fig. 5.** The FIRE trial. (*Top*) Cumulative frequency-distribution curves of peak postprocedural creatine kinase MB (CK-MB) for patients randomized to distal protection with the FilterWire EX (*closed circles*) versus the GuardWire (*open circles*). Each curve shows the percentage of patients whose CK-MB elevation (expressed as a multiple of institutional upper limit of normal) exceeds the value on the x-axis. (*Bottom*) Primary end-point major adverse cardiac events (MACE) rates at 30 days in patients randomized to the FilterWire EX (*black bars*) or the GuardWire (*white bars*), establishing noninferiority of the FilterWire EX. MI, myocardial infarction; TVR, target-vessel revascularization. (*From* Stone GW, Rogers C, Hermiller J, et al. Randomized comparison of distal protection with a filter-based catheter and a balloon occlusion and aspiration system during percutaneous intervention of diseased saphenous vein aorto-coronary bypass grafts. Circulation 2003; 108:551; with permission.)

### *Proximal Balloon Occlusive Devices*

The main characteristics of the proximal occlusive devices and the differences between them and distal devices were summarized in **Table 1**. The Proxis Embolic Protection System (St. Jude Medical, Maple Grove, MN) is the prototypical EPD in this class. The main advantage of this type of EPD is that the SVG culprit lesion is not crossed until the EPD is deployed and the distal circulation is protected. With distal EPDs, the lesion has to be crossed before deployment of an EPD, which in itself carries a risk of distal embolization. Once the proximal occlusion balloon is inflated in the proximal segment of the graft, antegrade flow is arrested. The lesion can then

be crossed with the angioplasty wire and PCI performed with no forward flow. Before deflation of the occlusive balloon, gentle aspiration is performed to remove any atherosclerotic debris or thrombi that may have accumulated in the body of the SVG as a result of the PCI (**Fig. 9**).

The major clinical trial in the Proxis history is the PROXIMAL trial published in 2007.[25] This trial randomized almost 600 patients to use of a Proxis device or either a FilterWire or GuardWire for embolic protection during SVG PCI. Specific exclusion criteria unique to this class of EPDs as opposed to other distal EPDs were lesions within 5 mm of the proximal anastomosis of the SVG. The primary end point was a composite of MACE events at 30 days, which included death, Q-wave or non–Q-wave MI, emergent CABG, or TVR, which occurred in 10.0% of control patients versus 9.2% of test patients ($P = .0061$). When analyzed by specific devices, the composite end point occurred in 11.7% of distal protection patients versus 7.1% of proximal protection patients ($P$ for superiority $= .10$, $P$ for noninferiority $= .001$). When analyzed by which lesions were amenable to treatment with either proximal or distal protection devices, the primary end point occurred in 7.4% of proximal protection patients versus 12.2% of distal protection patients ($P$ for superiority $= .14$, $P$ for noninferiority $= .001$). The Proxis system has recently been discontinued by the manufacturer.

## PLANNING FOR SVG PCI: TECHNICAL CONSIDERATIONS

When a hemodynamically significant stenosis is identified in an SVG, the decision and planning for SVG PCI entails several points: (1) selection of the guiding catheter, (2) feasibility of using an EPD, (3) optimal type of EPD(s) to be used, and (4) anticoagulation and adjunctive antiplatelet regimen.

In SVG PCI, selection of guiding catheter follows the general rules as in any other PCI: finding a catheter shape that is suitable to intubate the graft and provide adequate support for delivering the interventional devices to the lesion site. All EPDs can fit through a 6F guiding catheter with the exception of the Proxis system, so a larger guiding catheter is needed if Proxis is the EPD of choice. It is generally more important to have a very supportive guiding catheter when a distal EPD is used, to minimize the motion of the EPD in the graft during introduction and removal of balloons and stents into the graft.

Anatomic considerations are individualized for each EPD, and are described accordingly here.

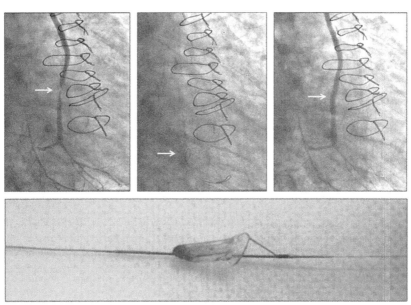

**Fig. 6.** Use of the FilterWire in Contemporary SVG PCI. Angiograms of an SVG to an obtuse marginal branch in a patient presenting with non–ST-segment elevation myocardial infarction. (*Left*) A subtotal lesion is noted in the body of the SVG (*arrow*). (*Middle*) The lesion is crossed with a FilterWire EZ, which is then deployed in the distal graft, as noted by the radiopaque nitinol ring at the base of the filter basket (*arrow*). The radiopaque spring coil tip is folded in the native vessel beyond the anastomosis. (*Right*) The final angiogram after stent deployment and removal of the FilterWire, with no residual stenosis within the stented segment (*arrow*) and good runoff into the distal obtuse marginal branch. (*Bottom*) The FilterWire contains macroscopic evidence of a thrombotic material and fatty debris from the degenerated lesion.

General considerations are a nontortuous vessel with a diameter between 3 and 6 mm containing a lesion located greater than 5 mm from the proximal aortic anastomosis and greater than 25 mm from the distal coronary arterial anastomosis (**Box 1**).[26]

There is some evidence that PCI for aorto-ostial lesions can be performed with distal-filter protection.

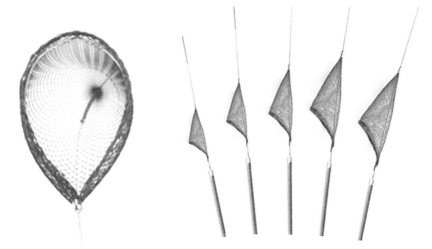

**Fig. 7.** The SpiderFX system. This distal-filter EPD is made of a nitinol braid (*left panel*) and has 2 significant differences that distinguish it from the FilterWire: It is separate from the angioplasty wire, thus the wire of choice can be used to cross the lesion and the SpiderFX filter can then be advanced distal to the lesion over the selected angioplasty wire. It also comes in different sizes between 3 and 7 mm (*right panel*). (*Courtesy of* Covidien AG. © Covidien. SpiderFX is a trademark of Covidien AG. All rights reserved; with permission.)

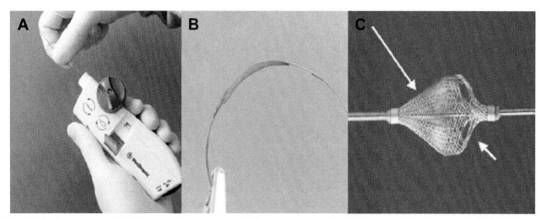

**Fig. 8.** The Interceptor PLUS system. Components of the Interceptor PLUS Coronary Filter System include (*A*) actuator handle for filter deployment and closure; (*B*) low-profile (2.7F) undeployed filter on a 0.014-inch wire; and (*C*) expanded filter with 1400- to 1800-μm proximal inflow openings (*long arrow*) and 100-μm distal pores (*short arrow*). (*From* Kereiakes DJ, Turco MA, Breall J, et al. A novel filter-based distal embolic protection device for percutaneous intervention of saphenous vein graft lesions: results of the AMEthyst randomized controlled trial. JACC Cardiovasc Interv 2008;1:250; with permission.)

Abdel-Karim and colleagues[27] described a series of patients in whom EPDs were used for these type of lesions. In this study, 113 aorto-ostial SVG lesions were retrospectively analyzed and 98 lesions (87%) were considered suitable for a distal-filter–based EPD strategy, which was implemented successfully in 70 lesions (71%). Proximal lesions are better suited for distal EPDs, whereas distal lesions with an inadequate landing zone may not be protected except by using a proximal occlusive balloon system. Extremely tight lesions may require crossing with a dedicated wire and advancing a SpiderFX filter over the wire. Although considered as off-label, the proximal occlusive balloon systems can be used in sequential grafts if the balloon can be inflated proximal to the origin of the second limb of the graft.

There has been no controlled trial addressing the role of bivalirudin versus heparin for anticoagulation during SVG PCI. National registry data indicate that bivalirudin is used in approximately 40% of SVG PCI.[28] There is no evidence of an interaction between the anticoagulation regimen and the use or type of EPD, although this aspect has not been adequately studied. On the other hand, there is some evidence that use of glycoprotein IIb/IIIa inhibitors offers no additional benefit in SVG PCI.[29] These agents are probably even less relevant with routine preloading with dual antiplatelet therapy.

One intriguing study, however, does suggest an interaction between the use of glycoprotein IIb/IIIa inhibitors and the type of EPD used. In a subgroup analysis of the FIRE trial, more than 50% of patients in both the FilterWire and the GuardWire groups received a glycoprotein IIb/IIIa inhibitor at the discretion of the operators. Examination of these results demonstrated a favorable interaction between the use of glycoprotein IIb/IIIa inhibitors and FilterWire use, but not with GuardWire use. This finding may be related to the improved flow seen with glycoprotein IIb/IIIa inhibitor administration in patients receiving FilterWire protection, probably attributable to reducing the degree of platelet aggregation and deposition on the surface of the filter.[30]

## CONTEMPORARY USE AND COST-EFFECTIVENESS OF EPDS

Based on the high risk of distal embolization with SVG PCI procedures and the significant reduction in MACE outcomes with EPD devices, it is logical that EPDs should be used in every SVG PCI when technically feasible. This approach is reflected in the Class 1B recommendation for use of these EPD devices during SVG PCI "when technically feasible" in the most recent update of the American College of Cardiology/American Heart Association (ACC/AHA) PCI guidelines from 2011.[31]

To evaluate modern-day practice patterns with EPD during SVG PCI, Mehta and colleagues[28] evaluated data from the American College of Cardiology—National Cardiovascular Data Registry (ACC-NCDR) to determine the frequency of EPD use from January 2004 through March 2006. Excluding primary PCI settings, data from more than 19,500 SVG PCI procedures was collected. In total, EPDs were used in 22% of all SVG PCIs. If one were to evaluate technical eligibility for EPD

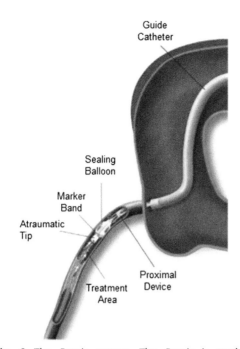

Guide
Catheter

Sealing
Balloon

Marker
Band

Atraumatic
Tip

Proximal
Device

Treatment
Area

**Fig. 9.** The Proxis system. The Proxis is tracked through the guide catheter and into the target vessel. Its atraumatic tip is positioned proximal to the treatment area. The guide wire and interventional device are inserted through Proxis and may be staged proximal to the treatment area before the inflation of the occlusive balloon. Balloon inflation seals the vessel and suspends blood flow, ensuring stagnation of blood and liberated embolic material during treatment of the lesion. During protection, a static column of contrast verifies adequate sealing and highlights the treatment area to facilitate placement of an interventional device. (*From* Mauri L, Cox D, Hermiller J, et al. The PROXIMAL trial: proximal protection during saphenous vein graft intervention using the Proxis Embolic Protection System: a randomized, prospective, multicenter clinical trial. J Am Coll Cardiol 2007;50:1443; with permission.)

use based on anatomic considerations in **Box 1** and **Table 2**, it is estimated that 50% of all SVG PCIs would be eligible for EPD use. This finding indicates that actual use is less than half of the estimated or potential use. EPDs were not used in 19% of centers participating in the registry, and were rarely used (<10% of cases) in another 41% of centers. More recently, analysis of the SOS (Stenting of Saphenous Vein Grafts) trial demonstrated that EPDs were used in 54% of cases.[32] Although some of the lack of use was dictated by anatomic considerations, there is evidence that operator preference still contributes to this underutilization of EPD. It is important to acknowledge that these data may be outdated and that recommendations to use EPDs in the national PCI guidelines in 2009

and 2011, in addition to more widespread availability and training, may have increased EPD use over the last few years.

In addition to establishing their value in improving clinical outcomes, cost-effectiveness of EPD use needed to be examined. It is clear that adverse events associated with distal embolism and periprocedural MI associated with SVG PCI increases length of stay and increases hospitalization costs. EPD use reduces these complications to a significant degree, leading to improved outcomes and reduced costs to the health care system. Two evaluations have been performed to examine EPD usage and cost-effectiveness. Cohen and colleagues[33] evaluated cost-effectiveness of the GuardWire system during SVG PCI as part of a planned subgroup analysis of the SAFER trial. Although the use of EPD increased the cost of the initial procedure, the reduced incidence of periprocedural MI resulted in savings attributable to the shorter length of stay in hospital. When the cost-effectiveness ratio was calculated based on the observed 30-day clinical outcomes and costs, the GuardWire-based PCI resulted in a cost-effectiveness ratio of $9342 per death or MI avoided. This figure translated into a lifetime incremental cost-effectiveness ratio for GuardWire-based PCI compared with standard SVG PCI without EPD of $3718 per year of life gained, based on statistical projections of long-term survival and life expectancy.[33]

A second more complex cost-effectiveness analysis of EPD use was performed by Senter and colleagues[34] on 126 consecutive patients in whom an EPD was used during SVG PCIs at a single institution. Patients were considered at high risk for distal embolism based on the presence of a bypass graft at least 8 years old or evidence of preprocedural thrombus. Three different distal embolic protection strategies were then compared: (1) no distal embolic protection (reference group); (2) routine distal embolic protection in all patients; and (3) selective distal embolic protection only in high-risk patients. Of the entire cohort, those at high risk included 70 (55%) patients with vein grafts 8 years of age and older, 28 (22%) patients with preprocedural thrombus, and 18 (14%) patients with both. Embolic complications occurred in 17% of patients, with a significant preponderance of events in the high-risk groups. Embolic complications significantly increased total procedure costs from $7228 to $9953 ($P$<.001) and increased total hospital costs by a median $2895 ($P$ = .015), which was twice the cost of the EPD ($1350). Using a routine EPD strategy, total procedure cost would theoretically increase in patients with an embolic complication by approximately $200 and those without an embolic complication by approximately $1350. Using an alternative strategy of selective EPD use in high-risk patients would theoretically decrease the total cost of the procedure for patients with an embolic complication by $2111 ($P$ = .003), without increasing the cost for patients without an embolic complication.

## SUMMARY

SVGs have a high rate of progressive atherosclerosis and graft failure. PCI for SVG is associated with a higher risk of distal embolization and periprocedural MI compared with native-vessel PCI. Many EPDs that have been developed over the past decade have consistently reduced the rate of 30-day MACE to less than 10%. Based on the results of randomized clinical trials, use of EPDs during SVG PCI has been given a Class 1b recommendation in the most recent 2011 ACC/AHA PCI guidelines. Not only do EPDs lower the rate of adverse events, they also have been shown to be cost-effective with both universal usage and selective usage in high-risk groups. Despite this, EPDs are used in only 22% to 50% of cases when they are technically feasible, mainly as a result of operator preference. With continued emphasis on national guideline recommendations and increasing familiarity and comfort of operators in using EPDs, the rate of EPD use and the subsequent improvement of outcomes of SVG PCI will continue to increase in the future.

## REFERENCES

1. Campeau L, Enjalbert M, Lesperance J, et al. The relation of risk factors to the development of atherosclerosis in saphenous-vein bypass grafts and the progression of disease in the native circulation. A study 10 years after aortocoronary bypass surgery. N Engl J Med 1984;311:1329–32.
2. Bourassa MG. Fate of venous grafts: the past, the present and the future. J Am Coll Cardiol 1991;17:1081–3.
3. Fitzgibbon GM, Kafka HP, Leach AJ, et al. Coronary bypass graft fate and patient outcome: angiographic follow-up of 5,065 grafts related to survival and reoperation in 1,388 patients during 25 years. J Am Coll Cardiol 1996;28:616–26.
4. Goldman S, Zadina K, Moritz T, et al. Long-term patency of saphenous vein and left internal mammary artery grafts after coronary artery bypass surgery: results from a Department of Veterans Affairs Cooperative Study. J Am Coll Cardiol 2004;44:2149–56.
5. Grube E, Teo SG, Buellesfeld L. Saphenous vein grafts and arterial conduits. In: Colombo A, Stankovic G, editors. Problem oriented approaches in interventional cardiology. London: Informa UK Ltd; 2007. p. 115–22.
6. Weintraub WS, Jones EL, Craver JM, et al. Frequency of repeat coronary bypass or coronary angioplasty after coronary artery bypass surgery using saphenous venous grafts. Am J Cardiol 1994;73:103–12.
7. Savage MP, Douglas JS Jr, Fischman DL, et al. Stent placement compared with balloon angioplasty for obstructed coronary bypass grafts. Saphenous Vein De Novo Trial Investigators. N Engl J Med 1997;337:740–7.
8. Piana RN, Paik GY, Moscucci M, et al. Incidence and treatment of 'no-reflow' after percutaneous coronary intervention. Circulation 1994;89:2514–8.
9. Hong MK, Mehran R, Dangas G, et al. Creatine kinase-MB enzyme elevation following successful saphenous vein graft intervention is associated with late mortality. Circulation 1999;100:2400–5.
10. Topol EJ, Yadav JS. Recognition of the importance of embolization in atherosclerotic vascular disease. Circulation 2000;101:570–80.
11. Rogers C, Huynh R, Seifert PA, et al. Embolic protection with filtering or occlusion balloons during saphenous vein graft stenting retrieves identical volumes and sizes of particulate debris. Circulation 2004;109:1735–40.
12. Prati F, Pawlowski T, Gil R, et al. Stenting of culprit lesions in unstable angina leads to a marked reduction in plaque burden: a major role of plaque embolization? A serial intravascular ultrasound study. Circulation 2003;107:2320–5.
13. Herrmann J. Peri-procedural myocardial injury: 2005 update. Eur Heart J 2005;26:2493–519.

14. Ziada KM, Mukherjee D. Peri-procedural myocardial infarction and embolism protection devices. In: Topol E, Tierstein P, editors. Textbook of interventional cardiology. 6th edition. Philadelphia: Saunders Elsevier; 2011. p. 372–87.

15. Gorog DA, Foale RA, Malik I. Distal myocardial protection during percutaneous coronary intervention: when and where? J Am Coll Cardiol 2005;46:1434–45.

16. Baim DS, Wahr D, George B, et al. Randomized trial of a distal embolic protection device during percutaneous intervention of saphenous vein aorto-coronary bypass grafts. Circulation 2002;105:1285–90.

17. Carrozza JP Jr, Caussin C, Braden G, et al. Embolic protection during saphenous vein graft intervention using a second-generation balloon protection device: results from the combined US and European pilot study of the TriActiv Balloon Protected Flush Extraction System. Am Heart J 2005;149:1136.

18. Kensey-Nash. TriActiv FX Embolic Protection System: 510(K) Summary. 2006: Letter from Kensey-Nash Corp to the FDA requesting approval for use of the TriActiv system in SVG PCI. Available at: http://www.accessdata.fda.gov/cdrh_docs/pdf6/K061772.pdf.

19. Lee MS, Park SJ, Kandzari DE, et al. Saphenous vein graft intervention. JACC Cardiovasc Interv 2011;4:831–43.

20. Stone GW, Rogers C, Hermiller J, et al. Randomized comparison of distal protection with a filter-based catheter and a balloon occlusion and aspiration system during percutaneous intervention of diseased saphenous vein aorto-coronary bypass grafts. Circulation 2003;108:548–53.

21. Cox DA, Liu H, Caputo R, et al. The combined BLAZE I and BLAZE II registries. Am J Cardiol 2005;96:5H.

22. ev3. SpiderFX Embolic Protection Device: instructions for use in saphenous vein graft (SVG) interventions. 2006. Available at: http://www.ev3.net/assets/007/5778.pdf.

23. Holmes DR, Coolong A, O'Shaughnessy C, et al. Comparison of the CardioShield filter with the Guard-Wire balloon in the prevention of embolisation during vein graft intervention: results from the CAPTIVE randomised trial. EuroIntervention 2006;2:161–8.

24. Kereiakes DJ, Turco MA, Breall J, et al. A novel filter-based distal embolic protection device for percutaneous intervention of saphenous vein graft lesions: results of the AMEthyst randomized controlled trial. JACC Cardiovasc Interv 2008;1:248–57.

25. Mauri L, Cox D, Hermiller J, et al. The PROXIMAL trial: proximal protection during saphenous vein graft intervention using the Proxis Embolic Protection System: a randomized, prospective, multicenter clinical trial. J Am Coll Cardiol 2007;50:1442–9.

26. Mehta SK, Stolker JM, Frutkin AD, et al. Suitability of saphenous vein graft lesions for the use of distal embolic protection devices. J Invasive Cardiol 2008;20:568–70.

27. Abdel-Karim AR, Papayannis AC, Mahmood A, et al. Role of embolic protection devices in ostial saphenous vein graft lesions. Catheter Cardiovasc Interv 2012;80(7):1120–6.

28. Mehta SK, Frutkin AD, Milford-Beland S, et al. Utilization of distal embolic protection in saphenous vein graft interventions (an analysis of 19,546 patients in the American College of Cardiology-National Cardiovascular Data Registry). Am J Cardiol 2007;100:1114–8.

29. Roffi M, Mukherjee D, Chew DP, et al. Lack of benefit from intravenous platelet glycoprotein IIb/IIIa receptor inhibition as adjunctive treatment for percutaneous interventions of aortocoronary bypass grafts: a pooled analysis of five randomized clinical trials. Circulation 2002;106:3063–7.

30. Jonas M, Stone GW, Mehran R, et al. Platelet glycoprotein IIb/IIIa receptor inhibition as adjunctive treatment during saphenous vein graft stenting: differential effects after randomization to occlusion or filter-based embolic protection. Eur Heart J 2006;27:920–8.

31. Levine GN, Bates ER, Blankenship JC, et al. 2011 ACCF/AHA/SCAI Guideline for Percutaneous Coronary Intervention. A report of the American College of Cardiology Foundation/American Heart Association Task Force on Practice Guidelines and the Society for Cardiovascular Angiography and Interventions. J Am Coll Cardiol 2011;58:e44–122.

32. Badhey N, Lichtenwalter C, de Lemos JA, et al. Contemporary use of embolic protection devices in saphenous vein graft interventions: insights from the stenting of saphenous vein grafts trial. Catheter Cardiovasc Interv 2010;76:263–9.

33. Cohen DJ, Murphy SA, Baim DS, et al. Cost-effectiveness of distal embolic protection for patients undergoing percutaneous intervention of saphenous vein bypass grafts: results from the SAFER trial. J Am Coll Cardiol 2004;44:1801–8.

34. Senter SR, Nathan S, Gupta A, et al. Clinical and economic outcomes of embolic complications and strategies for distal embolic protection during percutaneous coronary intervention in saphenous vein grafts. J Invasive Cardiol 2006;18:49–53.

# Pharmacotherapy During Saphenous Vein Graft Intervention

Willis M. Wu, MD[a], A. Michael Lincoff, MD[b],*

## KEYWORDS

- Saphenous vein graft • Percutaneous coronary intervention
- Heparin and glycoprotein IIb/IIIa inhibitor • Bivalirudin • No-reflow phenomenon
- Calcium channel blocker • Adenosine • Nitroprusside

## KEY POINTS

- Glycoprotein IIb/IIIa inhibition during vein graft intervention does not improve rates of ischemic end points but does confer a significantly increased risk of major bleeding.
- Compared with heparin plus glycoprotein IIb/IIIa inhibitors, bivalirudin is equally efficacious in preventing ischemic end points but is associated with a lower risk of bleeding.
- No-reflow, mediated by both distal embolization of debris and microvascular vasoconstriction, is a common complication of vein graft intervention.
- Data from small studies suggest that vasoactive agents such as nicardipine, adenosine, and nitroprusside are effective in treating the no-reflow phenomenon.

## INTRODUCTION

Coronary revascularization using coronary artery bypass grafting (CABG) is a fundamental treatment option for patients with severe coronary artery disease. However, the long-term patency of saphenous vein grafts (SVGs) that are used as surgical conduits is poor, and approximately half of grafts may be closed within 10 years of the surgery.[1,2] For patients who have already undergone prior surgical revascularization, repeat CABG carries a significant risk of morbidity and mortality. Therefore, percutaneous coronary intervention (PCI) remains a viable option for patients with diseased or degenerated SVGs. However, these procedures have had slow or no-reflow rates as high as 10% to 15%,[3] factors which can lead to myocardial infarction (MI) and other adverse clinical events. There are no universally recommended guidelines as to what concomitant pharmacotherapies should be used during vein graft interventions to prevent or diminish the risk of periprocedural adverse events. In general, the general considerations regarding pharmacotherapy relate to (1) anticoagulation and antiplatelet strategies, and (2) prevention and treatment of no-reflow during SVG PCI.

## ANTICOAGULANT THERAPY

### Unfractionated Heparin

Unfractionated heparin is a sulfated glycosaminoglycan whose anticoagulant properties work by binding to antithrombin III, which then leads to inactivation of thrombin. Because of its ease of administration, monitoring via activated clotting time (ACT), and reversal using protamine, heparin monotherapy was the fundamental anticoagulant

The authors report no disclosures.
[a] Department of Cardiovascular Medicine, Cleveland Clinic, 9500 Euclid Avenue Desk J2-3, Cleveland, OH 44195, USA; [b] Department of Cardiovascular Medicine, Cleveland Clinic Coordinating Center for Clinical Research, 9500 Euclid Avenue Desk J2-3, Cleveland, OH 44195, USA
* Corresponding author.
E-mail address: lincofa@ccf.org

Intervent Cardiol Clin 2 (2013) 273–282
http://dx.doi.org/10.1016/j.iccl.2012.12.004
2211-7458/13/$ – see front matter © 2013 Elsevier Inc. All rights reserved

interventional.theclinics.com

strategy in the early experience of SVG intervention. Heparin has never been compared with placebo in a randomized trial during PCI. The Saphenous Vein De Novo (SAVED) trial[4] evaluated balloon angioplasty versus bare metal stent placement in SVG in the era before routine use of glycoprotein (Gp) IIb/IIIa inhibitors (GPI) and thienopyridines during percutaneous intervention. Heparin was administered concomitantly with aspirin, dipyridamole, and warfarin. In both the angioplasty and stenting arms, there were low rates of in-hospital death (2% in each group), Q-wave MI (1% vs 2% respectively), and non–Q-wave MI (7% vs 2% respectively). The 30-day transfusion rate in the stenting group (15%) was significantly higher than in the angioplasty group (3%), which was attributable to the use of warfarin with stents. Similar rates of ischemic and bleeding end points were observed in other trials that used heparin monotherapy for anticoagulation, despite differences in techniques including balloon angioplasty, directional atherectomy, and stenting.[5,6]

### Unfractionated Heparin with Gp IIb/IIIa Inhibitors

#### Abciximab

Inhibition of the Gp IIb/IIIa receptor with abciximab is an effective means of suppressing platelet aggregation and has been shown to decrease clinical events when used adjunctively with unfractionated heparin during PCI.[7,8] Abciximab is a human-murine chimeric antibody Fab fragment that has a half-life of approximately 10 minutes, but it binds irreversibly to platelets, thus making its therapeutic effect longer. Overall, the literature on abciximab use compared with heparin in vein graft interventions shows modest angiographic benefit, little improvement in clinical outcomes, and an increased risk of bleeding.

In the Evaluation of IIb/IIIa Platelet Receptor Antagonist 7E3 in Preventing Ischemic Complications (EPIC) trial,[9] the subgroup of a small number of patients undergoing balloon angioplasty or directional atherectomy of aortocoronary SVGs had angiographic evidence of distal embolization in 3% of cases when abciximab was used concomitantly with heparin compared with 21% with placebo.[10] Despite this angiographic benefit, there was no difference in the 30-day composite end point of death, non-fatal MI, urgent revascularization, emergency stenting, or need for intra-aortic balloon pump counterpulsation. In addition, patients who received abciximab had higher rates of non–CABG-related major bleeding (16%) compared with those in the placebo group (0%). Observational data also indicate that, even during intervention for higher-risk vein graft lesions (older vein grafts, increased presence of thrombus, more complex lesions, and higher rates of Thrombolysis in Myocardial Infarction (TIMI) 0 grade flow before a procedure),[11] abciximab had no significant impact on angiographic success or in-hospital rates of death, Q-wave MI, or bypass surgery. Again, a higher incidence of major bleeding (19% vs 8%) was seen with abciximab use. Administration of abciximab was similarly shown to have little benefit on death, target vessel revascularization, and major adverse cardiac event (MACE) rates when administered during SVG intervention in high-risk diabetic patients, even when used concomitantly with a thienopyridine.[12] Local delivery of abciximab to the site of obstruction via an infusion catheter also does not seem to confer any advantage compared with systemic administration. In one small study, delivery of abciximab to the target lesion via an infusion catheter decreased thrombus burden but did not improve postprocedural TIMI flow grade.[13]

#### Other Gp IIb/IIIa inhibitors

Eptifibatide is a cyclic heptapeptide that binds to and reversibly inhibits the Gp IIb/IIIa receptor. Tirofiban is a small nonpeptide antagonist of the Gp IIb/IIIa receptor and, like eptifibatide, its action is reversible. Although it has been suggested that tirofiban may attenuate troponin release after SVG PCI[14] and decrease slow or no-reflow[15] in small studies, pooled data of abciximab and eptifibatide do not support the use of Gp IIb/IIIa inhibitors for SVG intervention. Given the similar mechanism of action, the overall data suggest little effect of any Gp IIb/IIIa inhibitor on clinical outcome after SVG PCI.

The largest analysis of Gp IIb/IIIa inhibition during PCI of vein grafts pooled 5 randomized trials involving Gp IIb/IIIa inhibitors and found no clinical benefit with Gp IIb/IIIa inhibitor use for SVG intervention at 30 days or 6 months.[16] The pooled trials, including the EPIC, Evaluation in PTCA to Improve Long-term Outcome with abciximab Gp IIb/IIIa blockade (EPILOG), Evaluation of Platelet IIb/IIIa Inhibitor for STENTing (EPISTENT),[17] Integrilin to Minimize Platelet Aggregation and Coronary Thrombosis-II (IMPACT II),[18] and Platelet Gp IIb/IIIa in Unstable Angina: Receptor Suppression Using Integrilin Therapy (PURSUIT)[19] trials, were mainly studies involving balloon angioplasty before the era of thienopyridine use, and the lack of benefit was observed across all 5 trials. Abciximab was used in 51% of cases and eptifibatide in 49%. At 30 days, the rates of the composite end point of death, MI, or urgent revascularization for the Gp IIb/IIIa group and placebo group were 16.5% and 12.6%, respectively. At 6 months, the rates were 39.4% and 32.7%, and there was no statistical difference between the 2 groups for either time point. Major bleeding also occurred more frequently in patients who were treated with Gp IIb/IIIa inhibitors than in those who received placebo (6.8% vs 1.4%) (**Table 1**).[16]

Although the reason for the consistent lack of efficacy of adjunctive Gp IIb/IIIa inhibition during SVG PCI is not certain, it may be related to the inability of the Gp IIb/IIIa inhibitors to protect the distal microvasculature against non–platelet-mediated embolization. Degenerated SVG plaques often consist of thrombus and friable atherosclerotic debris, both of which are not significantly affected by antiplatelet agents, which can plug the microcirculation when embolized during SVG PCI and lead to adverse events.[16]

### Gp IIb/IIIa inhibition and distal embolic protection

When used with a mechanical device to protect the microvasculature from embolic debris, Gp IIb/IIIa inhibition has been associated with improvement in angiographic end points, although clinical benefit has not been shown. The FilterWire EX Randomized Evaluation (FIRE) trial[20] randomized patients undergoing SVG intervention to distal embolization protection with either a filter device (FilterWire EX, Boston Scientific Corp, Natick, MA) or a balloon occlusion device (GuardWire balloon occlusion and aspiration device, Medtronic Inc, Santa Rosa, CA). Although the use of Gp IIb/IIIa inhibitors was not randomized, a secondary analysis of this trial showed improved flow with concomitant use of Gp IIb/IIIa inhibitors and the FilterWire EX (Boston Scientific Corp, Natick, MA) distal protection

device, but not with the balloon occlusion catheter.[21] Concomitant medical therapy included aspirin, a thienopyridine, and intracoronary vasodilators, including nitroglycerin (NTG) and nitroprusside (SNP). In that trial, when a Gp IIb/IIIa inhibitor was used, the operator's choice was eptifibatide in 56.8% of cases, abciximab in 33.9%, and tirofiban in 9.3%. When the FilterWire was deployed, there were lower rates of procedural complications including abrupt vessel closure, no-reflow, or distal embolization when a Gp IIb/IIIa inhibitor was given. In addition, use of a Gp IIb/IIIa inhibitor with the FilterWire decreased the incidence of TIMI 0 to 1 flow to 26.3% compared with 76.5% without its use. However, composite MACE, including death, MI, or target vessel revascularization, was not different at 30 days between patients who received the FilterWire and a Gp IIb/IIIa inhibitor compared with those without a Gp IIb/IIIa inhibitor.

### Bivalirudin

Bivalirudin is a short-acting, synthetic small molecule that directly inhibits both soluble and clot-bound thrombin. Bivalirudin has been shown to be associated with similar efficacy and less major bleeding compared with heparin monotherapy or heparin plus Gp IIb/IIIa blockade when used in patients undergoing PCI for stable coronary disease[22–24] or acute coronary syndromes.[8,25,26] Although there no randomized clinical trials have compared bivalirudin with other indirect thrombin inhibitors such as heparin or low-molecular-weight heparin specifically in patients undergoing vein graft intervention, subgroup analyses of the large-scale interventional trials suggest that bivalirudin is an effective antithrombotic choice for bypass graft interventions.

The Randomized Evaluation in PCI Linking Angiomax to Reduced Clinical Events (REPLACE)-1 and REPLACE-2 trials showed the efficacy and safety of bivalirudin use in PCI performed for both stable and unstable angina,[22,24] and, between these 2 trials, 423 patients underwent vein graft interventions. In REPLACE-1, patients were randomized to receive either heparin or bivalirudin, and the use of a GPI (abciximab, eptifibatide, or tirofiban) was left to the discretion of the interventional operator. This decision was made before randomization to bivalirudin or heparin and approximately 70% of patients in both arms received a Gp IIb/IIIa inhibitor. In REPLACE-2, patients were randomized to bivalirudin monotherapy (with provisional use of a Gp IIb/IIIa inhibitor in the event of ischemic complications) versus heparin plus a Gp IIb/IIIa inhibitor (abciximab or eptifibatide). In both trials, all patients received aspirin, and

**Table 1**
**Six-month ischemic event rates (%) of SVG PCI from pooled GPI trials**

|  | GPI (n = 389) | Placebo (n = 216) | P Value |
|---|---|---|---|
| Death | 5.9 | 2.9 | .08 |
| MI | 19.6 | 15.0 | .14 |
| Revascularization | 26.0 | 21.9 | .23 |
| Death/MI/ revascularization | 39.4 | 32.7 | .07 |

*Adapted from* Roffi M, Mukherjee D, Chew DP, et al. Lack of benefit from intravenous platelet glycoprotein IIb/IIIa receptor inhibition as adjunctive treatment for percutaneous interventions of aortocoronary bypass grafts: a pooled analysis of five randomized clinical trials. Circulation 2002;106(24):3065; with permission.

pretreatment with clopidogrel (300 mg loading dose followed by 75 mg daily for at least a month) was strongly encouraged.[27]

Retrospective analysis of these two trials showed no significant difference in the composite ischemic end points of death, MI, or urgent revascularization within 48 hours, which occurred in 9.4% of the patients receiving bivalirudin with or without a Gp IIb/IIIa inhibitor and in 10% of patients receiving heparin plus a Gp IIb/IIIa inhibitor. These findings were consistent even during longer-term follow-up, because the rates of MI (14.4% vs 14%), death (4.2% vs 7.8%), and target vessel revascularization (10.8% vs 12.8%) were not significantly different between the bivalirudin and heparin groups at 12 months in the REPLACE-2 trial (**Table 2**).[27] However, although the ischemic end point rates were similar in the bivalirudin and heparin groups, bleeding complications within 48 hours were seen less frequently with bivalirudin. Minor bleeding was significantly less frequent in the bivalirudin arm, occurring in 14.8% of patients in the bivalirudin group versus 22.7% of patients in the heparin group. Major bleeding was infrequent and occurred at similar rates in the bivalirudin arm (3.4%) and the heparin arm (3.2%).[27]

Concordant with the results seen in the REPLACE-1 and REPLACE-2 trials, subgroup analysis of The Acute Catheterization and Urgent Intervention Triage Strategy (ACUITY) trial suggested that bivalirudin alone is a safe and effective anticoagulant strategy for patients with non-ST elevation acute coronary syndromes undergoing vein graft intervention.[25] Of the total interventions in ACUITY, 4% were performed on vein grafts; broken down by pharmacologic strategy, this amounted to 114 patients in the bivalirudin alone group, 114 patients in the bivalirudin plus Gp IIb/IIIa inhibitor group, and 101 patients in the heparin (unfractionated heparin or enoxaparin) plus a Gp IIb/IIIa inhibitor group.

When a Gp IIb/IIIa inhibitor was used, eptifibatide was used most frequently (97%) and abciximab and tirofiban were used in the remainder of cases. Concurrent medications in this trial included aspirin and clopidogrel.[28]

In the patients undergoing SVG PCI in ACUITY, there was no significant difference in rates of MACE between the bivalirudin alone, bivalirudin plus Gp IIb/IIIa inhibitor, or heparin plus Gp IIb/IIIa inhibitor groups at 30 days, occurring in 19%, 20%, and 19% of patients, respectively. Death from any cause was also similar between the three groups at 1 year, occurring in 5% of patients in the bivalirudin group, 10% in the bivalirudin plus Gp IIb/IIIa inhibitor group, and 7% in the heparin plus Gp IIb/IIIa inhibitor group (**Table 3**). TIMI major and minor bleeding at 30 days occurred at a comparable rate in all three groups.[28]

### Bivalirudin and distal embolic protection

When used in conjunction with a distal embolic protection device, it has been suggested that bivalirudin may decrease periprocedural creatine kinase myocardial band (CK-MB) release compared with heparin. A single-center retrospective study evaluated 136 SVG lesions in 114 patients in which PCI was performed with either bivalirudin or heparin in addition to using either the GuardWire (Percusurge, Medtronic AVE, Sunnyvale, CA) distal balloon and occlusion system or the retrievable FilterWire EX (Boston Scientific, Natick, MA), a distal embolic filter protection system.[29] Choice of bivalirudin or heparin was not randomized. In this study, all patients received aspirin and a thienopyridine, and no patients received Gp IIb/IIIa inhibitors. Peak periprocedural CK-MB values greater than 5 times the upper limit of normal were observed in 3 out of 54 patients (5.6%) on bivalirudin and in 11 out of 60 (18.3%) patients on heparin alone. Clinical events such as in-hospital death, Q-wave MI, and repeat percutaneous transluminal coronary angioplasty occurred at similar rates in the bivalirudin and heparin arms.

### Enoxaparin

Enoxaparin is a low-molecular-weight heparin that has been shown to be safe and efficacious in PCI, performed both electively for angina and urgently for acute coronary syndromes.[30–35] It can be dosed using an intravenous bolus of 0.5, 0.75, or 1 mg/kg, or it can be given subcutaneously at 1 mg/kg every 12 hours. The major disadvantages of enoxaparin use during PCI compared with heparin is the lack of a reversal agent, such as protamine for heparin, in the event of a complication, as well as the difficulty of monitoring to ensure therapeutic anticoagulation in patients

**Table 2**
**Twelve-month ischemic event rates (%) of SVG PCI from the REPLACE-2 trial**

|  | Bivalirudin (n = 203) | Heparin + GPI (n = 220) | P Value |
|---|---|---|---|
| Death | 4.2 | 7.8 | .16 |
| MI | 14.4 | 14.0 | .91 |
| TVR | 10.8 | 12.8 | .55 |

*Abbreviation:* TVR, target vessel revascularization.

*Data from* Kao J, Lincoff AM, Topol EJ, et al. Direct thrombin inhibition appears to be a safe and effective anticoagulant for percutaneous bypass graft interventions. Catheter Cardiovasc Interv 2006;68(3):355.

**Table 3**
**One-year clinical event rates (%) of SVG PCI from the ACUITY trial**

|  | Heparin + GPI (n = 101) | Bivalirudin + GPI (n = 114) | P Value | Bivalirudin (n = 114) | P Value (vs Heparin + GPI) |
|---|---|---|---|---|---|
| Major adverse cardiac event | 43.0 | 37.0 | .74 | 37.0 | .89 |
| Death from any cause | 7.0 | 10.0 | .46 | 5.0 | .60 |
| MI | 21.0 | 22.0 | .75 | 25.0 | .57 |
| Unplanned ischemic TVR | 27.0 | 22.0 | .80 | 19.0 | .64 |

*Data from* Kumar D, Dangas G, Mehran R, et al. Comparison of bivalirudin versus bivalirudin plus glycoprotein IIb/IIIa inhibitor versus heparin plus glycoprotein IIb/IIIa inhibitor in patients with acute coronary syndromes having percutaneous intervention for narrowed saphenous vein aorto-coronary grafts (the ACUITY trial investigators). Am J Cardiol 2010;106(7):943.

dosed before PCI. However, the trials investigating enoxaparin use for both elective PCI and for acute coronary syndromes only incorporated small percentages of patients undergoing vein graft intervention,[31,32] so drawing definitive conclusions regarding its relative efficacy during SVG PCI is not possible.

### Thrombolytic Therapy

In some cases of chronically occluded or old and degenerated SVG, the pathophysiology includes a significant degree of thrombus burden in addition to atherosclerotic changes. Not only does the thrombus make PCI more difficult, it also increases the risk of stent thrombosis.[36] Early studies investigated the feasibility of using a thrombolytic agent, most commonly urokinase, to achieve enough patency to allow percutaneous intervention on these types of grafts.[37] However, this strategy of using adjunctive thrombolytics during SVG PCI is no longer commonly used in current practice because of marginal long-term outcomes and an increased risk of bleeding.[38] In addition, percutaneous intervention to a chronically occluded SVG is currently contraindicated according to the most recent American College of Cardiology/American Heart Association guidelines.

### NO-REFLOW PHENOMENON

No-reflow describes a phenomenon characterized by poor or absent antegrade coronary flow in an epicardial vessel without evidence of dissection, thrombus, or vessel closure. It occurs in up to 5% of patients undergoing PCI, and can approach 30% in those undergoing higher-risk procedures such as vein graft intervention, rotational atherectomy, or PCI for MI.[39] Various mechanisms for the pathophysiology of no-reflow have been

proposed, including distal embolization of plaque and/or thrombus, and increased microvascular vasoconstriction.[40] No-reflow carries an association with poor outcomes after PCI, including increased risk of death and MI.[40] Distal embolic protection devices have been shown to decrease the incidence of no-reflow, but there may be instances in which the lesion is too distal or other anatomic contraindications exist for a distal protection device to be safely used. Therefore, using pharmacologic agents may be the best available strategy to prevent or treat this complication. Commonly used drugs in this scenario include calcium channel blockers, adenosine, nitroprusside, and nitroglycerin. In general, only weak evidence exists to support the use of any of these medications, because the literature on this topic is limited by small trials or subgroup analyses showing small benefit, mostly in angiographic parameters rather than with more robust clinical end points.

### Calcium Channel Blockers

#### Nicardipine
Nicardipine is a dihydropyridine calcium channel blocker with high coronary selectivity, and it has potent vasodilating capacity for the microcirculation.[41] Unlike other calcium channel blockers, such as diltiazem and verapamil, it has few negative effects on myocardial contractility or atrioventricular conduction. It also has a long duration of effect (approximately 5–7 minutes), unlike other vasodilating agents such as adenosine or nitroprusside.[41] For these reasons, nicardipine has been shown to be an attractive drug to prevent and treat no-reflow.

When nicardipine is administered prophylactically, SVG PCI has been shown to be safe, with low rates of adverse events both immediately after a procedure and at 30 days.[41] One small, non-randomized trial showed the effectiveness of prophylactic administration of 200 to 300 µg of nicardipine via the guiding catheter to prevent no-reflow without adjunctive use of a distal protection device, even in grafts with a mean age of 11.9 years. Mean TIMI flow grade was maintained throughout the procedure, and CK levels were increased to twice normal in only 2.6% of patients and greater than 3 times normal in only 1.5% of patients 12 to 18 hours after the procedure. At 30 days, the total MACE rate was 4.4%. These results compare favorably with those noted in other studies evaluating the efficacy of distal protection devices.[42,43]

In addition to being used as an agent to prevent no-reflow, nicardipine has also been shown to be efficacious in reversing no-reflow if it occurs during SVG PCI. In a small, single-center, retrospective analysis of no-reflow during native vessel and SVG PCI, nicardipine was administered in 100-µg boluses either through the guide catheter or via a selective infusion catheter every 2 to 5 minutes if no-reflow developed. In all 23 cases of SVG PCI during which no-reflow was observed, it was successfully reversed with nicardipine without episodes of hypotension or atrioventricular conduction block.[39]

### Verapamil

Verapamil is a nondihydropyridine calcium channel blocker that promotes vasodilation via vascular smooth muscle relaxation. Intracoronary doses typically start at 100 or 200 µg, and the medication has potential to cause bradycardia and hypotension. Although total patient numbers are small, studies have suggested that intracoronary verapamil can be used to treat microvascular spasm[44] and no-reflow[45] during PCI of native vessels as well as for no-reflow during SVG PCI.

In a small randomized study, intragraft administration of 200 µg of verapamil was associated with an improvement in TIMI frame count[46] by 53.3% ± 22.4% compared with 11.5% ± 38.9% in the group that received placebo. There was also a trend toward reduction in the risk of no-reflow with verapamil, occurring in none of the patients taking verapamil compared with 4 out of 12 (33%) patients in the placebo group. Despite these findings, there was no difference in incidence of TIMI 2 or 3 grade flow, post-PCI CK, or troponin I release between groups.

### Adenosine

Adenosine is potent arterial vasodilator once bound to its receptors in the endothelium and smooth muscle cells of the coronary arteries, thus producing relaxation of the vascular wall.[47] It has a rapid onset of action within seconds, and it has a short half-life of less than 10 seconds. When administered via an intracoronary or intragraft route, a common starting dose is 24 µg, and escalating doses up to 120 µg may be required, depending on each dose response. Atrioventricular block can rapidly occur, especially at higher doses, but, because of its short half-life, the need for temporary pacing or use of a chronotropic agent is rare. The rationale for adenosine use is to treat microvascular vasospasm that may be contributing to no-reflow.

One small study showed the usefulness of rapid and forceful injections of adenosine followed by saline flushes using a 3-mL syringe.[48] The mean TIMI flow was $2.0 \pm 1.0$ in these cases before intervention and was reduced to TIMI $1.0 \pm 0.5$ initially after the stenting. The investigators used a mean of $12.1 \pm 3.4$ boluses of 18 µg of adenosine for each case followed by 3 to 4 saline flushes of 3 mL each. TIMI flow was subsequently increased to $2.9 \pm 0.31$ after adenosine. There were no adverse reductions in blood pressure during adenosine administration or episodes of heart block. There were also no Q-wave MIs or deaths. The investigators postulated that both the mechanical displacement of embolic debris from the high-velocity injections and the vasodilatory effects of adenosine contributed to the benefit that was observed.

A larger study confirmed the efficacy of adenosine in reversing no-reflow, but it also showed its inability to prevent this phenomenon.[3] In this retrospective study, patients received 24-µg boluses of adenosine followed by 2 to 3 saline flushes of 3 to 4 mL each, injected into the guide catheter before intervention. There was no significant difference in the incidence of slow or no-reflow, occurring in 10 out of 70 (14.2%) patients who received prophylactic adenosine compared with 10 out of 73 (13.6%) patients who did not. There was also no difference in final TIMI flow, with the group receiving prophylactic adenosine having $2.5 \pm 0.7$ TIMI grade flow, whereas the group that did not receive prophylactic adenosine had $2.3 \pm 0.9$ TIMI grade flow.

### Nitroprusside

Nitroprusside is a direct donor of nitric oxide (NO), which is an endothelium-derived compound that contributes to arteriolar vasodilation and platelet inhibition and has antiinflammatory properties.[49] Unlike nitroglycerin (NTG), which is more effective in the larger, nonresistance vessels, nitroprusside does not require metabolism from the vascular wall to produce NO and is therefore effective in dilating both epicardial vessels and resistance vessels such as arterioles and the microcirculation. Common starting doses of nitroprusside, when given via an intracoronary route, begin at 50 μg or 100 μg and can be increased at multiples thereof. The most frequent side effect of nitroprusside use is hypotension, but this is typically transient.

Most of the studies that support use of nitroprusside in the treatment of no-reflow enrolled a small number of patients, only a small percentage of whom underwent vein graft interventions, so conclusions on the benefit of nitroprusside in this SVG PCI must be extrapolated. Hillegass and colleagues[49] reported their experience of 20 instances of no-reflow associated with PCI, of which 9 were SVG interventions, treated with nitroprusside. After nitroprusside administration, TIMI flow was significantly increased on final angiography compared with after no-reflow was noted. No episodes of hypotension were observed. Similar findings of improved TIMI flow grade were also observed in other trials of nitroprusside treatment once no-reflow has been observed,[50,51] but results are less clear when prophylactic nitroprusside is given to prevent no-reflow.[52,53] There is some evidence to suggest that combining nitroprusside with adenosine has incremental benefits in improving TIMI flow grade after no-reflow.[54]

### Nitroglycerin

Similar to nitroprusside, nitroglycerin vasodilates coronary epicardial vessels via production of NO. However, because it is not readily converted to its active metabolite in the small arterioles of the heart, its potency in dilating the microvasculature is limited.[55] Intracoronary doses of nitroglycerin are typically given in increments of 100 μg and can cause brief hypotension. Although it is a commonly used medication to treat no-reflow during PCI, the data to support this are limited.

When directly compared with verapamil in vein graft interventions, nitroglycerin was inferior in its ability to reverse no-reflow.[56] In a small, prospective study, balloon angioplasty, stenting, extraction atherectomy, or any combination thereof were used to treat no-reflow in 32 SVG lesions with concomitant intracoronary nitroglycerin or verapamil. Nitroglycerin was given at 200-μg doses in 16 patients. Verapamil was given at doses ranging from 100 to 250 μg in the other 16 patients, and additional doses were given if there was no response to initial treatment. In patients receiving NTG, TIMI flow did not

significantly improve, going from $1.2 \pm 0.5$ before NTG use to $1.4 \pm 0.7$ afterward. In contrast, verapamil use was associated with an increase in TIMI flow from $1.4 \pm 0.8$ before verapamil to $2.8 \pm 0.5$ afterward. Despite the lack of improvement in TIMI flow in the nitroglycerin group, only 2 patients from both groups combined sustained a non–Q-wave MI, defined by CK-MB levels greater than 25 IU/L.

## SUMMARY

SVGs have poor long-term patency and often require percutaneous intervention once they develop severe lesions, because repeat bypass surgery carries increased risk of morbidity and mortality. Because there is potential for adverse events during SVG PCI, the effective adjunctive pharmacotherapy is of paramount importance. Gp IIb/IIIa inhibitors used concomitantly with heparin have only modest benefit, mostly with angiographic parameters, and significantly increase the risk of bleeding. In contrast, when chosen as the anticoagulant strategy during SVG PCI, bivalirudin has been shown in retrospective analyses to have equivalent rates of adverse clinical events compared with heparin, but it has the advantage of reduced risk of significant bleeding. Thrombolytic therapy with agents such as urokinase has been shown to have no, or at most only modest, benefit, with increased bleeding risk, and is therefore not commonly used in clinical practice. With regard to the treatment of no-reflow, vasodilators have been most commonly used given the contribution of microvascular vasospasm associated with the condition. Data are most robust with calcium channel blockers including nicardipine and verapamil. Adenosine is effective in the treatment of no-reflow, but likely has little capacity to prevent the phenomenon. In addition, the NO-donating agents such as nitroprusside and nitroglycerin are commonly used to treat no-reflow, but robust data to support such use are lacking. Randomized studies with each subclass of medications would be helpful in further elucidating which agents confer superior benefit in SVG PCI.

## REFERENCES

1. Bourassa MG, Enjalbert M, Campeau L, et al. Progression of atherosclerosis in coronary arteries and bypass grafts: ten years later. Am J Cardiol 1984;53(12):102C–7C.
2. Goldman S, Zadina K, Moritz T, et al. Long-term patency of saphenous vein and left internal mammary artery grafts after coronary artery bypass

surgery: results from a Department of Veterans Affairs cooperative study. J Am Coll Cardiol 2004; 44(11):2149–56.

3. Sdringola S, Assali A, Ghani M, et al. Adenosine use during aortocoronary vein graft interventions reverses but does not prevent the slow-no reflow phenomenon. Catheter Cardiovasc Interv 2000; 51(4):394–9.

4. Savage MP, Douglas JS Jr, Fischman DL, et al. Stent placement compared with balloon angioplasty for obstructed coronary bypass grafts. Saphenous Vein De Novo Trial Investigators. N Engl J Med 1997;337(11):740–7.

5. Holmes DR Jr, Topol EJ, Califf RM, et al. A multicenter, randomized trial of coronary angioplasty versus directional atherectomy for patients with saphenous vein bypass graft lesions. CAVEAT-II Investigators. Circulation 1995;91(7):1966–74.

6. Wong SC, Baim DS, Schatz RA, et al. Immediate results and late outcomes after stent implantation in saphenous vein graft lesions: the multicenter U.S. Palmaz-Schatz stent experience. The Palmaz-Schatz Stent Study Group. J Am Coll Cardiol 1995; 26(3):704–12.

7. Platelet glycoprotein IIb/IIIa receptor blockade and low-dose heparin during percutaneous coronary revascularization. The EPILOG Investigators. N Engl J Med 1997;336(24):1689–96.

8. Kastrati A, Neumann FJ, Schulz S, et al. Abciximab and heparin versus bivalirudin for non-ST-elevation myocardial infarction. N Engl J Med 2011;365(21): 1980–9.

9. Use of a monoclonal antibody directed against the platelet glycoprotein IIb/IIIa receptor in high-risk coronary angioplasty. The EPIC Investigation. N Engl J Med 1994;330(14):956–61.

10. Mak KH, Challapalli R, Eisenberg MJ, et al. Effect of platelet glycoprotein IIb/IIIa receptor inhibition on distal embolization during percutaneous revascularization of aortocoronary saphenous vein grafts. EPIC Investigators. Evaluation of IIb/IIIa platelet receptor antagonist 7E3 in preventing ischemic complications. Am J Cardiol 1997;80(8):985–8.

11. Mathew V, Grill DE, Scott CG, et al. The influence of abciximab use on clinical outcome after aortocoronary vein graft interventions. J Am Coll Cardiol 1999;34(4):1163–9.

12. Applegate RJ, Upadhya B, Little WC, et al. Late outcomes after intervention of vein grafts in diabetics with abciximab use. Int J Cardiol 2006; 111(1):136–41.

13. Barsness GW, Buller C, Ohman EM, et al. Reduced thrombus burden with abciximab delivered locally before percutaneous intervention in saphenous vein grafts. Am Heart J 2000;139(5):824–9.

14. Kurowski V, Toelg R, Jain D, et al. Effect of adjunctive treatment with tirofiban on troponin T elevation during stenting of critically stenosed aortocoronary saphenous vein grafts. Am J Cardiol 2005;96(5): 681–4.

15. Ozkan M, Sag C, Yokusoglu M, et al. The effect of tirofiban and clopidogrel pretreatment on outcome of old saphenous vein graft stenting in patients with acute coronary syndromes. Tohoku J Exp Med 2005;206(1):7–13.

16. Roffi M, Mukherjee D, Chew DP, et al. Lack of benefit from intravenous platelet glycoprotein IIb/IIIa receptor inhibition as adjunctive treatment for percutaneous interventions of aortocoronary bypass grafts: a pooled analysis of five randomized clinical trials. Circulation 2002;106(24):3063–7.

17. EPISTENT Investigators. Randomised placebo-controlled and balloon-angioplasty-controlled trial to assess safety of coronary stenting with use of platelet glycoprotein-IIb/IIIa blockade. Lancet 1998;352(9122):87–92.

18. Randomised placebo-controlled trial of effect of eptifibatide on complications of percutaneous coronary intervention: IMPACT-II. Integrilin to Minimise Platelet Aggregation and Coronary Thrombosis-II. Lancet 1997;349(9063):1422–8.

19. Inhibition of platelet glycoprotein IIb/IIIa with eptifibatide in patients with acute coronary syndromes. The PURSUIT Trial Investigators. Platelet glycoprotein IIb/IIIa in unstable angina: receptor suppression using integrilin therapy. N Engl J Med 1998;339(7): 436–43.

20. Stone GW, Rogers C, Hermiller J, et al. Randomized comparison of distal protection with a filter-based catheter and a balloon occlusion and aspiration system during percutaneous intervention of diseased saphenous vein aorto-coronary bypass grafts. Circulation 2003;108(5):548–53.

21. Jonas M, Stone GW, Mehran R, et al. Platelet glycoprotein IIb/IIIa receptor inhibition as adjunctive treatment during saphenous vein graft stenting: differential effects after randomization to occlusion or filter-based embolic protection. Eur Heart J 2006;27(8):920–8.

22. Lincoff AM, Bittl JA, Harrington RA, et al. Bivalirudin and provisional glycoprotein IIb/IIIa blockade compared with heparin and planned glycoprotein IIb/IIIa blockade during percutaneous coronary intervention: REPLACE-2 randomized trial. JAMA 2003;289(7):853–63.

23. Kastrati A, Neumann FJ, Mehilli J, et al. Bivalirudin versus unfractionated heparin during percutaneous coronary intervention. N Engl J Med 2008;359(7): 688–96.

24. Lincoff AM, Bittl JA, Kleiman NS, et al. Comparison of bivalirudin versus heparin during percutaneous coronary intervention (the Randomized Evaluation of PCI Linking Angiomax to Reduced Clinical Events [REPLACE]-1 trial). Am J Cardiol 2004;93(9):1092–6.

25. Stone GW, McLaurin BT, Cox DA, et al. Bivalirudin for patients with acute coronary syndromes. N Engl J Med 2006;355(21):2203–16.
26. Stone GW, Witzenbichler B, Guagliumi G, et al. Bivalirudin during primary PCI in acute myocardial infarction. N Engl J Med 2008;358(21):2218–30.
27. Kao J, Lincoff AM, Topol EJ, et al. Direct thrombin inhibition appears to be a safe and effective anticoagulant for percutaneous bypass graft interventions. Catheter Cardiovasc Interv 2006;68(3):352–6.
28. Kumar D, Dangas G, Mehran R, et al. Comparison of bivalirudin versus bivalirudin plus glycoprotein IIb/IIIa inhibitor versus heparin plus glycoprotein IIb/IIIa inhibitor in patients with acute coronary syndromes having percutaneous intervention for narrowed saphenous vein aorto-coronary grafts (the ACUITY trial investigators). Am J Cardiol 2010;106(7):941–5.
29. Rha SW, Kuchulakanti PK, Pakala R, et al. Bivalirudin versus heparin as an antithrombotic agent in patients who undergo percutaneous saphenous vein graft intervention with a distal protection device. Am J Cardiol 2005;96(1):67–70.
30. Madan M, Radhakrishnan S, Reis M, et al. Comparison of enoxaparin versus heparin during elective percutaneous coronary intervention performed with either eptifibatide or tirofiban (the ACTION Trial). Am J Cardiol 2005;95(11):1295–301.
31. Ferguson JJ, Califf RM, Antman EM, et al. Enoxaparin vs unfractionated heparin in high-risk patients with non-ST-segment elevation acute coronary syndromes managed with an intended early invasive strategy: primary results of the SYNERGY randomized trial. JAMA 2004;292(1):45–54.
32. Montalescot G, White HD, Gallo R, et al. Enoxaparin versus unfractionated heparin in elective percutaneous coronary intervention. N Engl J Med 2006;355(10):1006–17.
33. Dumaine R, Borentain M, Bertel O, et al. Intravenous low-molecular-weight heparins compared with unfractionated heparin in percutaneous coronary intervention: quantitative review of randomized trials. Arch Intern Med 2007;167(22):2423–30.
34. Bhatt DL, Lee BI, Casterella PJ, et al. Safety of concomitant therapy with eptifibatide and enoxaparin in patients undergoing percutaneous coronary intervention: results of the Coronary Revascularization Using Integrilin and Single bolus Enoxaparin Study. J Am Coll Cardiol 2003;41(1):20–5.
35. Gibson CM, Morrow DA, Murphy SA, et al. A randomized trial to evaluate the relative protection against post-percutaneous coronary intervention microvascular dysfunction, ischemia, and inflammation among antiplatelet and antithrombotic agents: the PROTECT-TIMI-30 trial. J Am Coll Cardiol 2006;47(12):2364–73.
36. Denardo SJ, Morris NB, Rocha-Singh KJ, et al. Safety and efficacy of extended urokinase infusion plus stent deployment for treatment of obstructed, older saphenous vein grafts. Am J Cardiol 1995;76(11):776–80.
37. Hartmann JR, McKeever LS, O'Neill WW, et al. Recanalization of chronically occluded aortocoronary saphenous vein bypass grafts with long-term, low dose direct infusion of urokinase (ROBUST): a serial trial. J Am Coll Cardiol 1996;27(1):60–6.
38. Cecena FA, Hoelzinger DH. Transcatheter therapy of thrombotic-occlusive lesions in saphenous vein grafts. Am J Cardiol 1996;78(1):31–6.
39. Huang RI, Patel P, Walinsky P, et al. Efficacy of intracoronary nicardipine in the treatment of no-reflow during percutaneous coronary intervention. Catheter Cardiovasc Interv 2006;68(5):671–6.
40. Habibzadeh MR, Thai H, Movahed MR. Prophylactic intragraft injection of nicardipine prior to saphenous vein graft percutaneous intervention for the prevention of no-reflow: a review and comparison to protection devices. J Invasive Cardiol 2011;23(5):202–6.
41. Fischell TA, Subraya RG, Ashraf K, et al. "Pharmacologic" distal protection using prophylactic, intragraft nicardipine to prevent no-reflow and non-Q-wave myocardial infarction during elective saphenous vein graft intervention. J Invasive Cardiol 2007;19(2):58–62.
42. Baim DS, Wahr D, George B, et al. Randomized trial of a distal embolic protection device during percutaneous intervention of saphenous vein aorto-coronary bypass grafts. Circulation 2002;105(11):1285–90.
43. Carrozza JP Jr, Mumma M, Breall JA, et al. Randomized evaluation of the TriActiv balloon-protection flush and extraction system for the treatment of saphenous vein graft disease. J Am Coll Cardiol 2005;46(9):1677–83.
44. Pomerantz RM, Kuntz RE, Diver DJ, et al. Intracoronary verapamil for the treatment of distal microvascular coronary artery spasm following PTCA. Cathet Cardiovasc Diagn 1991;24(4):283–5.
45. Werner GS, Lang K, Kuehnert H, et al. Intracoronary verapamil for reversal of no-reflow during coronary angioplasty for acute myocardial infarction. Catheter Cardiovasc Interv 2002;57(4):444–51.
46. Michaels AD, Appleby M, Otten MH, et al. Pretreatment with intragraft verapamil prior to percutaneous coronary intervention of saphenous vein graft lesions: results of the randomized, controlled vasodilator prevention on no-reflow (VAPOR) trial. J Invasive Cardiol 2002;14(6):299–302.
47. Freilich A, Tepper D. Adenosine and its cardiovascular effects. Am Heart J 1992;123(5):1324–8.
48. Fischell TA, Carter AJ, Foster MT, et al. Reversal of "no reflow" during vein graft stenting using high velocity boluses of intracoronary adenosine. Cathet Cardiovasc Diagn 1998;45(4):360–5.

49. Hillegass WB, Dean NA, Liao L, et al. Treatment of no-reflow and impaired flow with the nitric oxide donor nitroprusside following percutaneous coronary interventions: initial human clinical experience. J Am Coll Cardiol 2001;37(5):1335–43.

50. Wang HJ, Lo PH, Lin JJ, et al. Treatment of slow/no-reflow phenomenon with intracoronary nitroprusside injection in primary coronary intervention for acute myocardial infarction. Catheter Cardiovasc Interv 2004;63(2):171–6.

51. Pasceri V, Pristipino C, Pelliccia F, et al. Effects of the nitric oxide donor nitroprusside on no-reflow phenomenon during coronary interventions for acute myocardial infarction. Am J Cardiol 2005;95(11):1358–61.

52. Amit G, Cafri C, Yaroslavtsev S, et al. Intracoronary nitroprusside for the prevention of the no-reflow phenomenon after primary percutaneous coronary intervention in acute myocardial infarction. A randomized, double-blind, placebo-controlled clinical trial. Am Heart J 2006;152(5):e9–14.

53. Shinozaki N, Ichinose H, Yahikozawa K, et al. Selective intracoronary administration of nitroprusside before balloon dilatation prevents slow reflow during percutaneous coronary intervention in patients with acute myocardial infarction. Int Heart J 2007;48(4):423–33.

54. Barcin C, Denktas AE, Lennon RJ, et al. Comparison of combination therapy of adenosine and nitroprusside with adenosine alone in the treatment of angiographic no-reflow phenomenon. Catheter Cardiovasc Interv 2004;61(4):484–91.

55. Kurz MA, Lamping KG, Bates JN, et al. Mechanisms responsible for the heterogeneous coronary microvascular response to nitroglycerin. Circ Res 1991;68(3):847–55.

56. Kaplan BM, Benzuly KH, Kinn JW, et al. Treatment of no-reflow in degenerated saphenous vein graft interventions: comparison of intracoronary verapamil and nitroglycerin. Cathet Cardiovasc Diagn 1996;39(2):113–8.

# Drug-Eluting Stents Versus Bare Metal Stents in Saphenous Vein Graft Intervention

John R. Hoyt, MD[a], Hitinder S. Gurm, MD[b],*

## KEYWORDS

- Drug-eluting stent • Bare metal stent • Saphenous vein graft • Percutaneous intervention

## KEY POINTS

- Percutaneous coronary intervention (PCI) of saphenous vein graft (SVG) is technically challenging because of complex plaque morphology and has been associated with higher adverse event rates, lower procedural success, and inferior long-term patency rates compared with native vessel PCI.
- A patient's ability to comply with dual antiplatelet therapy and whether the patient will need an interruption in dual antiplatelet therapy should be taken into account when deciding whether to implant a drug-eluting stent (DES) or bare metal stent (BMS) in a SVG.
- DES use in SVG reduces target vessel revascularization (TVR) across observational and randomized studies. Meta-analyses provide evidence that DES use in SVGs reduces the composite of major adverse events driven mainly by TVR reduction, but DES do not conclusively reduce rates of future death and MI.
- It is the author's opinion that in the absence of contraindication, DES should be used for SVG PCI, because they appear to reduce TVR without increasing rates of adverse events. However, DES use for SVG lesions remains an off-label indication.

## INTRODUCTION

Coronary artery bypass graft (CABG) surgery remains one of the main treatments for coronary artery disease (CAD). Use of the reversed saphenous vein graft (SVG) as conduit for CABG was popularized by Favaloro[1] in 1969 and remains essential in the contemporary surgical treatment of CAD. Percutaneous coronary intervention (PCI) in SVG can be technically challenging because of the presence of complex friable plaque and thrombus, which may embolize and cause distal stasis and periprocedural myocardial infarction (MI).[2] SVG PCI has been associated with higher adverse event rates, lower procedural success, and inferior long-term patency rates compared with native vessel PCI.[3–8] Drug-eluting stents (DES) have been shown to reduce target vessel revascularization (TVR) in native coronary arteries; however, SVG PCI remains an off-label indication for DES use.[9,10] According to a study that analyzed the National Cardiovascular Data Registry from January 1, 2004 to March 31, 2009, SVG PCI represented 5.7% of total PCI volume and DES

No conflict of interest.
[a] Division of Cardiovascular Disease, Department of Internal Medicine, University of Michigan Cardiovascular Center, University of Michigan, 1500 East Medical Center Drive, 2381 CVC SPC 5853, Ann Arbor, MI 48109-5853, USA; [b] Division of Cardiovascular Disease, Department of Internal Medicine, University of Michigan Cardiovascular Center, University of Michigan, 1500 East Medical Center Drive, Room 2A394, Ann Arbor, MI 48109-5853, USA
* Corresponding author.
E-mail address: hgurm@med.umich.edu

Intervent Cardiol Clin 2 (2013) 283–305
http://dx.doi.org/10.1016/j.iccl.2012.11.007
2211-7458/13/$ – see front matter © 2013 Elsevier Inc. All rights reserved.

were used in 64.5% of cases.[11] This article reviews the evolution and contemporary evidence regarding use of DES versus bare metal stent (BMS) in SVG PCI.

## PATHOPHYSIOLOGY AND PATENCY RATES OF SVGS

A combination of physical, cellular, and humoral factors predispose the SVG toward intimal hyperplasia, smooth muscle proliferation, endothelial dysfunction, deposition of extracellular matrix, and accelerated atherosclerosis, which lead to inferior patency rates compared with arterial conduits.[12] SVG lesions may present with recurrent angina related to progressive stenosis or less commonly as an acute coronary syndrome (ACS) related to acute plaque rupture that is similar to native vessel plaque rupture.[13] A study analyzing culprit SVG lesions in an ACS setting by angiography and optical coherence tomography found a fibrofatty composition in 100% of lesions, calcification in 32%, plaque rupture in 60%, and thrombus in 46% of lesions, which suggests that the mechanism of ACS in SVG is similar to that found in native vessel ACS.[14,15]

Acute SVG closure has been attributed to thrombosis or surgical technical problems. Risk factors believed to confer an increased risk of SVG thrombosis within the first 6 months of CABG surgery include aspirin nonresponsiveness, small target vessel diameter, female gender, and low graft blood flow.[16,17] Although 1-year SVG patency graft rates have been reported as low as 58% at year 1,[18] most trials report 1-year patency rates from 64% to 81%.[16,19–22] Chronic patency rates vary approximately from 69% to 86%, 60%, and 32% to 50% at 5, 10, and 15 years, respectively.[19,20,23] In comparison, left internal mammary artery (LIMA) (n = 1482) patency rates are approximately 97%, 95%, and 93% at 5, 10, and 15 years.[23]

## PCI VERSUS REPEAT CABG IN OBSTRUCTIVE SVG DISEASE

Therapeutic options for obstructive SVG disease include PCI of the SVG or native vessel versus repeat CABG versus medical therapy alone. The clinical presentation, angiographic findings, amount of myocardium jeopardized by ischemia, and chances for therapeutic success should guide decision making in accordance with the 2011 American College of Cardiology Foundation (ACCF)/American Heart Association (AHA)/Society for Cardiovascular Angiography and Interventions (SCAI) PCI and ACCF/AHA CABG guidelines.[24,25]

Myocardial ischemia occurring in the setting of ACS may be life-threatening, and therefore an invasive assessment with revascularization procedure should be strongly considered.[24,26] Consideration for coronary angiography should also be given to patients with previous CABG presenting with new stable angina as well to detect lesions that may be amendable to PCI before total loss of the graft.

If the decision is made to proceed to PCI, stent choice is important (DES vs BMS). Stent thrombosis can lead to considerable morbidity and mortality.[27] Therefore, the patient's ability to comply with dual antiplatelet therapy and whether the patient will need an interruption in dual antiplatelet therapy should be taken into account when deciding whether to implant a DES or BMS in an SVG.

Redo CABG has been associated with good long-term survival in appropriate candidates, with cumulative survival rates as high as 90.1%, 74%, and 63.4% at 5-year, 10-year, and 15-year follow-ups, respectively.[28] However, redo CABG is associated with increased operative mortality and morbidity and carries approximately 2.5 to 3.5 times higher risk of postoperative mortality compared with primary CABG.[29,30] A contemporary report analyzed outcomes of 458 patients who underwent repeat CABG from 2001 to 2008 and found that operative mortality was 4.8% for repeat CABG versus 1.8% for primary CABG ($P<.001$), and repeat CABG carried a 2.8 times higher risk for postoperative MI.[30] Repeat CABG can be technically challenging, with lack of suitable conduit or identifying targets for grafting, longer perfusion and aortic cross-clamp times, increased risk of damaging existing grafts that are patent, redo sternotomy complications, prolonged mechanical ventilator/balloon pump support, and hemorrhagic complications.[29,31,32] Furthermore, many of the patients who present with high-grade SVG stenosis are poor repeat CABG candidates because of advanced age, multiple medical comorbidities, and limited amount of myocardium in jeopardy, which often makes PCI the rational therapeutic procedure.

### Summary

- In general, PCI is favored over repeat CABG if there are acceptable PCI target lesions, a patent graft to the left anterior descending (LAD), limited ischemic territory, poor graft targets, or unfavorably high surgical risk because of comorbid conditions.
- In general, factors favoring repeat CABG include availability of LIMA and other graft

conduits, vessels unsuitable for PCI, good graft targets, increased number of diseased grafts or jeopardized myocardium, and acceptable surgical risk.

- The patency status of the LAD coronary artery or its graft should influence revascularization decision making because patency is strongly associated with better survival.

## PRE-DES ERA
### Percutaneous Transluminal Coronary Angioplasty for SVG Lesions

Early trials in the 1980s using percutaneous transluminal coronary angioplasty (PTCA) to treat SVG lesions were generally small and observational but established that PTCA could be technically successful 86% to 98% of the time.[33–43] Plokker and colleagues[44] reported on 454 SVG PTCA procedures performed in the Netherlands from 1980 to 1989 (one of the larger cohorts reported). They reported a technical success rate of 90%, with 2.8% of patients having periprocedural MI and 1.3% undergoing emergent CABG. After 5 years, 74% of patients were alive overall and 26% of patients were alive without MI, surgical revascularization, or repeat PTCA. In general, SVG lesions treated with PTCA had substantial rates of restenosis, ranging from 33% to 53%, and therefore later trials incorporated use of stents in an effort to reduce restenosis rates.[45–48]

### PTCA Versus BMS in SVG Interventions

As with PTCA, early observational trials established that BMS could be placed with good immediate angiographic results; however, periodic early occlusion and late restenosis remained substantial.[49–54]

Introduction of stents for treatment of native CAD was associated with a dramatic reduction in acute closure and restenosis compared with PTCA alone. Early after the introduction of stents, the safety and efficacy of stenting for SVG intervention were evaluated in the SAVED (Saphenous Vein De Novo) trial by Savage and colleagues.[55] This trial randomized 220 patients with SVG lesions to Palmaz-Schatz BMS (n = 108) or PTCA (n = 107). Coronary angiography was performed at the initial procedure and 6 months later. There was no use of distal embolic protection devices. The outcome of death, MI, repeat CABG, or TVR was better in the stent group (73% vs 58%, P = .03) at 6 months. Patients receiving a stent had larger gains in immediate luminal diameter (1.92 ± 0.30 mm vs 1.21 ± 0.37 mm, P<.001) and 6-month diameter (0.85 ± 0.96 vs 0.54 ± 0.91 mm, P = .002). However, restenosis rates were not significantly different (37% with BMS vs 46% with PTCA, P = .24).[55] Major adverse cardiac events were not statistically significant between the BMS versus PTCA group; however, the study was underpowered for such a comparison: death (7% vs 9%, P = .44), Q-wave MI (5% vs 4%, P = .99), non-Q-wave MI (6% vs 11%, P = .13), CABG (7% vs 12%, P = .24), repeat PTCA (13% vs 16%, P = .54), and TVR (17% vs 26%, P = .09).[55]

Another randomized multicenter trial comparing BMS with PTCA was performed by Hanekamp and colleagues[47] using the Wiktor I BMS. A total of 150 patients were randomized to BMS (n = 77) versus PTCA (n = 73), with angiographic follow-up at 6 months. This trial included only de novo lesions in the body of a graft and excluded restenotic, ostial, and anastomotic lesions and diffusely diseased SVGs. No embolic protection devices were used. The BMS group had lower 6-month restenosis rates (19.1% vs 32.8%, P = .069), 1-year TVR rates (14.5% vs 31.4%, P<.05), and better event-free survival (73% vs 60%, P<.05). At 1 year, patients with BMS showed a trend toward lower rates of death (6.6% vs 7.1%, P = 1.0) and MI (10.5% vs 12.9%, P = .66). Together with the trials mentioned earlier, these studies solidified the BMS as a therapeutic option for SVG lesions; however, the risk for TVR and major adverse cardiac events remained clinically substantial.

### Summary

- BMS use over PTCA in SVG was associated with greater procedural success and greater gains in initial and follow-up luminal diameter.
- Randomized studies showed equivocal results regarding reduction in major adverse cardiac events with use of BMS over PTCA in SVG PCI.
- BMS were associated with persistently high rates of restenosis in SVG, ranging from 17% to 47%.[49–54]

### Covered Stents in SVG Intervention

Because of the friability of SVG plaques and higher risk of periprocedural plaque and thrombus embolization, covered stents have been studied as an alternative to BMS.[56–62] In a cohort study, Baldus and colleagues[57] followed 109 patients who received polytetrafluoroethylene (PTFE)-membrane-covered stents in 125 SVG lesions. All stents were successfully deployed, with the exception of a single patient. Death at follow-up occurred in 7% of patients, repeat CABG in 3%, and 8% required target lesion PTCA. Repeat angiography showed complete vessel occlusion in 9% and in-stent restenosis (ISR) in 8%.[57]

This study was followed by 3 randomized prospective multicenter trials of PTFE membrane covered stents compared with BMS in SVGs. The STING (Stents In Grafts) trial[58] randomized 211 patients with SVG lesions to receive a BMS or PTFE-covered Jostent Coronary Stentgraft (Jomed, Rangendingen, Germany). The primary end point was angiographic restenosis rate at 6 months defined as greater than 50% diameter stenosis. Restenosis rates were similar between the Flex (Jomed, Rangendingen, Germany) and Stentgraft (20% vs 29%, $P = .15$). Occlusion rates (defined as TIMI [Thrombolysis in Myocardial Infarction] score $\leq 1$ at time of follow-up angiography) showed a trend toward higher late occlusion rate in the Stentgraft group (7% vs 16%, $P = .069$). Major adverse cardiac events (MACE) were similar after a mean follow-up of 14 months (31% vs 31%, $P = .93$).

The RECOVERS (Randomized Evaluation of PTFE Covered Stent in Saphenous Vein Grafts) trial was a randomized, multicenter trial also comparing a PTFE-covered stent with a BMS in SVG lesions.[59] The trial randomized 301 patients to treatment with the PTFE-covered JoStent graft (n = 156) or the SS JoFlex (Jomed, Rangendingen, Sweden) BMS (n = 145). The primary end point was angiographic restenosis at 6 months, defined as stenosis of more than 50% at time of follow-up angiography. The primary end point of restenosis at 6 months was similar between the groups (24.2% vs 24.8%, $P = .237$). 30-day MACE were higher in the PTFE group (10.9% vs 4.1%, $P = .047$), driven by higher 30-day MI rates in the PTFE group (10.3% vs 3.4%, $P = .037$). Six-month non-Q-wave MI rates were also higher in the PTFE group (12.8% vs 4.1%, $P = .013$). The investigators concluded that 6-month restenosis rates were no different and that PTFE stents were associated with a higher incidence of nonfatal MI.

The third randomized controlled trial (RCT) was the Symbiot III trial, which compared the Symbiot (Boston Scientific Corporation, Natick, MA) self-expanding, nitinol PTFE-covered stent versus a BMS in SVG.[63] This trial randomized 201 patients to the Symbiot PTFE-covered stent and 199 patients to a BMS stratified based on intended use of glycoprotein IIbIIIa inhibitors and embolic protection device. The primary end point of percent diameter stenosis by quantitative coronary angiography at 8 months was no different between groups (30.9% Symbiot PTFE-covered stent, 31.9% BMS, $P = .80$). There was also no difference in the secondary end point of MACE composed of cardiac death, MI, and TVR (30.6% Symbiot PTFE-covered stent, 26.6% BMS, $P = .43$).[63]

The BARRICADE (Barrier Approach to Restenosis: Restrict Intima and Curtail Adverse Events) trial was halted after enrolling 243 of a goal 500 patients because of a higher total number of cases of occlusion in the JoMed stent compared with the BMS (20% vs 10%, $P = .09$) and higher restenosis rate (39% vs 28%, $P = .14$).[60]

## Summary

- Covered stents did not reduce restenosis rates or MACE compared with BMS.
- Covered stents are approved for use in SVG only in cases of perforation.

### DES for SVG Intervention

DES have shown remarkable antirestenotic efficacy, and soon after the approval of the first DES for clinical use, they were being used for SVG PCI in an off-label fashion.

## OBSERVATIONAL TRIALS OF DES VERSUS BMS IN SVG INTERVENTIONS

As one of the larger observational studies, the STENT[64] (Strategic Transcatheter Evaluation of New Therapies) trial used a multicenter registry to report outcomes of patients undergoing SVG PCI. A total of 785 patients received DES and 343 received BMS. In general, patients receiving a DES had smaller reference vessel diameters ($3.3 \pm 0.05$ vs $3.7 \pm 0.8$, $P<.001$) and longer lesions ($18.2 \pm 13.2$ vs $16.4 \pm 10.2$, $P = .003$). Rates of diabetes in patients with BMS and DES were similar (37.3% vs 38.1%, $P = .75$). Both groups had similar rates of distal embolic protection device use (33.7% of BMS vs 37.3% of DES, $P = .27$). Those receiving DES had lower rates of combined death and MI at 9 months of follow-up (8.7% vs 14.1%, hazard ratio [HR] 0.52, 95% confidence interval [CI] 0.33–0.83, $P = .006$). However, at 2 years, death and MI rates showed no statistical difference (17.0% vs 22.3%, HR 0.74, 95% CI 0.51–1.08, $P = .12$). DES reduced TVR at 9 months (7.2% vs 10.0%, HR 0.36, 95% CI 0.22–0.61, $P<.001$) but the benefit was lost by 2 years (18.3% vs 16.9%, $P = .86$).

Recently, clinical outcomes after SVG stenting with a TAXUS DES from the OLYMPIA registry were published.[65] This registry collected data on 21,954 patients between September 2005 and April 2007 receiving at least 1 TAXUS Liberté stent and included 345 patients with SVG lesions. These patients reflect real-world patients with no mandatory inclusion/exclusion criteria. SVG patients had higher baseline risk but similar 12-month clinical outcomes compared with patients receiving a TAXUS stent in a native vessel (death/MI/stroke 5.1% vs 4.4%, death 2% vs 2.2%, MI 1.3% vs 1%, target lesion revascularization [TLR] 1.8% vs 2.3%, TVR 3.8% vs 3.2%, and stent thrombosis 1.2% vs 0.8%). This study provides evidence that the TAXUS DES can be used safely in SVG PCI and is one of the larger cohorts of SVG PCI published. However, it does have several limitations, such as no control group, outcome monitoring was less complete than that of RCTs, there was no core laboratory analysis, and measurement of cardiac biomarkers was also not mandatory.

Table 1 lists observational studies comparing DES versus BMS in SVG interventions.[4,64,66–88] The observational studies can be summarized as follows:

## Summary

- Generally these trials were small, had a short trial period of 6 to 12 months, and because of their nonrandomized nature, bias may have been introduced when the decisions were made to implant a DES versus BMS.

## RANDOMIZED TRIALS OF DES VERSUS BMS IN SVG INTERVENTIONS

There have been only 3 RCTs,[89–91] 1 subgroup analysis[92] of a randomized trial comparing DES to BMS in SVG lesions, and post hoc analysis of the trials mentioned earlier (Table 2).[90,93,94]

The first RCT was the RRISC (Reduction of Restenosis in Saphenous Vein Grafts with Cypher Sirolimus-eluting Stent) conducted by Vermeersch and colleagues,[89] which compared sirolimus-eluting stents with BMS in SVGs. This was a single-center study that included 38 patients who received 60 sirolimus-eluting stents (SES) for 47 lesions and 37 patients who received 54 BMS for 49 lesions. The primary end point was 6-month angiographic in-stent late lumen loss. Follow-up angiography was performed in 37 (100%) patients with BMS and 35 (92%) patients with SES. Baseline characteristics were similar between both groups and no patients were lost to follow-up. Embolic protection devices were used in more than 80% of patents. Patients randomized to SES had significantly lower rates of binary ISR (11.3% vs 30.6%, relative risk [RR] 0.37; 95% CI 0.15–0.97, $P = .024$) and in-segment restenosis (13.6% vs 32.6%, RR 0.42; 95% CI 0.18–0.97, $P = .031$). In addition, TLR (5.3% vs 21.6%, RR 0.24; 95% CI 0.05–1.0,

$P = .047$) and TVR rates were significantly reduced (5.3% vs 27%, RR 0.19; 95% CI 0.05–0.83, $P = .012$). There was no difference in rates of death or MI. The main limitation of this study was that it was underpowered to detect differences in major clinical end points. The investigators conclude that SES reduced 6-month angiographic late lumen loss, binary restenosis, and repeat TVR and TLR compared with BMS.

The cumulative follow-up data for the RRISC trial were published in 2007, with a median follow-up time of 32 months. Rates of MI (5% vs 18%, $P = .15$) and TVR (38% vs 34%, $P = .74$) were not different between the BMS versus SES groups; however, there was higher mortality in those patients receiving SES (29% vs 0%, $P<.001$). Of the 11 deaths in the SES group, 7 deaths were considered cardiac in origin, with 3 presenting as sudden cardiac death. One of the cardiac deaths was caused by very late stent thrombosis 14.5 months after the index stent placement. The patient's antithrombotic therapy had been discontinued for knee surgery. The investigators concluded that the short-term benefits of lower TVR rates with SES were no longer evident at 32 months; however, the trial was not sufficiently powered to detect differences in mortality.

The second RCT was the SOS (Stenting of Saphenous Vein Grafts) trial,[90] which was a multicenter trial that randomized 80 patients to a TAXUS paclitaxel-eluting stent (PES) (41 patients, 45 grafts, 57 lesions) versus a BMS (29 patients, 43 grafts, 55 lesions). The primary outcome of binary angiographic restenosis was defined as a stenosis of 50% or more of the minimal lumen diameter. TVR and TLR were defined as repeat PCI or CABG because of restenosis of the target vessel/lesion. Target vessel failure (TVF) was defined as the composite end point of cardiac death, MI, and TVR. Baseline characteristics between the 2 groups were similar. Indications for stenting were ACS in 60% and stable angina in 31% of patients. The median follow-up was 18 months. Procedure success was 96%. The primary outcome of angiographic binary restenosis at 12 months was greater in the BMS group (51% vs 9%, RR 0.18, 95% CI 0.07–0.48, $P<.0001$). The use of PES in SVG was associated with less TLR (28% vs 5%, HR: 0.38; 95% CI 0.15–0.74, $P = .003$) and TVF (46% vs 22%, HR 0.65; 95% CI 0.42–0.96, $P = .03$).[90] PES showed trends of reducing rates of TVR (31% vs 15%, HR 0.66; 95% CI 0.39–1.05, $P = .08$), MI (31% vs 15%, HR 0.67; 95% CI 0.40–1.08, $P = .10$), and mortality (5% vs 12%, HR 1.56; 95% CI 0.72–4.11, $P = .27$); however, these differences did not reach

**Table 1**
Observational trials with a control group comparing DES versus BMS in SVG PCI

| References | Study Date | Study Size | Age (y) | DES | Duration Mean Follow/up (mo) | Results DES vs BMS | Author Conclusions |
|---|---|---|---|---|---|---|---|
| Ge et al,[66] 2005 | 2002–2004 | BMS 89 DES 61 | BMS 67 ± 8 DES 67 ± 8 | SES PES | 6 | Death: 0% vs 2.2%, $P = .85$ Q-wave MI: 0% vs 1.1%, $P = .85$ Non-Q MI: 8.2% vs 7.9%, $P = .82$ TVR: 4.9% vs 23.1%, $P = .003$ TLR: 3.3% vs 19.8%, $P = .003$ MACE: 11.5% vs 28.1%, $P = .016$ | PCI with DES in SVG lesions is associated with a reduction in the restenosis rate and a beneficial effect on MACE-free survival at 6-month follow-up |
| Lee et al,[67] 2005 | 2003–2004 | BMS 84 DES 139 | BMS 69.4 ± 11.2 DES 68.6 ± 10.5 | PES SES | 9 | Death: 1% vs 4%, $P = .03$ MI: 4% vs 20%, $P = .04$ TVR: 10% vs 37%, $P = .035$ MACE: 10% vs 37%, $P = .035$ | DES was associated with a lower incidence of death, MI, TVR compared with BMS in SVG PCI |
| Chu et al,[68] 2006 | 2001–2004 | BMS 57 DES 48 | BMS 71.4 ± 9.9 DES 68.6 ± 10.2 | SES | 12 | Death: 6% vs 7%, $P = .88$ Q wave MI: 4% vs 0%, $P = .12$ Non-Q MI: 4% vs 4%, $P = .86$ TVR: 13% vs 11%, $P = .75$ TLR: 6% vs 7%, $P = .88$ | SES in SVG PCI are safe and feasible but are not associated with decreased clinical events up to 1 y compared with BMS |
| Ellis et al,[69] 2007 | 2000–2003 | BMS 175 DES 175 | BMS 68.5 ± 10.0 DES 69.8 ± 9.0 | SES | 12 | Death: 4.7% vs 3.6%, $P = .79$ TVR: 6.8% vs 11.8%, $P = .14$ TLR: 6.8% vs 9.9%, $P = ns$ Restenosis: 7.4% vs 13.6%, $P = .07$ | SES seem to reduce TVR modestly |
| Hoffman et al,[4] 2007 | 2002–2004 | BMS 60 DES 60 | BMS 67 ± 7 DES 67 ± 11 | PES | 6 | MACE: 15% vs 37%, $P = .014$ Restenosis: 12% vs 33%, $P = .012$ TVFa: 18% vs 41%, $P = .019$ | Restenosis rates were lower in SVG lesions treated with PES. Target vessel failure and MACE rates remained substantial |
| Minutello et al,[70] 2007 | 2003–2005 | BMS 50 DES 59 | BMS 69.4 ± 11.0 DES 70.8 ± 12.7 | SES | 20 | Death: 6.8% vs 12%, $P = .51$ MI: 6.8% vs 2%, $P = .37$ TVR: 15.3% vs 36%, $P = .01$ TLR: 13.6% vs 22.0%, $P = .31$ Restenosis: 11.9% vs 36% $P = .01$ MACE: 25.4% vs 50%, $P = .01$ | SES appeared to be safe and were associated with less restenosis, target vessel failure, and better outcomes compared with BMS |

| Study | Years | N | Age | Stent | Duration (mo) | Outcomes | Conclusion |
|---|---|---|---|---|---|---|---|
| Wohrle et al,[71] 2007 | 2005–2005 | BMS 26<br>DES 13 | BMS 69.6 ± 6.4<br>DES 70.7 ± 4.1 | PES | 12 | 6-mo MACE: 0% vs 26.9%, $P = .039$<br>1-y MACE: 7.7% vs 38.5%, $P = .045$<br>6-mo restenosis: 34.6% vs 0%, $P = .016$ | PES have potential to superior clinical outcomes compared with BMS in treatment of SVG lesions |
| Assali et al,[72] 2008 | 2003–2005 | BMS 43<br>DES 68 | BMS 71 ± 9<br>DES 70 ± 8 | SES<br>PES | 24 | Death: 2.9% vs 4.7%, $P = .6$<br>MI: 8.8% vs 7%, $P = .6$<br>TVR: 10.3% vs 27.9%, $P = .02$<br>TLR: 14.7% vs 32.6%, $P = .03$<br>MACE FS: 79.4% vs 58.1%, $P = .02$ | DES implantation in SVG lesions had favorable outcomes after 2 y without excess cardiac mortality |
| Bansal et al,[73] 2008 | 2003–2005 | BMS 72<br>DES 37 | BMS 64.9 ± 1.1<br>DES 68.0 ± 1.6 | SES | 33 | Death: 19% vs 22%, $P = .68$<br>TVR: 35% vs 42%, $P = .47$<br>TLR: 30% vs 38%, $P = .39$<br>Restenosis: 30% vs 35%, $P = .60$<br>MACE: 46% vs 50%, $P = .63$ | No difference in the long-term outcomes of PCI on SVG, irrespective of the type of stent used |
| Gioia et al,[74] 2008 | 2002–2006 | BMS 119<br>DES 106 | BMS 70 ± 7<br>DES 71 ± 8 | SES<br>PES<br>TES | 24 | Death: 6% vs 6%, $P = .9$<br>STEMI: 2% vs 1%, $P = .8$<br>TVR: 14% vs 14%, $P = .9$<br>TLR: 13% vs 13%, $P = .9$<br>MACE: 19% vs 18%, $P = .9$<br>MACE FS: 81% vs 82%, $P = .9$ | No benefit of DES over BMS in SVG lesions at 2 y |
| Okabe et al,[75] 2008 | 2000–2006 | BMS 334<br>DES 138 | BMS 70 ± 11<br>DES 70 ± 11 | SES<br>PES | 12 | Death: 9% vs 12%, $P = .2$<br>Q-wave MI: 1% vs 0.3%, $P = 1.0$<br>TVR: 20% vs 13%, $P = .08$<br>TLR: 7% vs 14%, $P = .5$<br>MACE: 29% vs 24%, $P = .2$ | Both DES and BMS safe and efficacious; however, DES did not reduce need for repeat revascularization |
| Ramana et al,[76] 2008 | 2003–2007 | BMS 170<br>DES 141 | BMS 69.1<br>DES 70.0 | SES | 34 | Death: 6% vs 12%, $P = .06$<br>MI: 5% vs 9%, $P = .19$<br>TVR: 13% vs 16%, $P = .52$<br>TLR: 7% vs 14%, $P = .07$<br>MACE: 20% vs 28%, $P = .14$ | SES used in SVG lesions result in a reduction in TLR without an increased risk of mortality |

(continued on next page)

**Table 1**
*(continued)*

| References | Study Date | Study Size | Age (y) | DES | Duration Mean Follow/up (mo) | Results DES vs BMS | Author Conclusions |
|---|---|---|---|---|---|---|---|
| Kaplan et al,[77] 2008 | 2003–2006 | BMS 33 DES 37 | BMS 70.5 ± 8.7 DES 72.3 ± 9.0 | N/a | 12 | Cardiac death: 2.7% vs 3.0%, $P = 1.0$ Noncardiac death: 0% vs 0% Q-wave MI: 0% vs 3.0%, $P = .47$ Non-Q MI: 5.4% vs 12.1%, $P = .18$ TVR: 10.8% vs 33.3%, $P = .045$ TLR: 5.4% vs 30.3%, $P = .015$ MACE: 10.8% vs 36.4%, $P = .024$ | DES in SVG associated with better outcomes. High rates of repeat revascularization at 1 y remained |
| Van Twisk et al,[78] 2008 | 2000–2005 | BMS 128 DES 122 | BMS 69.3 DES 68.3 | SES PES | 48 | Death: 22.5% vs 27%, $P = .65$ MACE FS: 61.5% vs 46.8%, HR 0.77, 95% CI 0.51–1.16, $P = $ ns TVR: 18.4% vs 31%, $P = $ ns | There was a trend toward lower rates of TVR and MACE at 4 y with DES use in SVG compared with BMS |
| Vignali et al,[79] 2008 | 2003–2006 | BMS 288 DES 72 | BMS 71.4 ± 8.6 DES 72.5 ± 7.8 | SES PES | 12 | Death: 3.7% vs 7.8%, $P = .186$ MI: 8.2% vs 5.2%, $P = .478$ TVR: 8.1% vs 11.3%, $P = .41$ TLR: 4.3% vs 8.1%, $P = .256$ MACE: 17.8% vs 20.3%, $P = .461$ | MACE associated with the use of DES and BMS in SVGs are similar at 12 mo |

| Study | Years | N | Age | Stent | Follow-up (mo) | Results | Conclusions |
|---|---|---|---|---|---|---|---|
| Brodie et al,[64] 2009 | 2003–2006 | BMS 343<br>DES 785 | BMS 68.8 ± 10.2<br>DES 67.5 ± 10.3 | SES<br>PES | 24 | Death: 8.2% vs 14.7%, HR 0.60, 95% CI 0.36–0.98, $P = .041$<br>MI: 11.9% vs 11.3%, HR 0.95, 95% CI 0.58–1.56, $P = .83$<br>TVR 9 mo: 7.2% vs 10.0%, $P<.001$<br>TVR 2 y: 18.3% vs 16.9%, $P = .86$<br>MACE: 30.4% vs 33.8%, HR 0.68, 95% CI 0.51–0.92, $P = .011$ | Treatment of SVG lesions with DES reduces TVR at 9 mo, but advantage lost at 2 y |
| Lozano et al,[80] 2009 | 1999–2007 | BMS 130<br>DES 107 | BMS 66.4 ± 9<br>DES 70.6 ± 8.9 | SES<br>PES<br>ZES | 30 | Absence cardiac death ($P = .66$):<br>12 mo: 95% vs 95%<br>24 mo: 91% vs 90%<br>30 mo: 89% vs 87%<br>Absence TVR ($P = .49$):<br>12 mo: 94% vs 90%<br>24 mo: 87% vs 86%<br>30 mo: 87% vs 83% | DES was not associated with reduction in mortality or TVR compared with BMS in SVG lesions |
| Applegate et al,[81] 2008 | 2002–2005 | BMS 74<br>DES 74 | BMS 69 ± 10<br>DES 69 ± 11 | SES<br>PES | 24 | Cardiac death: HR 1.19, CI 0.32–4.45, $P = .79$<br>TVR: HR 0.54; CI 0.21–1.36, $P = .18$<br>MI + cardiac death: HR 0.68, CI 0.27–1.68, $P = .395$ | Safety profile of DES vs BMS in SVG was similar, with trend toward less need for reintervention |

(continued on next page)

**Table 1**
*(continued)*

| References | Study Date | Study Size | Age (y) | DES | Duration Mean Follow/up (mo) | Results DES vs BMS | Author Conclusions |
|---|---|---|---|---|---|---|---|
| Shishehbor et al,[82] 2009 | 2000–2007 | BMS 349 239 before 2003 –110 after 2003 DES 217 | BMS 68 ± 10 DES: 70 ± 10 | SES PES | 35 | MACE before 2003: 27% vs 51%, HR 0.61, 95% CI 0.28–1.35, P = .23) MACE after 2003: 27% vs 30%, HR 0.61, 95% CI 0.35–1.07, P = .08 | DES showed a trend toward fewer MACE compared with BMS after 2003 but not before 2003, which may reflect bias in observational registries |
| Goswami et al,[83] 2010 | 2003–2007 | BMS 95 DES 284 | BMS 69.5 ± 10.4 DES 70.7 ± 9.7 | SES PES | 36 | All-cause death: 9.2% vs 4.2%, P = ns Cardiac death: 5.3% vs 3.1%, P = ns MI: 4.2% vs 2.1%, P = ns TLR: 4.2% vs 2.1% MACE: 20.4% vs 18.9%, P = ns | DES in SVG PCI did not improve 3-y mortality or revascularization rates over BMS |
| Latib et al,[84] 2010 | 2002–2006 | BMS 131 DES 127 | BMS 66.5 ± 7.9 DES 67.6 ± 8.3 | SES PES | 24 | Death: 8.7% vs 7.8%, P = .99 MI: 6.3% vs 9.4%, P = .50 TVR: 19.7% vs 24.2%, P = .47 TLR: 15% vs 18.8%, P = .52 MACE: 26.8% vs 35.9%, P = .15 | No increase in mortality with DES vs BMS in SVGs despite DES group having more diabetes, older grafts, restenotic lesions, smaller stents, and longer stents |

| Study | Years | Patients | Age | Stent type | Follow-up (mo) | Outcomes | Conclusion |
|---|---|---|---|---|---|---|---|
| Baldwin et al,[85] 2010 | 1999–2006 | BMS 192 DES 203 | BMS 70.4 DES 69.7 | SES PES | 36 | Death: 16.8% vs 18.1%, $P = .73$<br>MI: 16.1% vs 18.6%, $P = .39$<br>Death: 23% vs 22.2%, $P = .88$<br>MACE: 40.9% vs 46.6%, $P = .16$ | No improved outcomes with DES over BMS in SVG lesions |
| Nair et al,[86] 2011 | | BMS 219 DES 169 | ILL | | 42 | Death: 11.8% vs 14.2%<br>MACE: 35.8% vs 37.6%<br>TVR/TLR: 21.6% vs 37.6% | DES and BMS in SVG PCI have similar mortality and MACE and revascularization rates |
| Nauta et al,[87] 2012 | 2000–2005 | BMS 128 DES 122 | BMS 69 ± 9.6 DES 68 ± 8.7 | SES PES | 87 | Death: 42% vs 46%, HR 0.84, CI 0.56–1.3, $P =$ ns<br>TVR: 29% vs 41%, HR 0.62, CI 0.38–0.99, $P<.05$<br>MACE: 68% vs 73%, HR 0.81, CI 0.59–1.1, $P =$ ns | DES in SVG appeared safe, with lower rates of TVR |
| Chakravarty et al,[88] 2012 | 2002–2008 | BMS 113 DES 133 | BMS 77.0 ± 10.7 DES 76.0 ± 11.3 | SES PES EES | 46 | Death: 23% vs 29.4%, $P = .60$<br>MI: 11.3% vs 13.3%, $P = .70$<br>TVR: 23.9% vs 22.9%, $P = .33$<br>TLR: 10% vs 14.8%, $P = .05$<br>MACE: 42.5% vs 43.2%, $P = .70$ | No mortality difference between DES and BMS for SVG lesions. BMS associated with increased risk of revascularization |
| Pasceri et al,[108] 2012 | 2006–2008 | BMS 173 DES 138 | BMS 68.4 ± 8.5 DES 68.3 ± 8.0 | SES PES ZES EES | 24 | Death: 7.2% vs 6.9%, $P = .91$<br>MI: 9.4% vs 9.2%, $P = .88$<br>TVR: 23.2% vs 28.9%, $P = .39$<br>TLR: 19.6% vs 25.4%, $P = .28$<br>MACE: 29.7% vs 37.0%, $P = .29$ | DES associated with lower MACE and TVR at 9 mo but the early benefit of DES in SVG may be lost at longer-term follow-up |

*Abbreviations:* EES, everolimus-eluting stent; ILL, in-stent late lumen loss; MACE FS, major adverse cardiac event-free survival; N/a; not applicable; ns, nonsignificant; PES, paclitaxel-eluting stent; SES, sirolimus-eluting stent; TES, tacrolimus-eluting stent; TVF, target vessel failure; ZES, zotarolimus-eluting stent.

[a] TVF = need for recurrent target vessel revascularization, restenosis >50% or complete vessel occlusion.

**Table 2**
Randomized trials and follow-up analysis of DES versus BMS in SVG PCI

| References Trial | Study Type | Study Period | Study Size | Age (y) | DES Type | Follow-up (mo) | Results (DES vs BMS) | Author Conclusions |
|---|---|---|---|---|---|---|---|---|
| Vermeersch et al,[89] 2006 RRISC | RCT | 2003–2004 | BMS 54 37 patients 49 lesions DES 60 38 patients 47 lesions | BMS 72 ± 8 DES 73 ± 7 | SES | 6 | In-stent late[a] lumen loss: 0.38 ± 0.51 mm vs 0.79 ± 0.66 mm, $P = .001$ ISR: 11.3% vs 30.6% RR 0.37; 95% CI 0.15–0.97, $P = .024$ TVR: 5.3% vs 27%, RR 0.19; 95% CI 0.05–0.83, $P = .012$ TLR: 5.3% vs 21.6%, RR 0.24; 95% CI 0.05–1.0, $P = .047$ Death: 2.6% vs 0%, $P = .99$ MI: 2.6% vs 0%, $P = .99$ Death: 15.8% vs 29.7%, $P = .15$ | At 6 mo, SES reduce late lumen loss, restenosis rates, and repeat TLR/ TVR procedures vs BMS in SVGs |
| Vermeersch et al,[93] 2007 DELAYED RRISC | RCT follow/up | 2003–2006 | BMS 37 DES 38 | BMS 72 ± 8 DES 73 ± 7 | SES | 32 | Death[a]: 29% vs 0%, $P<.001$ MI[a]: 18% vs 5%, $P = .15$ TVR[a]: 34% vs 38%, $P = .74$ TLR: 24% vs 30%, $P = .55$ MACE: 58% vs 41%, $P = .13$ | BMS were associated with lower long-term mortality than SES for SVG disease. The 6-mo reduction in repeated revascularization procedures with SES was lost at longer-term follow-up |
| Jeger et al,[92] 2009 | RCT Subgroup | 2003–2004 | BMS 13 DES 34 | 71 ± 8 | SES PES | 18 | MACE[a]: 21 vs 62%, $P = .007$ MI: 0% vs 6%, $P = 1.0$ TVR: 18% vs 46%, $P = .045$ | Treatment with DES reduced TVR at 18 mo |

| Study | Design | Years | No. | Age | Stent | Follow-up (mo) | Outcomes | Conclusion |
|---|---|---|---|---|---|---|---|---|
| Brilakis et al,[90] 2009 SOS | RCT | 2005–2007 | BMS 39 DES 41 | BMS 67 ± 9 DES 66 ± 9 | PES | 12 | Restenosis[a] at 12 mo: 9% vs 51%, RR 0.18, CI 0.07–0.48, $P<.0001$)<br>Death: 12% vs 5%, HR 1.56; CI 0.72–4.11, $P = .27$<br>MI: 15% vs 31%, HR 0.67; CI 0.40–1.08, $P = .10$<br>TVR: 15% vs 31%, HR 0.66; CI 0.39–1.05, $P = .08$<br>TVF: 22% vs 46%, HR 0.65; CI 0.42–0.96, $P = .03$<br>TLR: 5% vs 28%; HR 0.38; CI 0.15–0.74, $P = .003$<br>MACE: 37% vs 49%, HR 0.80; CI 0.57–1.12, $P = .07$ | PES are associated with lower rates of angiographic restenosis and target vessel failure, target lesion revascularization compared with BMS in SVG lesions |
| Brilakis et al,[94] 2011 SOS (follow-up) | RCT follow/up | 2005–2007 | BMS 39 DES 41 | BMS 67 ± 9 DES 66 ± 9 | PES | 35 | Death: 24% vs 13%, HR 2.04, CI 0.70–6.0, $P = .19$<br>MI: 17% vs 46%, HR 0.32, CI 0.13–0.76, $P = .01$<br>TVR: 22% vs 49%, HR 0.41, CI 0.19–0.90, $P = .03$<br>TLR: 10% vs 41%, HR 0.20, CI 0.07–0.60, $P = .004$<br>MACE: 54% vs 77%, HR 0.82, CI 0.47–1.44, $P = .49$ | PES were associated with significantly better clinical outcomes than BMS in SVG lesions |
| Mehilli et al,[91] 2011 ISAR-CABG | RCT | 2007–2010 | BMS 307 DES 303 | BMS 71 DES 74 | SES PES | 12 | MACE[a]: 15% vs 22.1%, HR 0.64, CI 0.44–0.94, $P = .02$<br>Death: 5.1% vs 4.7%, HR 1.08, CI 0.52–2.23, $P = .83$<br>MI: 4.1% vs 6%, HR 0.66, CI 0.32–1.37, $P = .27$<br>TVR: 9.6% vs 15.5%, HR 0.59, CI 0.36–0.95, $P = .03$<br>TLR: 6.8% vs 13.1%, HR 0.49, CI 0.28–0.86, $P = .01$ | DES are associated with better clinical and angiographic outcomes compared with BMS in SVG lesions at 1 y |

Abbreviations: PES, paclitaxel-eluting stent; RR, relative risk; SES, sirolimus-eluting stent.
[a] Primary end point.

statistical significance.[90] The main limitations of the SOS trial were that it was underpowered for major clinical outcomes and all participants were male. The trial also had an 18% loss to angiographic follow-up, which is similar to that of other trials. However, if more patients had undergone angiographic follow-up, this might have increased the rate of repeat revascularization in both study groups and likely relatively more in the BMS group.

A nonprespecified, post hoc analysis of the SOS trial was published in 2011, with a median follow-up of 35 months.[94] Patients who received a PES had lower rates of MI (46% vs 17%, HR 0.32, $P$ = .01), TLR (41% vs 10%, HR 0.20, $P$ = .004), TVR (49% vs 22%, HR 0.41, $P$ = .03), and TVF (72% vs 34%, HR 0.34, $P$ = .001). Cardiac mortality (13% vs 7%, HR 0.62, $P$ = .51) and all-cause mortality (13% vs 24%, HR 2.04, $P$ = .19) were not statistically different between groups.

The third RCT studying DES versus BMS in SVG was conducted by Mehilli and colleagues.[91] In their study, 610 patients were randomized in a 1:1:1:3 fashion to receive 1 of 3 types of DES (permanent-polymer PES, permanent-polymer SES, or biodegradable-polymer SES) or a BMS. DES were used in 303 patients and 307 received a BMS. As a group, DES reduced the primary composite end point of death, MI, and TLR at 1 year (15% vs 22%; HR 0.64, 95% CI 0.44–0.94, $P$ = .02), but this was driven primarily by a reduction in TLR (7% vs 13%, HR 0.49, 95% CI 0.28–0.86; $P$ = .01) (**Fig. 1**). Individually, neither all-use death (5% vs 14.5%; HR 1.08, 95% CI 0.52–2.24; $P$ = .83) nor MI (4% vs 6%; HR 0.66, 95% CI 0.32–1.37; $P$ = .27) was different between groups. Rates of definite or probable stent thrombosis were similar as well (1% vs 1%; HR 1.00, 95% CI 0.14–7.10; $P$ = .99).[91] The investigators concluded that DES provide better clinical and angiographic outcomes up to 1 year in SVGs.

## Summary

- There have been only 3 dedicated RCTs and 1 subgroup analysis of an RCT comparing DES with BMS in SVG
- Use of DES has been associated with a reduction in angiographic restenosis and TLR in patients undergoing SVG PCI.

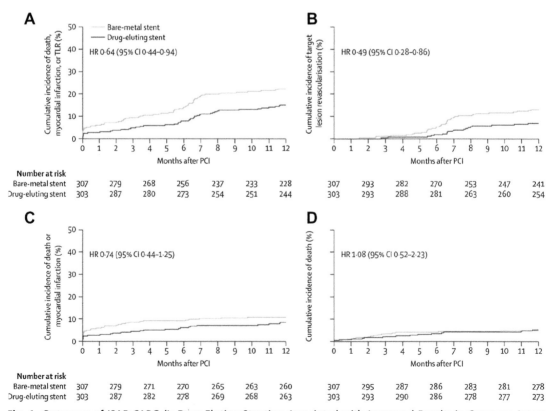

**Fig. 1.** Outcomes of ISAR-CABG (Is Drug-Eluting-Stenting Associated with Improved Results in Coronary Artery Bypass Grafts?) trial comparing patients randomized to DES versus BMS for SVG PCI. (*From* Mehilli J, Pache J, Abdel-Wahab M, et al. Drug-eluting vs bare-metal stents in saphenous vein graft lesions (ISAR-CABG): a randomised controlled superiority trial. Lancet 2011;378(9796):1071–8; with permission.)

**Table 3**
Pooled outcomes of DES versus BMS in SVG PCI

| End Point | Study Characteristic | Studies | Number of Patients | Mean Follow-up (mo) | Risk Ratio RE (95% CI) | P | Risk Ratio FE (95% CI) | P | I² (%) | Heterogeneity (P) |
|---|---|---|---|---|---|---|---|---|---|---|
| Death | Overall | 28 | 7862 | 21 | 0.82 (0.7–0.97) | .02 | 0.85 (0.73–0.99) | .03 | 8 | .34 |
| | ≥1 y FU | 24 | 5634 | 23 | 0.83 (0.67–1.03) | .1 | 0.85 (0.72–1.01) | .06 | 21 | .23 |
| | ≥2 y FU | 13 | 3101 | 32 | 0.81 (0.61–1.08) | .14 | 0.82 (0.67–1.00) | .05 | 37 | .09 |
| MACE | Overall | 26 | 6867 | 21 | 0.7 (0.6–0.8) | <.00001 | 0.69 (0.64–0.76) | <.00001 | 54 | .0005 |
| | ≥1 y FU | 22 | 5030 | 23 | 0.76 (0.65–0.88) | <0.008 | 0.75 (0.67–0.83) | <.00001 | 49 | .008 |
| | ≥2 y FU | 12 | 2851 | 32 | 0.77 (0.65–0.91) | .003 | 0.74 (0.65–0.83) | <.00001 | 49 | .03 |
| MI | Overall | 24 | 6886 | 21 | 0.72 (0.57–0.91) | .007 | 0.74 (0.61–0.88) | .001 | 26 | .12 |
| | ≥1 y FU | 20 | 4537 | 24 | 0.86 (0.65–1.14) | .30 | 0.85 (0.68–1.06) | .16 | 21 | .19 |
| | ≥2 y FU | 10 | 2354 | 30.5 | 0.82 (0.57–1.18) | .28 | 0.82 (0.62–1.10) | .18 | 24 | .22 |
| TVR | Overall | 26 | 7103 | 21 | 0.71 (0.59–0.85) | .0002 | 0.73 (0.65–0.82) | <.00001 | 56 | .0003 |
| | ≥1 y FU | 23 | 5550 | 24 | 0.76 (0.63–0.91) | .004 | 0.78 (0.69–0.88) | <.0001 | 47 | .008 |
| | ≥2 y FU | 13 | 3381 | 31 | 0.84 (0.68–1.03) | .09 | 0.84 (0.73–0.97) | .02 | 48 | .03 |

*Abbreviations:* FE, fixed effect model; FU, follow-up; RE, random effect model.
*From* Hakeem A, Helmy T, Munsif S, et al. Safety and efficacy of drug eluting stents compared with bare metal stents for saphenous vein graft interventions: a comprehensive meta-analysis of randomized trials and observational studies comprising 7994 patients. Catheter Cardiovasc Interv 2011;77(3):351; with permission.

**Table 4**
Future and ongoing trials involving SVG PCI

| Trial Name/ClinicalTrials.gov Identifier | Objectives | Study Type | Start/Finish[a] | Size[a] | Primary End Point |
|---|---|---|---|---|---|
| Drug-eluting Stents vs Bare Metal Stents in Saphenous Vein Graft Angioplasty (DIVA trial) NCT01121224 | To compare outcomes of DES vs BMS in PCIs of SVGs | RCT | 5/2011–5/2014 | 520 | Target vessel failure defined as composite of cardiac death, target vessel MI, TVR at 12 mo |
| Basel Stent Kosten Effektivitäts Trial–Saphenous Venous Graft Angioplasty Using Glycoprotein IIb/IIIa Receptor Inhibitors and Drug-Eluting Stents NCT00595647 | To compare the safety and efficacy of DES vs BMS in PCIs of SVG | RCT | 2/2008–3/2014 | 240 | MACE (death, nonfatal MI, TVR) at 12 mo |
| Comparison of Safety and Efficacy of Two Different Drug Eluting Stents: TAXUS vs LUC-Chopin Stent Implanted Into Saphenous Vein Grafts. Study With Serial Intravascular Ultrasounds. NCT00766129 | To compare safety and efficacy of implantation of 2 different types of PES from stable vs biodegradable polymer (TAXUS stent vs LUC-CHOPIN stent) into coronary artery bypass grafts | RCT | 2/2008–4/2011 | 50 | Neointima hyperplasia volume by IVUS at 9 mo |

| Study | Description | Design | Dates | Size | Primary Outcome |
|---|---|---|---|---|---|
| Sealing Moderate Coronary Saphenous Vein Graft Lesions With Paclitaxel-eluting Stents as a New Approach to Maintaining Vein Graft Patency and Reducing Cardiac Events (VELETI II trial) NCT01223443 | To determine the effect of stenting moderate SVG lesions compared with medical treatment on limiting SVG disease progression as evaluated by IVUS To evaluate by IVUS the effect of stenting moderate SVG lesions with PES compared with medical treatment on atherosclerosis progression in angiographically nondiseased SVG segments | RCT | 10/2010–1/2016 | 450 | MACE (cardiac death, MI, coronary revascularization related to target SVG) over 60 mo |
| Prospective Evaluation of the Xience V Everolimus-eluting Stent In Saphenous Vein Graft Atherosclerosis: the Stenting Of Saphenous Vein Grafts Xience V Angiographic Study (SOS-Xience V trial) NCT00911976 | To examine the 12-mo incidence of binary angiographic in-stent restenosis after implantation of the Xience V stent in aortocoronary saphenous vein bypass graft lesions | Cohort | 5/2009–8/2011 | 40 | Binary angiographic in-stent restenosis at 12 mo assessed by coronary angiography |
| Over and Under/Aneugraft Pericardium Covered Stent Long-term Follow-up Registry NCT01307553 | To track the clinical safety and effectiveness of the pericardium covered stent in real-world use | Cohort | 9/2010–4/2015 | 75 | MACE (cardiac death, MI, TVR) |

*Abbreviation:* IVUS, intravascular ultrasonography.
[a] Anticipated start/finish dates and study size.

## META-ANALYSIS OF DES VERSUS BMS IN SVG INTERVENTIONS

Several meta-analyses have been conducted comparing DES with BMS in SVG lesions.[95–106] Again, most of the data included in these meta-analyses come from nonrandomized trials and therefore bias may exist.

Hakeem and colleagues meta-analysis from 2011[104] has been the largest to date and numbered 7994 patients, including 4187 patients who underwent DES and 3807 patients who underwent BMS to SVG lesions. The study included 26 observational trials and 2 randomized trials, with a mean follow-up duration of 21 ± 11 months (range 6–48) months. The investigators stratified the data by overall pooled results and duration of follow-up and also reported risk ratios computed by a random effect model and fixed effect model (**Table 3**). DES compared with BMS in SVG were found to decrease the risk of MACE (19% vs 28%, RR 0.7, $P<.00001$), death (7.8% vs 9%, RR 0.82, $P = .02$), MI (5.7% vs 7.6%, RR 0.72, $P = .007$), and TVR (12% vs 17%, RR 0.71, $P = .0002$).

A meta-analysis including only the 4 RCTs[89–94] comparing DES versus BMS in SVG intervention was recently published.[107] At a median follow-up of 25 months, patients with SVG lesions treated with DES had lower rates of repeat revascularization (odds ratio [OR] 0.40, 95% CI 0.22–0.75). DES and BMS groups had similar rates of death (OR 1.63, 95% CI 0.45–5.92), MI (OR 0.83, 95% CI 0.27–2.60), and MACE (OR 0.58, 95% CI 0.25–1.32).[107]

## ONGOING/FUTURE TRIAL OF DES VERSUS BMS IN SVG INTERVENTIONS

At the time of this writing, there are 2 RCTs specifically comparing DES with BMS in SVG intervention. The DIVA trial (Drug-eluting Stents vs Bare Metal Stents in Saphenous Vein Graft Angioplasty) (NCT01121224) is a randomized multicenter trial with an estimated enrollment of 520 patients. The primary end point will be TVF, defined as the composite of cardiac death, target vessel MI, and TVR at 12 months. In patients who require angiography, in-segment binary restenosis and angiographic late in-segment luminal loss will be assessed. Secondary end points include individual components of the primary outcome, cost-effectiveness of DES versus BMS, procedural success/complications, stent thrombosis, cerebrovascular accident, and in-stent neointimal proliferation by intravascular ultrasonography.

The second RCT comparing DES (TAXUS Liberté) with BMS in SVG is the BASKET-SAVAGE trial (Basel Stent Kosten Effektivitäts Trial–Saphenous Venous Graft Angioplasty Using Glycoprotein IIb/IIIa Receptor Inhibitors and Drug-eluting Stents), based in Switzerland. It has a goal enrollment of 240 patients undergoing SVG PCI with documented ischemia, angina, or ACS. The primary outcome measure will be MACE (a composite of cardiac and noncardiac death, nonfatal MI, and TVR) at 12 months.

Additional trials are studying a stable versus biodegradable PES in SVG (NCT00766129), another is looking at whether stenting of moderate SVG lesions (30%–60% by visual estimation) with PES prevents SVG atherosclerosis progression and cardiac events (NCT01223443), and another is studying everolimus-eluting stents in SVG (NCT00911976) (**Table 4**).

## IMPLICATIONS FOR CARE AND FUTURE DIRECTIONS

- A patient's ability to comply with dual antiplatelet therapy and whether the patient will need an interruption in dual antiplatelet therapy should be taken into account when deciding whether to implant a DES or BMS in an SVG.
- Because observational studies account for most of the studies included in the meta-analyses of DES versus BMS in SVG, there is potential for bias introduction. Many of the trials have had a limited duration of clinical follow-up and variable use of embolic protection devices.
- There are only 3 RCTs comparing DES with BMS in SVG intervention.
- There is heterogeneity in the type of DES and BMS used in the trials, some stent types are no longer in clinical use, and there are limited data and follow-up regarding use of contemporary DES and BMS stents.
- DES use in SVG reduces TVR across observational and randomized studies. Recent meta-analyses provide evidence that DES use in SVGs reduces the composite of major adverse events driven mainly by TVR reduction, but DES do not conclusively reduce rates of future death and MI.
- In the absence of contraindication, DES should be used for SVG PCI, because they seem to reduce TVR without increasing rates of adverse events.

## REFERENCES

1. Favaloro RG. Saphenous vein graft in the surgical treatment of coronary artery disease. Operative

technique. J Thorac Cardiovasc Surg 1969;58(2): 178–85.

2. Hong MK, Mehran R, Dangas G, et al. Creatine kinase-MB enzyme elevation following successful saphenous vein graft intervention is associated with late mortality. Circulation 1999;100(24):2400–5.

3. Al-Lamee R, Ielasi A, Latib A, et al. Clinical and angiographic outcomes after percutaneous recanalization of chronic total saphenous vein graft occlusion using modern techniques. Am J Cardiol 2010;106(12):1721–7.

4. Hoffmann R, Pohl T, Köster R, et al. Implantation of paclitaxel-eluting stents in saphenous vein grafts: clinical and angiographic follow-up results from a multicentre study. Heart 2007;93(3):331.

5. Gaglia MA, Torguson R, Xue Z, et al. Outcomes of patients with acute myocardial infarction from a saphenous vein graft culprit undergoing percutaneous coronary intervention. Catheter Cardiovasc Interv 2011;78(1):23–9.

6. Keeley EC, Velez CA, O'Neill WW, et al. Long-term clinical outcome and predictors of major adverse cardiac events after percutaneous interventions on saphenous vein grafts. J Am Coll Cardiol 2001;38(3):659–65.

7. Pucelikova T, Mehran R, Kirtane AJ, et al. Short- and long-term outcomes after stent-assisted percutaneous treatment of saphenous vein grafts in the drug-eluting stent era. Am J Cardiol 2008;101(1):63–8.

8. Roffi M, Mukherjee D, Chew DP, et al. Lack of benefit from intravenous platelet glycoprotein IIb/IIIa receptor inhibition as adjunctive treatment for percutaneous interventions of aortocoronary bypass grafts. Circulation 2002;106(24):3063–7.

9. Marroquin OC, Selzer F, Mulukutla SR, et al. A comparison of bare-metal and drug-eluting stents for off-label indications. N Engl J Med 2008;358(4):342–52.

10. Kirtane AJ, Gupta A, Iyengar S, et al. Safety and efficacy of drug-eluting and bare metal stents. Circulation 2009;119(25):3198–206.

11. Brilakis ES, Wang TY, Rao SV, et al. Frequency and predictors of drug-eluting stent use in saphenous vein bypass graft percutaneous coronary interventions: a report from the American College of Cardiology National Cardiovascular Data CathPCI registry. JACC Cardiovasc Interv 2010;3(10):1068–73.

12. Davies MG, Hagen PO. Reprinted article "pathophysiology of vein graft failure: a review". Eur J Vasc Endovasc Surg 2011;42(Suppl 1):S19–29.

13. Pregowski J, Tyczynski P, Mintz GS, et al. Comparison of ruptured plaques in native coronary arteries and in saphenous vein grafts: an intravascular ultrasound study. Am J Cardiol 2006;97(5):593–7.

14. Davlouros P, Damelou A, Karantalis V, et al. Evaluation of culprit saphenous vein graft lesions with optical coherence tomography in patients with acute coronary syndromes. JACC Cardiovasc Interv 2011;4(6):683–93.

15. Libby P. Molecular and cellular mechanisms of the thrombotic complications of atherosclerosis. J Lipid Res 2009;50(Suppl):S352–7.

16. Gluckman TJ, McLean RC, Schulman SP, et al. Effects of aspirin responsiveness and platelet reactivity on early vein graft thrombosis after coronary artery bypass graft surgery. J Am Coll Cardiol 2011;57(9):1069–77.

17. McLean RC, Nazarian SM, Gluckman TJ, et al. Relative importance of patient, procedural and anatomic risk factors for early vein graft thrombosis after coronary artery bypass graft surgery. J Cardiovasc Surg (Torino) 2011;52(6):877–85.

18. Alexander JH, Hafley G, Harrington RA, et al. Efficacy and safety of edifoligide, an E2F transcription factor decoy, for prevention of vein graft failure following coronary artery bypass graft surgery: PREVENT IV: a randomized controlled trial. JAMA 2005;294(19):2446–54.

19. Fitzgibbon GM, Kafka HP, Leach AJ, et al. Coronary bypass graft fate and patient outcome: angiographic follow-up of 5,065 grafts related to survival and reoperation in 1,388 patients during 25 years. J Am Coll Cardiol 1996;28(3):616–26.

20. Goldman S, Zadina K, Moritz T, et al. Long-term patency of saphenous vein and left internal mammary artery grafts after coronary artery bypass surgery: results from a Department of Veterans Affairs Cooperative Study. J Am Coll Cardiol 2004;44(11): 2149–56.

21. Khot UN, Friedman DT, Pettersson G, et al. Radial artery bypass grafts have an increased occurrence of angiographically severe stenosis and occlusion compared with left internal mammary arteries and saphenous vein grafts. Circulation 2004;109(17): 2086–91.

22. Shroyer AL, Grover FL, Hattler B, et al. On-pump versus off-pump coronary-artery bypass surgery. N Engl J Med 2009;361(19):1827–37.

23. Tatoulis J, Buxton BF, Fuller JA. Patencies of 2,127 arterial to coronary conduits over 15 years. Ann Thorac Surg 2004;77(1):93–101.

24. Levine GN, Bates ER, Blankenship JC, et al. 2011 ACCF/AHA/SCAI Guideline for Percutaneous Coronary Intervention: executive summary a report of the American College of Cardiology Foundation/American Heart Association Task Force on Practice Guidelines and the Society for Cardiovascular Angiography and Interventions. J Am Coll Cardiol 2011;58(24):2550–83.

25. Hillis LD, Smith PK, Anderson JL, et al. 2011 ACCF/AHA Guideline for Coronary Artery Bypass Graft Surgery. A report of the American College of Cardiology Foundation/American Heart Association Task Force on Practice Guidelines. Developed in

collaboration with the American Association for Thoracic Surgery, Society of Cardiovascular Anesthesiologists, and Society of Thoracic Surgeons. J Am Coll Cardiol 2011;58(24):e123–210.

26. Fox KA, Clayton TC, Damman P, et al. Long-term outcome of a routine versus selective invasive strategy in patients with non–ST-segment elevation acute coronary syndrome: a meta-analysis of individual patient data. J Am Coll Cardiol 2010; 55(22):2435–45.

27. Iakovou I, Schmidt T, Bonizzoni E, et al. Incidence, predictors, and outcome of thrombosis after successful implantation of drug-eluting stents. JAMA 2005;293(17):2126.

28. Shapira I, Isakov A, Heller I, et al. Long-term follow-up after coronary artery bypass grafting reoperation. Chest 1999;115(6):1593–7.

29. Christenson JT, Schmuziger M, Simonet F. Reoperative coronary artery bypass procedures: risk factors for early mortality and late survival. Eur J Cardiothorac Surg 1997;11(1):129–33.

30. Yap CH, Sposato L, Akowuah E, et al. Contemporary results show repeat coronary artery bypass grafting remains a risk factor for operative mortality. Ann Thorac Surg 2009;87(5):1386–91.

31. Schmuziger M, Christenson J, Maurice J, et al. Reoperative myocardial revascularization: an analysis of 458 reoperations and 2645 single operations. Cardiovasc Surg 1994;2(5):623.

32. Salomon N, Page US, Bigelow J, et al. Reoperative coronary surgery. Comparative analysis of 6591 patients undergoing primary bypass and 508 patients undergoing reoperative coronary artery bypass. J Thorac Cardiovasc Surg 1990;100(2): 250.

33. Douglas JS Jr, Gruentzig AR, King SB III, et al. Percutaneous transluminal coronary angioplasty in patients with prior coronary bypass surgery. J Am Coll Cardiol 1983;2(4):745–54.

34. Ford W, Wholey M, Zikria E, et al. Percutaneous transluminal angioplasty in the management of occlusive disease involving the coronary arteries and saphenous vein bypass grafts: preliminary results. J Thorac Cardiovasc Surg 1980;79(1):1.

35. El Gamal M, Bonnier H, Michels R, et al. Percutaneous transluminal angioplasty of stenosed aortocoronary bypass grafts. Br Heart J 1984;52(6):617.

36. Block PC, Cowley MJ, Kaltenbach M, et al. Percutaneous angioplasty of stenoses of bypass grafts or of bypass graft anastomotic sites. Am J Cardiol 1984;53(6):666–8.

37. Corbelli J, Franco I, Hollman J, et al. Percutaneous transluminal coronary angioplasty after previous coronary artery bypass surgery. Am J Cardiol 1985;56(7):398–403.

38. Dorros G, Johnson W, Tector A, et al. Percutaneous transluminal coronary angioplasty in patients with prior coronary artery bypass grafting. J Thorac Cardiovasc Surg 1984;87(1):17.

39. Dorros G, Lewin RF, Mathiak LM, et al. Percutaneous transluminal coronary angioplasty in patients with two or more previous coronary artery bypass grafting operations. Am J Cardiol 1988; 61(15):1243–7.

40. Reed DC, Beller GA, Nygaard TW, et al. The clinical efficacy and scintigraphic evaluation of post-coronary bypass patients undergoing percutaneous transluminal coronary angioplasty for recurrent angina pectoris. Am Heart J 1989;117(1):60–71.

41. Platko WP, Hollman J, Whitlow PL, et al. Percutaneous transluminal angioplasty of saphenous vein graft stenosis: long-term follow-up. J Am Coll Cardiol 1989;14(7):1645–50.

42. Tan KH, Henderson RA, Sulke N, et al. Percutaneous transluminal coronary angioplasty in patients with prior coronary artery bypass grafting: ten years' experience. Cathet Cardiovasc Diagn 1994;32(1):11–7.

43. Webb JG, Myler RK, Shaw RE, et al. Coronary angioplasty after coronary bypass surgery: initial results and late outcome in 422 patients. J Am Coll Cardiol 1990;16(4):812–20.

44. Plokker H, Meester BH, Serruys PW. The Dutch experience in percutaneous transluminal angioplasty of narrowed saphenous veins used for aorto-coronary arterial bypass. Am J Cardiol 1991;67(5): 361–6.

45. Fischman DL, Leon MB, Baim DS, et al. A randomized comparison of coronary-stent placement and balloon angioplasty in the treatment of coronary artery disease. N Engl J Med 1994; 331(8):496–501.

46. de Feyter PJ, van Suylen RJ, de Jaegere PP, et al. Balloon angioplasty for the treatment of lesions in saphenous vein bypass grafts. J Am Coll Cardiol 1993;21(7):1539–49.

47. Hanekamp CE, Koolen JJ, Den Heijer P, et al. Randomized study to compare balloon angioplasty and elective stent implantation in venous bypass grafts: the Venestent study. Catheter Cardiovasc Interv 2003;60(4):452–7.

48. Brener SJ, Ellis SG, Apperson-Hansen C, et al. Comparison of stenting and balloon angioplasty for narrowings in aortocoronary saphenous vein conduits in place for more than five years. Am J Cardiol 1997;79(1):13–8.

49. Ellis S, Savage M, Fischman D, et al. Restenosis after placement of Palmaz-Schatz stents in native coronary arteries. Initial results of a multicenter experience. Circulation 1992;86(6):1836–44.

50. de Scheerder IK, Strauss BH, de Feyter PJ, et al. Stenting of venous bypass grafts: a new treatment modality for patients who are poor candidates for reintervention. Am Heart J 1992;123(4):1046–54.

51. Piana RN, Moscucci M, Cohen DJ, et al. Palmaz-Schatz stenting for treatment of focal vein graft stenosis: immediate results and long-term outcome. J Am Coll Cardiol 1994;23(6):1296–304.

52. Fenton SH, Fischman DL, Savage MP. Long-term angiographic and clinical outcome after implantation of balloon-expandable stents in aortocoronary saphenous vein grafts. Am J Cardiol 1994;74(12): 1187–91.

53. Wong SC, Baim DS, Schatz RA, et al. Immediate results and late outcomes after stent implantation in saphenous vein graft lesions: the multicenter US Palmaz-Schatz stent experience. J Am Coll Cardiol 1995;26(3):704–12.

54. Eeckhout E, Goy JJ, Stauffer JC, et al. Endoluminal stenting of narrowed saphenous vein grafts: long-term clinical and angiographic follow-up. Cathet Cardiovasc Diagn 1994;32(2):139–46.

55. Savage MP, Douglas JS Jr, Fischman DL, et al. Stent placement compared with balloon angioplasty for obstructed coronary bypass grafts. N Engl J Med 1997;337(11):740–7.

56. Abizaid A, Weiner B, Bailey SR, et al. Use of a self-expanding super-elastic all-metal endoprosthesis; to treat degenerated SVG lesions: the SESAME first in man trial. Catheter Cardiovasc Interv 2010;76(6): 781–6.

57. Baldus S, Köster R, Elsner M, et al. Treatment of aortocoronary vein graft lesions with membrane-covered stents: a multicenter surveillance trial. Circulation 2000;102(17):2024–7.

58. Schachinger V, Hamm CW, Munzel T, et al. A randomized trial of polytetrafluoroethylene-membrane-covered stents compared with conventional stents in aortocoronary saphenous vein grafts. J Am Coll Cardiol 2003;42(8):1360.

59. Stankovic G, Colombo A, Presbitero P, et al. Randomized evaluation of polytetrafluoroethylene-covered stent in saphenous vein grafts: the Randomized Evaluation of polytetrafluoroethylene COVERed stent in Saphenous vein grafts (RECOVERS) Trial. Circulation 2003;108(1):37–42.

60. Stone G, Goldberg S, Mehran R. A prospective, randomized US trial of the PTFE-covered Jostent for the treatment of diseased saphenous vein grafts: the BARRICADE trial [abstract]. J Am Coll Cardiol 2005;45(Suppl A):27A.

61. Kaluski E, Hauptmann KE, Müller R, et al. Coronary stenting with MGuard: first-in-man trial. J Invasive Cardiol 2008;20(10):511–5.

62. Vaknin-Assa H, Assali A, Kornowski R. Preliminary experiences using the MGuard stent platform in saphenous vein graft lesions. Catheter Cardiovasc Interv 2009;74(7):1055–7.

63. Turco MA, Buchbinder M, Popma JJ, et al. Pivotal, randomized U.S. study of the Symbiottrade mark covered stent system in patients with saphenous vein graft disease: eight-month angiographic and clinical results from the Symbiot III trial. Catheter Cardiovasc Interv 2006;68(3):379–88.

64. Brodie BR, Wilson H, Stuckey T, et al. Outcomes with drug-eluting versus bare-metal stents in saphenous vein graft intervention results from the STENT (strategic transcatheter evaluation of new therapies) group. JACC Cardiovasc Interv 2009; 2(11):1105–12.

65. Mendiz OA, Ahmed WH, Fava CM, et al. Clinical outcome after saphenous vein stenting with Taxus Liberté stent: results from the OLYMPIA Registry (TAXUS Liberté Postapproval Global Program). Angiology 2012;63(8):574–8.

66. Ge L, Iakovou I, Sangiorgi GM, et al. Treatment of saphenous vein graft lesions with drug-eluting stents: immediate and midterm outcome. J Am Coll Cardiol 2005;45(7):989–94.

67. Lee MS, Shah AP, Aragon J, et al. Drug-eluting stenting is superior to bare metal stenting in saphenous vein grafts. Catheter Cardiovasc Interv 2005; 66(4):507–11.

68. Chu WW, Kuchulakanti PK, Wang B, et al. Efficacy of sirolimus-eluting stents as compared to paclitaxel-eluting stents for saphenous vein graft intervention. J Interv Cardiol 2006;19(2):121–5.

69. Ellis SG, Kandzari D, Kereiakes DJ, et al. Utility of sirolimus-eluting Cypher stents to reduce 12-month target vessel revascularization in saphenous vein graft stenoses: results of a multicenter 350-patient case-control study. J Invasive Cardiol 2007; 19(10):404–9.

70. Minutello RM, Bhagan S, Sharma A, et al. Long-term clinical benefit of sirolimus-eluting stents compared to bare metal stents in the treatment of saphenous vein graft disease. J Interv Cardiol 2007;20(6):458–65.

71. Wohrle J, Nusser T, Kestler HA, et al. Comparison of the slow-release polymer-based paclitaxel-eluting Taxus-Express stent with the bare-metal Express stent for saphenous vein graft interventions. Clin Res Cardiol 2007;96(2):70–6.

72. Assali A, Raz Y, Vaknin-Assa H, et al. Beneficial 2-years results of drug-eluting stents in saphenous vein graft lesions. EuroIntervention 2008;4(1):108–14.

73. Bansal D, Muppidi R, Singla S, et al. Percutaneous intervention on the saphenous vein bypass grafts–long-term outcomes. Catheter Cardiovasc Interv 2008;71(1):58–61.

74. Gioia G, Benassi A, Mohendra R, et al. Lack of clinical long-term benefit with the use of a drug eluting stent compared to use of a bare metal stent in saphenous vein grafts. Catheter Cardiovasc Interv 2008;72(1):13–20.

75. Okabe T, Lindsay J, Buch AN, et al. Drug-eluting stents versus bare metal stents for narrowing in

saphenous vein grafts. Am J Cardiol 2008;102(5): 530–4.

76. Ramana RK, Ronan A, Cohoon K, et al. Long-term clinical outcomes of real-world experience using sirolimus-eluting stents in saphenous vein graft disease. Catheter Cardiovasc Interv 2008;71(7): 886–93.

77. Kaplan S, Barlis P, Kiris A, et al. Immediate procedural and long-term clinical outcomes following drug-eluting stent implantation to ostial saphenous vein graft lesions. Acute Card Care 2008;10(2):88–92.

78. van Twisk PH, Daemen J, Kukreja N, et al. Four-year safety and efficacy of the unrestricted use of sirolimus- and paclitaxel-eluting stents in coronary artery bypass grafts. EuroIntervention 2008;4(3): 311–7.

79. Vignali L, Saia F, Manari A, et al. Long-term outcomes with drug-eluting stents versus bare metal stents in the treatment of saphenous vein graft disease (results from the REgistro Regionale AngiopLastiche Emilia-Romagna registry). Am J Cardiol 2008;101(7):947–52.

80. Lozano I, Garcia-Camarero T, Carrillo P, et al. Comparison of drug-eluting and bare metal stents in saphenous vein grafts. Immediate and long-term results. Rev Esp Cardiol 2009;62(1):39–47 [in Spanish].

81. Applegate RJ, Sacrinty M, Kutcher M, et al. Late outcomes of drug-eluting versus bare metal stents in saphenous vein grafts: propensity score analysis. Catheter Cardiovasc Interv 2008;72(1):7–12.

82. Shishehbor MH, Hawi R, Singh IM, et al. Drug-eluting versus bare-metal stents for treating saphenous vein grafts. Am Heart J 2009;158(4): 637–43.

83. Goswami NJ, Gaffigan M, Berrio G, et al. Long-term outcomes of drug-eluting stents versus bare-metal stents in saphenous vein graft disease: results from the Prairie "Real World" Stent Registry. Catheter Cardiovasc Interv 2010;75(1):93–100.

84. Latib A, Ferri L, Ielasi A, et al. Comparison of the long-term safety and efficacy of drug-eluting and bare-metal stent implantation in saphenous vein grafts. Circ Cardiovasc Interv 2010;3(3):249–56.

85. Baldwin DE, Abbott JD, Trost JC, et al. Comparison of drug-eluting and bare metal stents for saphenous vein graft lesions (from the National Heart, Lung, and Blood Institute Dynamic Registry). Am J Cardiol 2010;106(7):946–51.

86. Nair S, Fath-Ordoubadi F, Clarke B, et al. Late outcomes of drug eluting and bare metal stents in saphenous vein graft percutaneous coronary intervention. EuroIntervention 2011;6(8):985–91.

87. Nauta ST, Van Mieghem NM, Magro M, et al. Seven-year safety and efficacy of the unrestricted use of drug-eluting stents in saphenous vein bypass grafts. Catheter Cardiovasc Interv 2012;79(6):912–8.

88. Chakravarty T, Morrissey RP, Wertman B, et al. Comparison of long-term outcomes of drug-eluting stents and bare metal stents for saphenous vein graft stenosis. Catheter Cardiovasc Interv 2012;79(6):903–9.

89. Vermeersch P, Agostoni P, Verheye S, et al. Randomized double-blind comparison of sirolimus-eluting stent versus bare-metal stent implantation in diseased saphenous vein grafts: six-month angiographic, intravascular ultrasound, and clinical follow-up of the RRISC trial. J Am Coll Cardiol 2006;48(12):2423–31.

90. Brilakis ES, Lichtenwalter C, de Lemos JA, et al. A randomized controlled trial of a paclitaxel-eluting stent versus a similar bare-metal stent in saphenous vein graft lesions the SOS (Stenting of Saphenous Vein Grafts) trial. J Am Coll Cardiol 2009;53(11):919–28.

91. Mehilli J, Pache J, Abdel-Wahab M, et al. Drug-eluting versus bare-metal stents in saphenous vein graft lesions (ISAR-CABG): a randomised controlled superiority trial. Lancet 2011;378(9796):1071–8.

92. Jeger RV, Schneiter S, Kaiser C, et al. Drug-eluting stents compared with bare metal stents improve late outcome after saphenous vein graft but not after large native vessel interventions. Cardiology 2009;112(1):49–55.

93. Vermeersch P, Agostoni P, Verheye S, et al. Increased late mortality after sirolimus-eluting stents versus bare-metal stents in diseased saphenous vein grafts: results from the randomized DELAYED RRISC trial. J Am Coll Cardiol 2007;50(3):261–7.

94. Brilakis ES, Lichtenwalter C, Abdel-Karim AR, et al. Continued benefit from paclitaxel-eluting compared with bare-metal stent implantation in saphenous vein graft lesions during long-term follow-up of the SOS (Stenting of Saphenous Vein Grafts) trial. JACC Cardiovasc Interv 2011;4(2):176–82.

95. Coolong A, Baim DS, Kuntz RE, et al. Saphenous vein graft stenting and major adverse cardiac events: a predictive model derived from a pooled analysis of 3958 patients. Circulation 2008;117(6):790–7.

96. Testa L, Agostoni P, Vermeersch P, et al. Drug eluting stent versus bare metal stent in the treatment of saphenous vein graft disease: a systematic review and meta-analysis. EuroIntervention 2010; 6(4):527–36.

97. Joyal D, Filion KB, Eisenberg MJ. Effectiveness and safety of drug-eluting stents in vein grafts: a meta-analysis. Am Heart J 2010;159(2):159–169.e4.

98. Meier P, Brilakis ES, Corti R, et al. Drug-eluting versus bare-metal stent for treatment of saphenous vein grafts: a meta-analysis. PLoS One 2010;5(6): e11040.

99. Navarese EP, Buffon A, De Luca G, et al. Effectiveness and safety of drug-eluting stents in vein grafts: a meta-analysis. Am Heart J 2010;160(2):e9.

100. Paradis JM, Belisle P, Joseph L, et al. Drug-eluting or bare metal stents for the treatment of saphenous vein graft disease: a Bayesian meta-analysis. Circ Cardiovasc Interv 2010;3(6):565–76.
101. Sanchez-Recalde A, Jimenez Valero S, Moreno R, et al. Safety and efficacy of drug-eluting stents versus bare-metal stents in saphenous vein grafts lesions: a meta-analysis. EuroIntervention 2010; 6(1):149–60.
102. Testa L, Agostoni P, Vermeersch P, et al. Drug eluting stents versus bare metal stents in the treatment of saphenous vein graft disease: a systematic review and meta-analysis. EuroIntervention 2010; 6(4):527–36.
103. Wiisanen ME, Abdel-Latif A, Mukherjee D, et al. Drug-eluting stents versus bare-metal stents in saphenous vein graft interventions: a systematic review and meta-analysis. JACC Cardiovasc Interv 2010;3(12):1262–73.
104. Hakeem A, Helmy T, Munsif S, et al. Safety and efficacy of drug eluting stents compared with bare metal stents for saphenous vein graft interventions: a comprehensive meta-analysis of randomized trials and observational studies comprising 7,994 patients. Catheter Cardiovasc Interv 2011;77(3): 343–55.
105. Lupi A, Navarese EP, Lazzero M, et al. Drug-eluting stents vs. bare metal stents in saphenous vein graft disease. Insights from a meta-analysis of 7,090 patients. Circ J 2011;75(2):280–9.
106. Mamas MA, Foley J, Nair S, et al. A comparison of drug-eluting stents versus bare metal stents in saphenous vein graft PCI outcomes: a meta-analysis. J Interv Cardiol 2011;24(2):172–80.
107. Alam M, Bandeali SJ, Virani SS, et al. Clinical outcomes of percutaneous interventions in saphenous vein grafts using drug-eluting stents compared to bare-metal stents: a comprehensive meta-analysis of all randomized clinical trials. Clin Cardiol 2012;35(5):291–6.
108. Pasceri V, Tarsia G, Niccoli G, et al. Early beneficial effects of drug-eluting stents in vein grafts wane during long term follow-up: A Case-Control Study. Catheter Cardiovasc Interv 2012;80(7):1112–7.

# Optimal Stenting in Saphenous Vein Graft Intervention

Gabriel Maluenda, MD, Augusto D. Pichard, MD*

## KEYWORDS

- Saphenous vein graft • Percutaneous coronary intervention • Stenting • Clinical outcomes

## KEY POINTS

- Saphenous vein graft disease is usually present as early as 1 year after grafting and is characterized by diffuse, concentric, and friable plaques with a poorly developed fibrous cap.
- Most symptomatic patients after coronary bypass surgery present with extensive native and graft disease and revascularization strategy must be based on a careful risk/benefit assessment.
- In view of the latest clinical evidence, drug-eluting stents seem to be the preferred treatment option. Further follow-up is needed to confirm long-term safety.
- Embolic protection devices remain the standard approach to prevent distal embolization.
- Direct and small-sized stenting may play major roles in improving acute and long-term outcomes, particularly when embolic protection devices are not used.

## INTRODUCTION

Durability of saphenous vein grafts (SVG) is limited due to the progressive atherosclerosis process initiated early after grafting.[1] Only 50% of SVGs remain patent after 10 years.[2] Ischemic symptoms due to SVG disease usually occur ≥3 years after grafting[1] and are associated with a degenerative atherosclerotic process characterized by diffuse, concentric, and friable plaques with poorly developed fibrous cap and little calcification.[3] Degenerated SVGs represent a clinical dilemma. Repeat coronary artery bypass grafting (CABG) results in higher rates of mortality, less relief of angina, and more frequent graft failure as compared with the first surgery.[4] On the other hand, percutaneous coronary intervention (PCI) of SVGs also results in higher rates of mortality, periprocedural myocardial infarction (MI), and restenosis when compared with native vessel PCI.[5,6]

Poorer outcomes following PCI in SVGs have been associated with embolization of atherothrombotic debris into the native coronary circulation, often resulting in periprocedural MI or the "no-reflow" phenomenon. Strategies to prevent distal embolization include the use of both proximal and distal protection devices as well as adjunctive pharmacology and new stenting approaches. Despite these advances, restenosis and target vessel rates of failure in degenerated SVGs remain relatively high. Here the strategies aimed at optimizing acute and long-term results in patients undergoing SVG stenting are reviewed.

## ASSESSING RISK/BENEFIT RATIO

In general, PCI of a native grafted vessel is usually preferred over PCI of a degenerated SVG because of the increased risk of periprocedural MI.[7] If PCI of the native vessel is not possible, the clinical benefit of a high-risk SVG PCI should be balanced against the risk of repeating the surgical revascularization.[8]

Limited studies have compared the efficacy of PCI to repeat CABG. The Angina With Extremely Serious Operative Mortality Evaluation (AWESOME) registry of 142 patients with refractory post-CABG ischemia who were reasonable candidates for

Division of Cardiology, Department of Internal Medicine, Washington Hospital Center, 110 Irving Street, Northwest, Suite 4B-1, Washington, DC 20010, USA
* Corresponding author.
*E-mail address:* Augusto.D.Pichard@medstar.net

Intervent Cardiol Clin 2 (2013) 307–313
http://dx.doi.org/10.1016/j.iccl.2012.11.006
2211-7458/13/$ – see front matter © 2013 Elsevier Inc. All rights reserved.

either PCI or CABG addressed this issue.[9] Arterial grafts were used in 75% of repeat CABG, whereas bare metal stents (BMS) were used in 54% of PCIs. Initial in-hospital mortality was higher in the CABG group (8 vs 0%), but after 3-year follow-up there was no difference in overall survival. A larger retrospective study described the results on 2191 patients from 1995 to 2000 with prior CABG who underwent multivessel revascularization: 1487 repeat CABG and 704 PCI.[10] Complete revascularization was achieved more frequently in the PCI group (89 vs 71%, P<.001). Periprocedural Q-wave MI was significantly higher in the CABG group (1.4 vs 0.3%, P = .01); however, similar rates of mortality were observed at 30-day follow-up (2.8% in the CABG group vs 1.7% in the PCI group, P = .34). At 5-year follow-up, PCI was associated with a nonsignificant increase in the adjusted rate of mortality (HR 1.47, CI 0.94–2.28, P = .09).

Based on the described evidence, the last updated American College of Cardiology/American Heart Association/Society for Cardiovascular Angiography and Interventions guidelines (2005) recommend PCI in the following circumstances[11]:

1. Early ischemia (usually within 30 days) after CABG, when technically feasible (class I).
2. Ischemia that occurs 1 to 3 years after CABG in patients with discrete lesions and preserved left ventricular function. It is also reasonable in patients with diseased SVG older than 3 years, and if feasible, in patients with patent left internal mammary artery and significant obstruction in other vessels (class IIa).
3. PCI is not recommended in patients with total SVG occlusions, or multiple target lesions (native/SVG disease), and impaired left ventricular function, unless repeat CABG poses excessive risk (class III).

In addition, CABG is usually reserved for patients who cannot have adequate percutaneous revascularization, or who may gain additional benefit from CABG, such as an unused left internal mammary artery to left anterior descending (LAD) graft. Indeed the 2004 American College of Cardiology/American Heart Association guidelines recommend repeat CABG in the following settings[12]:

1. Disabling ischemia, despite optimal medical therapy (class I).
2. Prior CABG without patent grafts and with a class I indication for surgery due to native disease: left main disease, left main equivalent, or 3-vessel disease (class I).
3. Atherosclerotic vein grafts with greater than 50% stenosis in vessels that supply the LAD or large areas of myocardium (class IIa).

In summary, PCI is usually preferred over repeat CABG for early recurrent symptoms after CABG (<3 years). Most symptomatic post-CABG patients present with extensive native and graft disease; however, the revascularization strategy must be based on careful procedural risk/benefit assessment and on local experience.

## STENT-TYPE SELECTION

Drug-eluting stent (DES) use is associated with a significant restenosis rate decrease in selected native coronary artery lesions when compared with BMS. Several DES types are currently available: sirolimus-eluting, paclitaxel-eluting, zotarolimus-eluting, everolimus-eluting, and biolimus-eluting. Large randomized trials have shown considerable reduction in angiographic restenosis and target lesion revascularization (TLR) with respect to standard interventional devices.[13-15] However, in almost all randomized trials, SVG lesions were excluded.

The mechanisms of in-stent restenotic processes in SVG are different when compared with native arteries. Further, the problem of higher local prothrombotic conditions in the vein graft and the expected delay in endothelial healing after DES placement are claimed as possible downsides of DES implantation in SVG, as they can potentially lead to a higher risk of late thrombosis.

Two randomized studies have initially tested the benefit of DES versus BMS in SVG: the Reduction of Restenosis In Saphenous Vein Grafts With Cypher Sirolimus-Eluting Stent (RRISC) trial, which included 75 patients,[16] and the Stenting Of Saphenous vein grafts (SOS) trial, in which 80 patients were assigned to either paclitaxel-eluting stents or BMS.[17] The primary end point of both trials was based on angiographic measures of restenosis at 6 to 12 months. Clinical outcomes over 3 years are also available in 2 separate reports.[18,19]

Both RRISC and SOS trials showed significant restenosis reduction with DES compared with BMS. However, their 3-year clinical outcomes revealed conflicting results. The SOS trial reported sustained benefit, with DES significantly reducing major adverse cardiac events. This profit was mostly driven by reduction of MI (46% vs 17%, HR: 0.32 [0.13–0.76], P = .01), TLR (41% vs 10%, HR: 0.20 [0.07–0.60], P = .004) and target vessel failure (72% vs 34%, HR: 0.34 [0.18–0.66], P = .001) without any significant difference in mortality.[19] The RRISC trial showed no significant difference in major adverse cardiac event rates between DES and BMS, but a notable increase in mortality with DES (29% vs 0%).[18]

Nonetheless, results from Is Drug-Eluting-Stenting Associated with Improved Results in

Coronary Artery Bypass Grafts? (ISAR-CABG),[20] a large randomized controlled superiority trial, bring new insights into the current evidence. In this randomized superiority trial, patients with de novo SVG lesions were assigned (1:1:1:3) to receive either DES (1 of 3 types: permanent-polymer paclitaxel-eluting stents, permanent-polymer sirolimus-eluting stents, or biodegradable-polymer sirolimus-eluting stents) or BMS. The primary end point was the composite of 1-year death-MI-TLR. Six hundred ten (n = 610) patients were allocated to treatment groups (n = 303, DES; n = 307, BMS). DES reduced the incidence of the primary end point compared with BMS (44 [15%] vs 66 [22%]; HR 0.64, P = .02), primarily driven by a reduction in TLR by DES (19 [7%] vs 37 [13%]; HR 0.49, P = .01) (**Fig. 1**). No significant differences were seen among DES types and BMS regarding all-cause mortality (15 [5%] vs 14 [5%]; HR 1.08, P = .83), MI (12 [4%] vs 18 [6%]; HR 0.66, P = .27), or definite or probable stent thrombosis (2 [1%] in both groups; HR 1.00, P = .99). Although long-term data are still needed, the results of ISAR-CABG support the use of DES as the preferred treatment option for patients undergoing PCI for de novo SVG lesions.[20]

## INTERVENTIONAL STRATEGIES FOR OPTIMAL STENTING RESULTS

The use of stents to treat SVG has demonstrated clear outcome benefit over conventional balloon angioplasty alone.[21,22] As a result, stenting is currently the standard practice to intervene SVG.

### Predilation Versus Direct Stenting

Compared to predilation with balloon angioplasty, direct stenting has the potential benefit of trapping debris and decreasing distal embolization that may occur from repeated balloon inflations, as shown during acute MI treatment.[23] We analyzed the clinical benefit of direct stenting in a retrospective series of 527 patients undergoing SVG interventions.[24] In this cohort, 170 patients with 229 lesions were treated with direct stenting and 357 patients with 443 lesions were treated with predilation. Patients treated with direct stenting had less creatine kinase (CK)-myocardial isoform (MB) release (P<.001), and less non-Q-wave MI (P = .024). At 1 year follow-up, the rate of the combined death-MI-TLR was significantly lower in patients treated with direct stenting (P = .021). In addition, the authors communicated in a separate retrospective report the excellent clinical outcome using this strategy and suggested that direct stenting could be considered an alternative treatment to PCI with distal protection devices for selected SVG lesions.[25] As a result, the authors recommend the direct stenting approach for treating SVG stenosis when technically feasible.

### Undersized Stenting Approach

The theoretical concept of "undersized" stenting intends to prevent plaque intrusion, a mechanism likely linked to distal embolization when treating degenerated SVG (**Fig. 2**). As illustrated in **Fig. 3**, this approach usually implies adequate expansion of an intentionally undersized stent, which may leave areas of malapposition that is better demonstrated by optical coherence tomography technology.

We recently reported the results of SVG lesions treated with DESs (n = 209) in 3 groups according to the ratio of the stent diameter to the

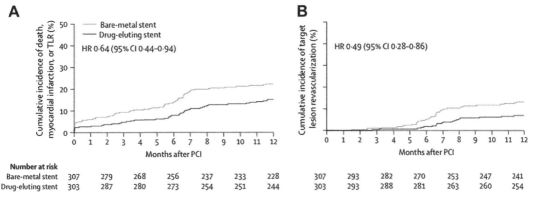

**Fig. 1.** One-year results of the ISAR-CABG trial. Kaplan-Meier curves are shown for (A) the primary endpoint (composite of death, myocardial infarction, and ischemia-driven target lesion revascularization). (B) The secondary efficacy endpoint of ischemia-driven target lesion revascularization. (From Mehilli J, Pache J, Abdel-Wahab M, et al. for the Is Drug-Eluting-Stenting Associated with Improved Results in Coronary Artery Bypass Grafts? (ISAR-CABG) Investigators. Drug-eluting versus bare-metal stents in saphenous vein graft lesions (ISAR-CABG): a randomised controlled superiority trial. Lancet 2011;378(9796):1071–8; with permission.)

## Undersized stenting for saphenous vein graft concept

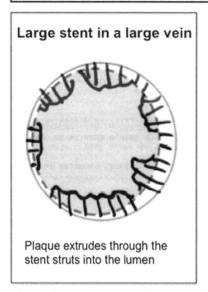

**Large stent in a large vein**

Plaque extrudes through the stent struts into the lumen

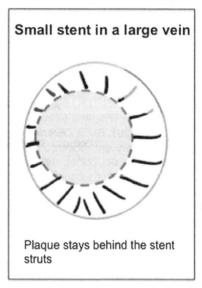

**Small stent in a large vein**

Plaque stays behind the stent struts

**Fig. 2.** The "undersized" stenting concept for saphenous vein grafts.

average intravascular ultrasound (IVUS) reference lumen diameter (group I: <0.89, group II: 0.9–1.0, and group III: >1.0).[26] Plaque intrusion volume, defined as the amount of tissue extrusion through the stent struts after SVG intervention, was smallest in group I (group I: 0.25 ± 0.68 $mm^3$, group II: 0.40 ± 0.68 $mm^3$, and group III: 0.75 ± 1.34 $mm^3$; $P$ = .007). The incidence of CK-MB elevation greater than 3 times normal was 6% in group I, 9% in group II, and 19% in group III ($P$ = .03) without an increase in clinical events at 1 year. The incidence of 1-year TLR (group I: 13%, group II: 9%, and group III: 15%; $P$ = .5) and target vessel revascularization (group I: 13%, group II: 13%, and group III: 15%; $P$ = .9) was similar.

We therefore recommend the "undersized stenting" strategy to treat SVG, which could be particularly attractive when embolic protection devices (EPD) are not available or cannot be used for technical reasons.

### Pharmacologic Methods to Prevent the No-Reflow Phenomenon

Pharmacologic methods for treating SVG atherosclerosis and disease progression, in comparison to native vessel atherosclerosis, are relatively limited. It does seem that aggressive low-density lipoprotein–lowering therapy with statins reduces progression of SVG atherosclerosis, as evaluated by both angiography and IVUS.[27,28] Other treatments, however, have been less successful.

Glycoprotein IIb/IIIa inhibitors might be expected to improve outcomes in patients undergoing SVG PCI, given their potent effects on platelet aggregation. Studies have consistently shown, however, that glycoprotein IIb/IIIa inhibitors increase rates of bleeding in SVG PCI, without any benefit in regard to periprocedural MI or to survival.[7,29–31] Similarly, intracoronary vasodilators (eg, adenosine, sodium nitroprusside) would be expected to improve microvascular spasm associated with the no-reflow phenomenon. Although studies have shown that such vasodilators can improve angiographic flow, they do not seem to improve ischemic outcomes.[32,33]

### Embolic Protection Devices

Multiple randomized clinical trials have demonstrated the significant benefit of EPDs in improving the outcomes of SVG interventions.[34] Three strategies for embolic protection, distal occlusion, distal filtering, and proximal occlusion, are available. EPDs of nearly every type seem to have similar outcomes. A pooled analysis of these devices, including distal, filter, and proximal combined, in nearly 4000 patients showed benefit of the device in both low-risk and high-risk strata undergoing SVG PCI.[34] It must be emphasized, however, that despite the improvement in outcomes with EPDs, rates of major adverse cardiac outcomes remain around 10% at 30 days. For detailed information regarding each device, see later discussion.

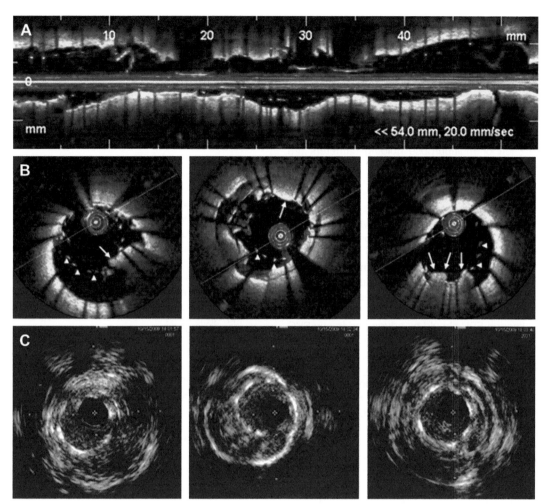

**Fig. 3.** Intravascular ultrasound and optical coherence tomography imaging of an undersized stenting strategy to treat a totally occluded SVG. Complete long run view of the optical coherence tomography (OCT) of the stented saphenous vein graft (distal segment at the left, and proximal segment at the right) (A). Cross-sectional view of OCT from distal to proximal, from left to right, respectively, showing areas of incomplete stent apposition (*triangles*) and areas of definite plaque prolapse (*arrows*) (B). Corresponding IVUS cross-sectional views, showing well-expanded stents, with circular lumen, but less areas of stent malapposition and no plaque prolapsed, contrasting with the OCT result (C).

## Intravascular Ultrasound Value in Vein Graft Interventions

Conventional angiography underestimates the severity of vein graft remodeling and athermanous plaque development compared with IVUS.[35] It has been demonstrated that the time course of TLR following successful SVG angioplasty appears differently from native vessels and continues after 1 year.[36] As a result, it has been suggested that intermediate lesions, better identified with IVUS, might be treated, avoiding early recurrence of symptoms attributed to those lesions.

As a general rule IVUS is not used before stenting in degenerated grafts to prevent embolization. If the lesion is distal in a vein graft, IVUS can be used proximally to assess vessel size. At the authors' institution, IVUS is always performed after stenting to assess results. Lack of apposition of undersized stents is frequent and is not associated with any clinical adverse event.[26]

## TECHNICAL ASPECTS

When dealing with an SVG lesion, pharmacologic pretreatment of the patient is extremely important. Dual antiplatelet therapy (given upfront) and statins are mandatory. Glycoprotein IIb/IIIa inhibitors, as previously mentioned, seem not to be effective in SVG interventions. However, in cases of acute MI due to acute graft closure, they may still play a role.

Choosing the correct guiding catheter is key. When approaching these bypasses via the radial approach, the authors strongly recommend avoiding the right radial artery and instead choosing the left radial artery. Guiding catheters of choice can be extra backup shaped, multipurpose with a long distal arm, or Amplatz left catheters. Sometimes vein grafts to the circumflex originate from the posterior surface of the aorta. In this case, Amplatz left or multipurpose guiding catheters are preferred. For the vein graft to the right coronary artery, originating most of the time from the right anterior surface of the aorta, the multipurpose catheter has the best alignment and support when performing the procedure via the femoral or radial artery. For vein grafts originating from the left anterior surface (usually to the LAD/diagonal or marginal arteries), the authors prefer left coronary bypass catheters in case of femoral access. If additional support is needed, Amplatz left catheters can be used.

Although EPD should be advocated in any SVG procedure, they are frequently unable to be used because of anatomic or economical reasons. In these cases, a soft-tip coronary guide wire and direct "undersized" stenting without predilation and postdilation should be the recommended strategy. Once the stenting procedure is finished, attention should be paid to the collection of debris from the protection device. With proximal device placement, direct aspiration of at least 5 cc blood from the device should be performed before releasing the occlusion. In case a distal occlusion device is used, the specific manual aspiration device should be used, and 2 syringes of 20 cc blood should be aspirated. If a filter is used, careful, complete closure of the filter is necessary before retrieval. Final angiographic evaluation of the stenting procedure without a device in place is mandatory in at least 2 orthogonal views. We highly recommend IVUS to assess the final result.

## SUMMARY

Percutaneous revascularization of diseased, usually degenerated saphenous vein grafts must be based on careful procedural risk/benefit assessment and on the local experience. It seems clear, however, that the variety of protection devices for distal embolization improves outcomes in this particularly difficult setting. Nonetheless, in many cases those devices are not used or cannot be used. In this particular situation the authors believe that novel stenting strategies, including direct stenting and small-sized stenting, may play major roles in improving acute and long-term outcomes. Further research is required in this evolving field.

## REFERENCES

1. Motwani JG, Topol EJ. Aortocoronary saphenous vein graft disease: pathogenesis, predisposition, and prevention. Circulation 1998;97:916–31.
2. Goldman S, Zadina K, Moritz T, et al. Long-term patency of saphenous vein and left internal mammary artery grafts after coronary artery bypass surgery: results from a Department of Veterans Affairs Cooperative Study. J Am Coll Cardiol 2004;44:2149–56.
3. Kalan JM, Roberts WC. Morphologic findings in saphenous veins used as coronary arterial bypass conduits for longer than 1 year: necropsy analysis of 53 patients, 123 saphenous veins, and 1865 five-millimeter segments of veins. Am Heart J 1990;119:1164–84.
4. Loop FD, Lytle BW, Cosgrove DM, et al. Reoperation for coronary atherosclerosis. Changing practice in 2509 consecutive patients. Ann Surg 1990;212:378–85.
5. Frimerman A, Rechavia E, Eigler N, et al. Long-term follow-up of a high risk cohort after stent implantation in saphenous vein grafts. J Am Coll Cardiol 1997;30:1277–83.
6. Pucelikova T, Mehran R, Kirtane AJ, et al. Short- and long-term outcomes after stent-assisted percutaneous treatment of saphenous vein grafts in the drug-eluting stent era. Am J Cardiol 2008;101:63–8.
7. Keeley EC, Velez CA, O'Neill WW, et al. Long-term clinical outcome and predictors of major adverse cardiac events after percutaneous interventions on saphenous vein grafts. J Am Coll Cardiol 2001;38:659–65.
8. Salomon NW, Page US, Bigelow JC, et al. Reoperative coronary surgery. Comparative analysis of 6591 patients undergoing primary bypass and 508 patients undergoing reoperative coronary artery bypass. J Thorac Cardiovasc Surg 1990;100:250–9.
9. Morrison DA, Sethi G, Sacks J, et al. Percutaneous coronary intervention versus repeat bypass surgery for patients with medically refractory myocardial ischemia: AWESOME randomized trial and registry experience with post-CABG patients. J Am Coll Cardiol 2002;40:1951–4.
10. Brener SJ, Lytle BW, Casserly IP, et al. Predictors of revascularization method and long-term outcome of percutaneous coronary intervention or repeat coronary bypass surgery in patients with multivessel coronary disease and previous coronary bypass surgery. Eur Heart J 2006;27:413–8.
11. Smith SC Jr, Feldman TE, Hirshfeld JW Jr, et al. ACC/AHA/SCAI 2005 Guideline Update for Percutaneous Coronary Intervention—summary article: a report of the American College of Cardiology/American Heart Association Task Force on Practice Guidelines (ACC/AHA/SCAI Writing Committee to Update the 2001 Guidelines for Percutaneous Coronary Intervention). Circulation 2006;113:156–75.
12. Eagle KA, Guyton RA, Davidoff R, et al. ACC/AHA 2004 guideline update for coronary artery bypass

graft surgery: a report of the American College of Cardiology/American Heart Association Task Force on Practice Guidelines (Committee to Update the 1999 Guidelines for Coronary Artery Bypass Graft Surgery). Circulation 2004;110:e340–437.

13. Moses JW, Leon MB, Popma JJ, et al. Sirolimus-eluting stents versus standard stents in patients with stenosis in a native coronary artery. N Engl J Med 2003;349:1315–23.

14. Stone GW, Ellis SG, Cox DA, et al. A polymer-based, paclitaxel-eluting stent in patients with coronary artery disease. N Engl J Med 2004;350:221–31.

15. Fajadet J, Wijns W, Laarman GJ, et al. Randomized, double-blind, multicenter study of the Endeavor zotarolimus-eluting phosphorylcholine-encapsulated stent for treatment of native coronary artery lesions: clinical and angiographic results of the ENDEAVOR II trial. Circulation 2006;114:798–806.

16. Vermeersch P, Agostoni P, Verheye S, et al. Randomized double-blind comparison of sirolimus-eluting stent versus bare-metal stent implantation in diseased saphenous vein grafts. Six-month angiographic, intravascular ultrasound, and clinical follow-up of the RRISC trail. J Am Coll Cardiol 2006;48:2423–31.

17. Brilakis ES, Lichtenwalter C, de Lemos JA, et al. A randomized controlled trial of a paclitaxel-eluting stent versus a similar bare-metal stent in saphenous vein graft lesions the SOS (Stenting of Saphenous Vein Grafts) trial. J Am Coll Cardiol 2009;53:919–28.

18. Vermeersch P, Agostoni P, Verheye S, et al. Increased late mortality after sirolimus-eluting stents versus bare-metal stents in diseased saphenous vein grafts: results from the randomized DELAYED RRISC Trial. J Am Coll Cardiol 2007;50:261–7.

19. Brilakis ES, Lichtenwalter C, Abdel-karim AR, et al. Continued benefit from paclitaxel-eluting compared with bare-metal stent implantation in saphenous vein graft lesions during long-term follow-up of the SOS (Stenting of Saphenous Vein Grafts) trial. JACC Cardiovasc Interv 2011;4:176–82.

20. Mehilli J, Pache J, Abdel-Wahab M, et al. Drug-eluting versus bare-metal stents in saphenous vein graft lesions (ISAR-CABG): a randomised controlled superiority trial. Lancet 2011;378:1071–8.

21. Savage MP, Douglas JS Jr, Fischman DL, et al. Stent placement compared with balloon 78 angioplasty for obstructed coronary bypass grafts. Saphenous Vein De Novo Trial Investigators. N Engl J Med 1997;337:740–7.

22. Hanekamp CE, Koolen JJ, Den Heijer P, et al. Randomized study to compare balloon angioplasty and elective stent implantation in 80 venous bypass grafts: the Venestent study. Catheter Cardiovasc Interv 2003;60:452–7.

23. Loubeyre C, Morice MC, Lefevre T, et al. A randomized comparison of direct stenting with conventional stent implantation in selected patients with acute myocardial infarction. J Am Coll Cardiol 2002;39:15–21.

24. Leborgne L, Cheneau E, Pichard A, et al. Effect of direct stenting on clinical outcome in patients treated with percutaneous coronary intervention on saphenous vein graft. Am Heart J 2003;146:501–6.

25. Okabe T, Lindsay J, Torguson R, et al. Can direct stenting in selected saphenous vein graft lesions be considered an alternative to percutaneous intervention with a distal protection device? Catheter Cardiovasc Interv 2008;72:799–803.

26. Hong YJ, Pichard AD, Mintz GS, et al. Outcome of undersized drug-eluting stents for percutaneous coronary intervention of saphenous vein graft lesions. Am J Cardiol 2010;105:179–85.

27. The effect of aggressive lowering of low-density lipoprotein cholesterol levels and low-dose anticoagulation on obstructive changes in saphenous-vein coronary-artery bypass grafts. The Post Coronary Artery Bypass Graft Trial Investigators. N Engl J Med 1997;336:153–62.

28. Hong YJ, Mintz GS, Kim SW, et al. Disease progression in non-intervened saphenous vein graft segments a serial intravascular ultrasound analysis. J Am Coll Cardiol 2009;53:1257–64.

29. Mak KH, Challapalli R, Eisenberg MJ, et al. Effect of platelet glycoprotein IIb/IIIa receptor inhibition on distal embolization during percutaneous revascularization of aorto- coronary saphenous vein grafts. EPIC Investigators. Evaluation of IIb/IIIa platelet receptor antagonist 7E3 in Preventing Ischaemic Complications. Am J Cardiol 1997;80:985–8.

30. Mathew V, Grill DE, Scott CG, et al. The influence of abciximab use on clinical outcome after aorto-coronary vein graft interventions. J Am Coll Cardiol 1999;34:1163–9.

31. Karha J, Gurm HS, Rajagopal V, et al. Use of platelet glycoprotein IIb/IIIa inhibitors in saphenous vein graft percutaneous coronary intervention and clinical outcomes. Am J Cardiol 2006;98:906–10.

32. Fischell TA, Carter AJ, Foster MT, et al. Reversal of "no reflow" during vein graft stenting using high velocity boluses of intracoronary adenosine. Cathet Cardiovasc Diagn 1998;45:360–5.

33. Resnic FS, Wainstein M, Lee MK, et al. No-reflow is an independent predictor of death and myocardial infarction after percutaneous coronary intervention. Am Heart J 2003;145:42–6.

34. Coolong A, Baim DS, Kuntz RE, et al. Saphenous vein graft stenting and major adverse cardiac events: a predictive model derived from a pooled analysis of 3958 patients. Circulation 2008;117:790–7.

35. Nase-Hueppmeier S, Uebis R, Doerr R, et al. Intravascular ultrasound to assess aorto-coronary venous bypass grafts in vivo. Am J Cardiol 1992;70:455–8.

36. Hong MK, Mehran R, Dangas G, et al. Comparison of time course of target lesion revascularization following successful saphenous vein graft angioplasty versus successful native coronary angioplasty. Am J Cardiol 2000;85:256–8.

# Intervention of Saphenous Vein Graft Chronic Total Occlusion

Evan Lau, MD, Patrick Whitlow, MD*

## KEYWORDS

- Saphenous vein graft • Chronic total occlusion • Vein graft intervention

## KEY POINTS

- Intervention of saphenous vein graft chronic total occlusion carries significant periprocedural and long-term risks.
- Saphenous vein graft chronic total occlusion intervention carries a class III indication, but there may be a limited number of circumstances where it may be warranted.
- There are several procedure-specific considerations when undertaking saphenous vein graft chronic total occlusion intervention.

## CASE 1

A 75-year-old man with a history of coronary artery bypass surgery (performed 25 years ago, left internal mammary artery to left anterior descending artery [LIMA-LAD], and saphenous vein graft to right coronary artery [SVG-RCA]), type 2 diabetes mellitus, and hypertension, presented with unstable angina. Stress testing showed hibernating myocardium involving the left circumflex and right coronary artery distributions. Coronary angiography found severe obstruction of the native left main coronary artery and the proximal left circumflex artery. The vein graft to the right coronary artery showed a stump occlusion. There was significant calcification of the right aortic sinus, and the native right coronary artery could not be selectively engaged. Root injection found flush occlusion at its ostium.

The patient underwent uncomplicated intervention to the native left circumflex and left main arteries. The SVG-RCA was engaged with a 7F Amplatz right 1 (AR1) guide, and a polymer jacketed wire of moderate tip stiffness was advanced into the midgraft using a microcatheter. The wire was exchanged for a nonpolymer jacketed, stiff wire, which was used to traverse the most difficult portion of the graft occlusion. The distal vessel could not be well visualized, so contrast injection was performed through the microcatheter to confirm appropriate, intraluminal distal vessel placement of the wire. The graft was dilated with a compliant, 1.5 × 20mm over-the-wire (OTW) balloon, but the distal portion of the graft would not allow the balloon to cross. A 2.6F Tornus catheter (Asahi Intecc, Nagoya, Japan) was used to cross the distal graft lesion, and this was followed again with dilation of the entire graft using a compliant, 1.5 × 20mm OTW balloon. The graft was further dilated with a compliant 2.5 × 30mm balloon. Intravascular ultrasound (IVUS) was used to determine the extent of diseased graft segments as well as size the diameter of the graft. Predilation was with a compliant 3.5 × 30mm balloon. Endoluminal reconstruction of the graft was performed with 3 overlapping 3.5 × 38mm drug-eluting stents. The stents were postdilated with a noncompliant 3.75 × 20mm balloon (**Fig. 1**).

## CASE 2

A 66-year-old man with a history of hypertension, hyperlipidemia, and coronary artery bypass surgery (performed 2 years ago, LIMA-LAD, saphenous vein graft to the first diagonal (SVG-D1), and sequential saphenous vein graft to the posterior

Robert and Suzanne Tomsich Department of Cardiology, Cleveland Clinic Foundation, Cleveland, OH 44195, USA
* Corresponding author.
E-mail address: whitlop@ccf.org

Intervent Cardiol Clin 2 (2013) 315–321
http://dx.doi.org/10.1016/j.iccl.2012.12.002
2211-7458/13/$ – see front matter © 2013 Elsevier Inc. All rights reserved.

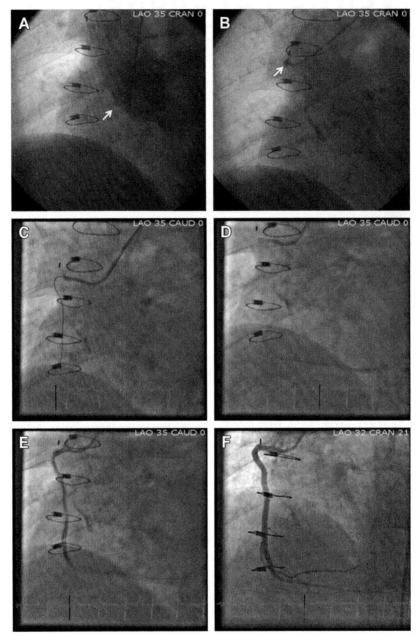

**Fig. 1.** (A) Flush occlusion of the native right coronary artery (*white arrow*). (B) Stump occlusion of the SVG-RCA (*white arrow*). (C) Soft-tipped, polymer jacketed coronary wire advanced midway through occluded vein graft. (D) Confirmation of distal wire placement using injection of contrast through microcatheter. (E) After balloon angioplasty. (F) After placement of 3 overlapping drug-eluting stents and post-dilation.

descending artery and posterolateral branch [SVG-PDA-RPLV]) presented with Canadian Cardiovascular Society Class III angina. Angiography showed a patent LIMA-LAD as well as SVG-RCA. The SVG-D1 was completely occluded in a proximal stented segment. The distal vessel was not well visualized, but on prior angiograms, it appeared that the SVG was grafted to a small, medial subdivision of D1. The larger, lateral subdivision of D1 was

jeopardized by severe disease in the retrograde limb between the SVG-D1 anastamosis and the bifurcation of the lateral subdivision. The native left main showed a complete occlusion of the proximal LAD before the D1 take-off.

The decision was made to attempt recanalization of D1. The antegrade approach through the native left main (LM)/LAD was unfavorable, in part, because of an ambiguous occlusion course and poor distal vessel filling via collaterals. The anatomy had been well delineated on prior angiography, but successful native LAD chronic total occlusion (CTO) recanalization would require better visualization. It was decided to attempt native CTO recanalization using assistance from a retrograde access through the occluded the bypass graft. Dual access was obtained, and a short Amplatz left guide was used to engage the LM, and a short left coronary bypass guide was used to engage the D1 bypass ostium. The SVG-D1 occlusion was successfully wired using a hydrophilic wire. An aspiration catheter was advanced over the wire, and an injection through the OTW port was used to confirm intraluminal wire placement and delineate the vessel anatomy beyond the occlusion. The wire was advanced retrograde through the occlusion into the native left main. Several balloons could not be passed retrograde through the vein graft into the LAD occlusion. Using the retrograde wire as a roadmap, an antegrade wire was brought through the native LM and used to wire into the distal D1. Once the antegrade wire was placed successfully, the retrograde wire was removed completely from the vein graft. Working over the antegrade wire, the occlusion was successfully dilated and stented with a 3.0 × 32mm drug-eluting stent (**Fig. 2**).

## INTRODUCTION

CTO of SVGs is a commonly encountered entity. Unfortunately, SVGs are often accompanied by acceleration of atherosclerotic disease in the proximal, native coronary arteries. This combination often creates anatomy that is difficult to approach percutaneously. This is why opening saphenous vein graft CTO is contemplated. Although the guidelines label revascularization of SVG CTO as a class III indication, there are a limited number of circumstances in which this may be considered. This article examines the rationale for doing so and the data for evaluating such interventions as well as discusses some of the technical issues surrounding these procedures.

## BACKGROUND

Saphenous vein graft interventions have substantially higher risk of periprocedural myocardial infarction than those performed in native coronary arteries. The atherosclerotic process in a vein graft is a diffuse and accelerated process that can lead to build-up of a substantial volume of plaque and friable material over a relatively short period. In autopsy studies, histology shows 3 distinct patterns of morphologic changes in vein grafts,

including typical atherosclerosis, fibro-intimal proliferation, and fibrotic changes, which are probably sequelae of thrombotic occlusions.[1] Aspirates retrieved from embolic protection devices show residue of atherosclerotic plaque, including fibrous caps and lipid laden necrotic cores.[2] If the age of occlusion has been misjudged and is actually subacute in nature, one should expect there to be significant thrombus burden in the graft.

In addition to the heightened periprocedural risk, the long-term patency of vein graft interventions is substantially worse when compared with that of native coronary intervention. Even in the drug-eluting stent era, the risk of target vessel failure was 22% over 1.5 years.[3] Most of this represents progression of disease outside of the stented area, which has been a phenomenon seen in several studies.[4,5]

The harsh realities of SVG percutaneous coronary intervention (PCI) make an SVG CTO an unattractive option for intervention. The outcomes of published case series of SVG CTO PCI have had mixed results. Berger and colleagues[6] published a series of 77 patients demonstrating a 71% procedural success rate but an 11.7% rate of distal embolization and a 30-day mortality rate of 5.2%.[7] Al-Lamee and colleagues,[8] published a series of 34 patients undergoing SVG CTO recanalization using contemporary techniques, including frequent embolic protection device (EPD) use and drug-eluting stent (DES) implantation. Procedural success was achieved in only 68% of patients, but there was a myocardial infarction rate of only 3%. Of those grafts that could be successfully opened, there was a 61% target lesion revascularization (TLR) over an 18-month follow-up period. The limited data show feasibility of performing recanalization, although procedural success rates are low. Compared with conventional SVG PCI, there is comparable risk of periprocedural complication; likewise, the need for repeat revascularization is high. Long-term patency of SVG CTO intervention is not well established.

## RISKS

Conventional vein graft intervention has a high rate of periprocedural myocardial infarction mostly because of distal embolization. This holds true, even in the era of embolic protection devices. In randomized, controlled trials of EPD, the device arms still demonstrated an incidence of 8.6%–11.3% risk of major adverse cardiac events.[9,10] Furthermore, these are not usually asymptomatic increases in cardiac biomarkers but clinically significant events that result in chest pain, electrocardiographic changes, no reflow,

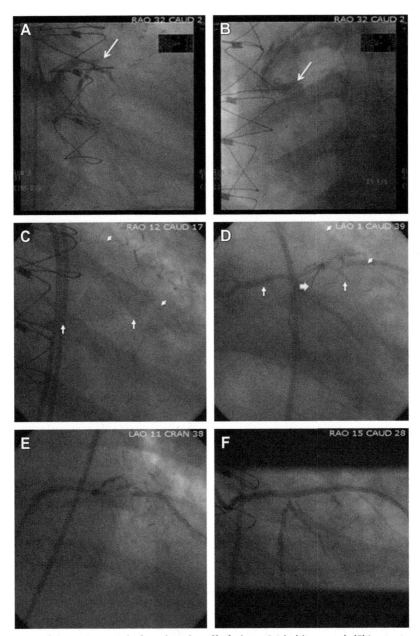

**Fig. 2.** (*A*) Occlusion of the native LAD, before the take-off of a large D1 (*white arrow*). (*B*) In-stent occlusion of the SVG-D1 (*white arrow*). (*C*) Passage of wire through the occluded SVG-D1, retrograde through the LAD occlusion, into the native left main (*white arrows*). (*D*) Using retrograde wire as a road map (*white arrows*), antegrade wire is advanced into the occlusion toward D1 (*block arrow*). (*E*) Successful placement of antegrade wire into distal D1 and removal of retrograde wire. (*F*) After single, drug-eluting stent extending from native left main into D1.

and sometimes hemodynamic instability. Once encountered, it is difficult to predict how well the situation can be salvaged with the limited resources available. To what degree this phenomenon applies to completely occluded vein grafts is not completely understood; however, it should be expected that there should be at least comparable risk of this complication. Our best protection against this complication, namely distal embolic protection, may not be feasible in many cases. Several of the distal EPD systems are built on-the-wire, with the wire attached distal to the basket. These are not nearly as facile as the wide array of available coronary wires, and it would be unlikely that one would be able to cross an occlusion with one of these systems alone. Furthermore, the EPD has a comparatively rigid delivery system that would be difficult to pass through a long segment of occlusion without predilation or debulking. An additional problem is the need for a distal landing zone, or a healthy, disease-free distal graft segment in which to deploy the basket. If the graft occlusion is long, or is accompanied by heavy, severe distal disease, there may not be a place to deploy the EPD.

Another important complication to consider is perforation, particularly wire perforation. This is a known complication of CTO interventions, which may require the use of stiff or hydrophilic wires to cross. These interventions are not common enough in vein grafts to know the true incidence of this complication. Aortocoronary grafts begin extrapericardial but then enter the pericardium along its distal segment. Perforation in its extrapericardial segment will lead to mediastinal bleeding, whereas intrapericardial perforation could lead to tamponade. Common wisdom suggests that patients with prior coronary bypass have significant mediastinal/pericardial scarring, making tamponade unlikely. However, this truism in any given patient cannot be predicted a priori, and even mediastinal bleeding can lead to significant blood loss or clinically significant compression of surrounding structures.

An important consideration involves the special situation of SVG occlusion that occurs as a result of in-stent restenosis. This may be identified when the SVG occlusion is confined to the stented portion of the SVG, with sparing of significant disease in nonstented portions of the graft. The pathology of these occlusions is likely to be quite different from diffuse degeneration of the graft. Although we can only postulate the implications of this situation compared with degenerative SVG occlusions, the risk of distal embolization and periprocedural myocardial infarction is probably lower, and the patency of intervention is likely to be better.

## BENEFITS/RATIONALE

There is a high bar set for undertaking a CTO intervention in a native coronary artery. This is a summation of the usual risk/benefit calculation for these specialized procedures. The same would hold true of a vein graft CTO intervention, particularly with the enhanced risk profile and suspected poor patency rate. The usual criteria of intractable anginal symptoms, failed medical management, and demonstrated ischemic burden should also hold true. However, there should also be a prerequisite of poor native coronary artery access to the target vessel.

One additional, albeit unconventional, rationale would be the use of the opened vein graft as a retrograde avenue to help with a native, antegrade intervention. If the proximal, native coronary artery is a total occlusion, an opened vein graft may be of great utility in helping to open the native CTO, by allowing for distal visualization, as well as a retrograde channel for wiring, should an antegrade approach be unfavorable or unsuccessful. With this reasoning in mind, one may proceed with recanalizing and stenting a vein graft, with the intention of bringing the patient back for a second procedure to tackle the native coronary CTO. Alternatively, one could also perform a partial recanalization, enough to pass a wire and equipment, with the goal of opening and stenting the native coronary artery occlusion as illustrated in case 2.

In tackling a case of SVG occlusion, the operator must seriously weigh the presumed benefits in any given patient against the technical difficulties, intraprocedural risk, and long-term patency of such an endeavor.

## INTERVENTIONAL TECHNIQUE

Many of the principles and techniques used for native coronary CTO interventions apply when approaching a vein graft occlusion.

### Angiography

Preprocedural angiography should identify the critical features of the occlusion, including the proximal cap, length of occlusion, course of the vessel, quality of the distal graft and native vessel, and collateral filling of the distal, native vessel. A thorough understanding of these anatomic facets will help in case selection and planning. Because most vein graft occlusions will be approached in an antegrade fashion, the entry shape of the proximal cap will strongly dictate the likelihood of success: beaked entries being most favorable, whereas ambiguous/convex caps are least favorable. Most grafts will be diffusely diseased, if not occluded, along their entire length. However, in some cases, particularly, when the occlusion occurs within a previously stented segment, the occlusion may be short. The course of the graft may be ambiguous if the entire graft is occluded; this will present a problem in identifying the appropriate direction for wiring and avoiding perforation of the graft. Finally, understanding the distal graft and native vessel are essential to a successful intervention. If the native vessel fills distally via collaterals, it would be strongly encouraged to perform the intervention using dual access, so that intraluminal wire placement can be confirmed by contralateral injection and filling of the native vessel.

## Guide

Most graft CTOs will involve short stumps from the aortic anastamosis. This makes guide selection critical, because adequate support will be provided mainly by the guide shape and size, as deep-seating guide manipulation is not an option. Usually, for grafts with horizontal or upward take-offs, the authors prefer Amplatz left shapes, with curves large enough to reach the contralateral wall of the aorta. If the graft has a downward take-off, a Williams style curve may be more appropriate. Multiple guide shapes may need to be attempted empirically before optimal support is achieved.

## Wiring

Antegrade wiring is performed with a variety of coronary wires, using the support of a microcatheter. The authors use a similar wire escalation strategy typically used in native coronary CTOs: a soft, polymer jacketed wire, followed by a polymer jacketed wire with moderate tip stiffness, then a stiff, non-jacketed wire. The soft, polymer-jacketed wire, particularly if it has a tapered tip, is suited for finding microchannels within the occluded vessel. The polymer-jacketed wire with moderate tip strength provides greater pushability for traversing long segments of occlusion. Stiff wires are particularly helpful when the proximal cap is tough to puncture or has an ambiguous entry. Ideally, the stiffest wires should be used to traverse as short a segment as possible, until the microcatheter can be delivered forward far enough to switch for a less traumatic wire.

For cases in which the course of the graft is highly ambiguous, the risk of perforation may be minimized by using a subintimal technique, such as knuckle-wiring or the CrossBoss microcatheter. The major limitation of a subintimal technique in this arena is the need for re-entry into the true lumen. Re-entry will need to occur in the distal graft, before the anastamosis with the native vessel. Ideally, this would require a large lumen in the distal portion of the vein, which may not be available if the entire graft is occluded.

## Embolic Protection Device

In SVG intervention, the ideal situation would be to use a distal EPD; however, as previously mentioned, there are significant limitations to doing this in vein graft occlusions. There will need to be sufficient, healthy, landing zone to deploy the EPD in the distal graft. In the absence of this, it would be possible to place the EPD in the native coronary bed, but this is will only provide partial protection, particularly if the native vessel bifurcates or has significant branches off of the antegrade and retrograde limbs.

Delivery of the EPD also presents a significant challenge. Once the occlusion is successfully crossed, the graft will usually have to be predilated before EPD delivery. Because most distal EPD systems are built on the wire, it is impossible to perform an exchange of the pre-existing wire for the EPD. The simplest solution is to wire the EPD, through the balloon-dilated channel, using the initial wire as a reference. There are distal EPD systems in which the basket and wire can be separated, such as the Emboshield NAV6 system (Abbott, Abbott Park, IL). However, the wire on this device has a larger diameter than a conventional 0.014-inch coronary wire, precluding a simple wire exchange with one of the commonly used coronary microcatheters or over-the-wire balloons.

## Intravascular Ultrasound Scan

The use of IVUS is strongly recommended during SVG CTO intervention. In a heavily diseased graft, it can be difficult to accurately define the size of the graft and choose the appropriate stent diameter. IVUS will also help to define the extent of disease along the length of the graft. This may help to minimize stent length by avoiding deployment in areas in which there is only mild disease.

## Stenting

Although there is some controversy as to the benefit of DES over BMS in SVG PCI, the randomized, controlled trial examining a paclitaxel eluting stent versus its bare metal platform in conventional SVG PCI suggests lower rates of in-stent restenosis and need for target lesion revascularization.[3] Extrapolating from these data, it would be preferable to use DES when performing extensive vein graft reconstruction of long graft occlusions. The major limitation for DES would be the patient's ability to tolerate prolonged dual antiplatelet therapy. On some occasions, the luminal diameter of the graft is larger than the maximal expansion diameter of the available DES. This is unlikely in a heavily diseased vein graft occlusion but should be taken into consideration. One final point in stenting would be careful attention toward stent placement at the distal anastomosis. If the graft intervention is to be used as a conduit for a CTO intervention of the native coronary artery, access to the retrograde limb of the native coronary must be maintained. Difficulty in wiring or passing equipment often is encountered because of an unfavorable angle from the graft into the retrograde limb.

If a stent is placed protruding into the native coronary, it may be impossible to negotiate an already difficult turn.

## SUMMARY

The cases presented represent 2 strategies using vein graft occlusion intervention. The first case shows a situation in which there are 2 approaches to a jeopardized right coronary artery: an unfavorable native CTO of the ostial RCA and a more favorable occluded vein graft to the RCA. The choice was made to target the vein graft occlusion. The procedure highlights several difficulties in opening vein graft CTOs, including the need for wire escalation, the inability to deploy an EPD, and difficulty in passage of equipment. The successful opening of the graft may be left as a stand-alone result, or the patient could be brought back to use the now-opened graft as a retrograde channel for opening a difficult, native ostial RCA CTO.

The second case illustrates the use of a graft occlusion as a retrograde channel for opening a native CTO of the LAD. In this instance, the graft occlusion was crossed with a wire, but the graft was not recanalized with angioplasty or stent. Instead, using injections through an aspiration catheter and the wire position, the course of the native vessel was delineated for assistance in antegrade wiring of the LAD CTO. After successful recanalization over the antegrade channel, the graft occlusion was left as is.

Interventions on vein graft occlusions are technically feasible procedures but carry significant risk for periprocedural complications and demonstrate questionable long-term patency. For those circumstances in which recanalization of a graft occlusion is warranted, the authors have highlighted some of the procedural considerations and available techniques that may help maximize chances for success. This should not be mistaken for a wholesale endorsement of vein graft CTO interventions. Before undertaking a procedure of this complexity, the operator must put strong consideration into the risks, benefits, and alternatives for a given patient.

## REFERENCES

1. Atkinson JB. Morphologic changes in long-term saphenous vein bypass grafts. Chest 1985;88(3):341. Available at: http://journal.publications.chestnet.org/article.aspx?doi=10.1378/chest.88.3.341. Accessed December 5, 2012.

2. Webb JG, Carere RG, Virmani R, et al. Retrieval and analysis of particulate debris after saphenous vein graft intervention. J Am Coll Cardiol 1999;34(2): 468–75. Available at: http://www.ncbi.nlm.nih.gov/pubmed/10440161.

3. Brilakis ES, Rao SV, Banerjee S, et al. Percutaneous coronary intervention in native arteries versus bypass grafts in prior coronary artery bypass grafting patients: a report from the National Cardiovascular Data Registry. JACC Cardiovasc Interv 2011;4(8): 844–50. Available at: http://www.ncbi.nlm.nih.gov/pubmed/21851896. Accessed December 5, 2012.

4. Laham RJ, Carrozza JP, Berger C, et al. Long-term (4- to 6-year) outcome of Palmaz-Schatz stenting: paucity of late clinical stent-related problems. J Am Coll Cardiol 1996;28(4):820–6. Available at: http://www.ncbi.nlm.nih.gov/pubmed/8837554.

5. Ellis SG, Brener SJ, DeLuca S, et al. Late myocardial ischemic events after saphenous vein graft intervention–importance of initially "nonsignificant" vein graft lesions. Am J Cardiol 1997;79(11):1460–4. Available at: http://www.ncbi.nlm.nih.gov/pubmed/9185633.

6. Berger PB, Bell MR, Grill DE, et al. Influence of procedural success on immediate and long-term clinical outcome of patients undergoing percutaneous revascularization of occluded coronary artery bypass vein grafts. J Am Coll Cardiol 1996;28(7):1732–7. Available at: http://linkinghub.elsevier.com/retrieve/pii/S0735109796004147. Accessed December 5, 2012.

7. Kahn JK, Rutherford BD, McConahay DR, et al. Initial and long-term outcome of 83 patients after balloon angioplasty of totally occluded bypass grafts. J Am Coll Cardiol 1994;23(5):1038–42. Available at: http://www.ncbi.nlm.nih.gov/pubmed/8144765.

8. Al-Lamee R, Ielasi A, Latib A, et al. Clinical and angiographic outcomes after percutaneous recanalization of chronic total saphenous vein graft occlusion using modern techniques. Am J Cardiol 2010; 106(12):1721–7. Available at: http://www.ncbi.nlm.nih.gov/pubmed/21126616. Accessed December 5, 2012.

9. Baim DS. Percutaneous treatment of saphenous vein graft disease. J Am Coll Cardiol 2003;42(8):1370–2. Available at: http://linkinghub.elsevier.com/retrieve/pii/S0735109703010398. Accessed December 5, 2012.

10. Stone GW, Rogers C, Hermiller J, et al. Randomized comparison of distal protection with a filter-based catheter and a balloon occlusion and aspiration system during percutaneous intervention of diseased saphenous vein aorto-coronary bypass grafts. Circulation 2003;108(5):548–53. Available at: http://www.ncbi.nlm.nih.gov/pubmed/12874191. Accessed December 5, 2012.

# Degenerated Saphenous Vein Graft Intervention
## Should We Target the Native Vessel instead?

Corey Foster, MD, Alan Zajarias, MD*

## KEYWORDS

- Saphenous vein graft • Complex percutaneous coronary intervention • Embolic protection device

## KEY POINTS

- Percutaneous interventions of saphenous vein grafts are associated with a higher rate of periprocedural major adverse cardiac events that can be mitigated by the use of embolic protection devices.
- Deciding to intervene on SVGs or native coronary arteries will depend on the lesion location, vessel angulation, presence of a chronic total occlusion, catheter shaft length, deliverability of the stents, amount of myocardium at risk, ability to place embolic protection devices, degree of ischemia, and patient symptoms.
- Appropriate selection of guide catheters, guide wires, and other equipment will facilitate procedural and clinical success when performing high-risk percutaneous intervention.

## INTRODUCTION

Saphenous vein graft (SVG) remains one of the most widely used conduits for coronary artery bypass graft (CABG) surgery. Its major advantage is that it is plentiful, easily harvested, can accommodate various lengths, and is technically easy to use. Despite these favorable characteristics, its durability and longevity remain less than ideal when compared with arterial grafts. One-year occlusion rates have been documented between 25%–45%.[1–4] At 15 years, only about half of vein grafts are patent and, of those, only half are free of angiographic arteriosclerosis.[5] Early graft failure (<6 months) is predominately caused by technical errors, thrombosis, and intimal hyperplasia, whereas arteriosclerosis is primarily responsible for late (>1year) SVG failure.[6]

Stenosed or occluded SVGs can be treated by percutaneous coronary intervention (PCI) or by repeat CABG. Despite improvement in surgical techniques, repeat-CABG poses a significant surgical challenge, is not performed for one-vessel intervention if arterial revascularization is not an option, and remains a significant risk factor for operative mortality in contemporary practice.[7,8] As a result, PCI remains the preferred treatment of SVG lesions. Currently, there is a lack of consensus on the treatment strategy for patients with severe stenosis of SVGs: PCI of the vein graft or target the native circulation. Percutaneous revascularization of SVGs is associated with worse clinical outcomes, including higher rates of in-stent restenosis, target vessel revascularization, myocardial infarction, and death compared with percutaneous coronary intervention of native coronary arteries.

If feasible, PCI of native coronary arteries is another treatment alternative for patients who present with angina and SVG disease. In cases in which percutaneous revascularization can be

Cardiovascular Division, Department of Internal Medicine, Washington University School of Medicine, 660 South Euclid Avenue, St Louis, MO 63110, USA
* Corresponding author. 660 South Euclid Avenue, Campus Box 8086, St Louis, MO 63110.
E-mail address: AZajaria@DOM.wustl.edu

Intervent Cardiol Clin 2 (2013) 323–337
http://dx.doi.org/10.1016/j.iccl.2012.11.005

accomplished via the both approaches, deciding on the treatment strategy will influence patient outcomes and procedural risks.

In this review, we describe the characteristics of native coronary versus SVG disease and risk factors for complications after SVG intervention and discuss the procedural treatment strategies imperative to the decision of which therapeutic strategy to follow: in the venous graft itself or in the native coronary artery. The measures to mitigate the risks of periprocedural complications in both approaches are discussed.

## FACTORS INFLUENCING VEIN GRAFT INTERVENTIONS
### Characteristics of Atherosclerotic Plaque of Saphenous Vein Grafts

Atherosclerosis of the SVGs differs from native coronary atherosclerosis. Several morphologic risk factors have been associated with reduced graft patency. These include native vessel diameter, grafted vessel, severity of bypass-grafted proximal stenosis, graft age, and sex. Traditional risk factors for coronary artery disease also play a significant role. In addition, lipoprotein (a), homocysteine, and fibrinogen have each been studied, to a varying degree, in the context of vein graft disease.[6]

All SVGs experience endothelial damage during harvesting and initial exposure to arterial pressure. This intimal injury leads to platelet adherence that may result in graft thrombosis and acute occlusion. Platelet adherence to the intimal surface is also the initial event in the development of intimal hyperplasia. After adhering to the intima, platelets release mitogenic proteins, stimulating smooth muscle cell migration, resulting in intimal proliferation and hyperplasia. More recently, it has been discovered that severe vascular wall degeneration and collagen deposition together with overexpressed transforming growth factor–β signaling cytokines may provide preliminary evidence for the failure of the saphenous vein and radial arterial grafts.[9]

To date, no therapeutic intervention has proved successful in treating late vein graft failure.[10] SVGs have friable plaque that represents degenerated, loose, fibrocellular atheromatous debris lining on the internal surface of the vessel. This is frequently found in vein grafts after bypass surgery, however, is rarely found in native coronary disease.[11] The histopathologic composition of atherosclerotic plaques at necropsy in SVGs and native coronary arteries vary; the atherosclerotic plaques of SVGs are rich in friable material, whereas friability

is absent in the native coronary arteries of the same patients.[12]

Diagnostic coronary angiography shows an irregular or serrated luminal border. More sensitive testing such as angioscopy shows fragmented, loosely adherent plaque lining the vessel wall.[13] One study comparing the in vivo assessment of the angioscopic morphology difference in the setting of unstable angina found that other than a high incidence of plaque friability in vein grafts, the surface morphology of culprit lesions in unstable angina patients is similar for SVGs and native coronary arteries.[14]

The atherosclerotic debris in SVGs is prone to embolization into the native coronary circulation causing periprocedural myocardial infarctions and leading to no-reflow phenomenon.[15] Degenerated grafts with high plaque burden or thrombus content are more prone to distal embolization. The use of proximal or distal embolic protection devices has been shown to decrease risk of procedural complications. The feasibility of safely using such a device influences the treatment approach: it is preferred to use such a device if intervening via the SVG.

### Diameter

Graft flow rate and diameter of the lumen of the target coronary arteries and the conduit vessel are important factors in predicting the outcome of the grafts, irrespective of the method of vein harvesting used. Observational studies have found that 1-year vein graft patency was 90% if grafted vessel diameter was greater than 1.5 mm at operation but only 65% if the diameter was ≤1.5 mm.[16,17] Other studies have found that the best results were obtained when large-caliber arteries were grafted with a small-diameter vein, suggesting that better graft patency was associated with smaller conduit size.[18–20] Stent patency has been found to depend on vessel diameter and flow into and out of the stent. Flow into and out of the stent will depend on the lesion length and characteristics of the vessel runoff. Vessel diameter mismatch when stenting from the graft into the native vessel can precipitate state thrombosis. In addition, the use of coronary stents is limited by the maximal diameter available, which may be a concern in an ectatic graft. Postdilatation to treat reference vessel diameter mismatch may predispose to plaque protrusion through the stent struts or plaque embolization leading to no-flow phenomenon.[21]

### Lesion Angulation

Stent implantation alters the geometric framework of coronary arteries and imparts the geometric effects of stents on the vessel wall. Radial stretch increases the lumen diameter but does not change the angles between the lumen axis and the tangents, whereas longitudinal straightening decreases the curvature of the vessel but does not necessarily affect the lumen diameter. The beneficial effect of the radial stretching effect of a stent may come at the cost of increased longitudinal straightening effects of a stent on an artery.[22]

The geometric changes that occur after stent implantation also provoke mechanical longitudinal stretching of the smooth muscle cells and intimal cells. This leads to the secretion of inflammatory mediators, which has been shown to stimulate the proliferative response to vascular injury.[23–25] Moreover, straightening of curved segments can cause more plaque disruption and promote distal embolization. Overall, this leads to alteration in flow dynamics and wall shear stress within the stented segment, triggering an exacerbated neointimal response.[26]

Angulation also interferes with stent delivery. Tortuous SVGs or those that have segments adhered to the sternum interfere with stent manipulation and increases the risk of dissection or disruption. The use of multiple stents of shorter length can be used to address this problem, however, at the risk of higher rates of stent thrombosis.

### Lesion Length and Reference Vessel Diameter

Lesion length and reference vessel diameter are well-known predictors of adverse events after percutaneous coronary intervention and may influence the decision for target vessel intervention. Coronary lesion length has been identified as a significant predictor of restenosis after balloon angioplasty.[27,28] Long lesions (>15 mm) are associated with higher maximum balloon pressure, greater number of stents implanted, a longer stented segment, and a higher proportion of overlapping stents when compared with short (<15 mm) lesions. This may lead to greater arterial injury, resulting in exaggerated neointimal hyperplasia.[29] Initial investigation evaluating outcomes in patients based on reference vessel diameter found that patients with small vessels present a higher risk for an adverse outcome after coronary stent placement because of a higher incidence of restenosis, especially in patients who have concomitant risk factors such as diabetes and complex lesions.[29]

Because of the nature of degenerated SVGs, atherosclerotic plaque progresses rapidly. In addition, a healthy segment abutting the stenosed area may not exist, making it complicated to use shorter stents, increasing the risk of restenosis. Stenting segments that appear moderate may

decrease the risk of further degeneration, as moderate lesions progress rapidly in SVGs.[30]

### Calcification

Treatment of calcified coronary artery lesions continue to present a management challenge. Fibrocalcific deposition enhances lesion rigidity, subsequently complicating device delivery and deployment. Technical failure owing to inability to pass stents occurs more frequently in patients with calcified lesions than in those with noncalcified lesions.[31] Lesion calcification, combined with geometric changes within the vessel, impede the approach to the lesion with the balloon and make successful stent deployment and implantation technically difficult.[32] Moreover, the use of balloon dilatation in this setting, especially at high pressures, can increase risk of dissection or perforation.[33] Coronary calcification is also associated with stent underexpansion, which can contribute to increased risk of restenosis, thrombosis, and target-lesion revascularization after PCI.

### Lesion Location Within a Saphenous Vein Graft

PCI of degenerated SVGs remains relatively high risk when compared with native vessel intervention. Distal embolization can lead to periprocedural myocardial infarction and no-reflow.[34] The occurrence of these events is associated with increased incidence of acute myocardial infarction and about 15% rate of mortality.[35] Lesions located in the shaft of an SVG are more likely to occur in patients with diabetes and hypercholesterolemia. They are associated with a larger plaque burden, more soft plaque, and more plaque ruptures and are more likely to undergo positive remodeling more frequently when compared with lesions located at the ostium of an SVG. These findings suggest that the mechanism of SVG shaft lesions is similar to that of native coronary artery atherosclerosis (particularly unstable native artery lesions in patients with an acute coronary syndrome) in which there is also an association of soft plaque, a larger plaque burden, more plaque ruptures, more positive remodeling, and hyperlipidemia.[36] Although lesion location may have accounted for some of the location-specific differences in interventional complications, there was no evaluation of the exact differences in short- and long-term complications after stent implantation according to the lesion location after PCI for SVG lesions. Hong and colleagues[37] reported that vulnerable plaque characteristics, including positive remodeling, hypoechoic plaque, plaque rupture, multiple plaque rupture, and an intraluminal mass, were significantly more common, and ruptured plaque cavity area was significantly greater in shaft lesions than in aorto-ostial lesions. In addition, post-PCI no-reflow and post-PCI creatine kinase-MB elevation more than 3 times normal were more frequently observed after PCI for shaft lesions than for aorto-ostial lesions. More than 300 lesions were identified with most (79%) of lesions located in the shaft. The overall incidences of death and myocardial infarction were significantly higher in patients with shaft lesion compared with those with aorto-ostial lesion at 5-year follow-up. Several studies have documented that PCI of SVG aorto-ostial lesions is less likely to be associated with postprocedural complications.

Lesion location interferes with the ability to place embolic protection devices (EPD). Lesions close to the origin cannot be protected with proximal occlusion devices, and lesions that are close to the anastomotic segment to the native coronary artery will interfere with position of the distal protection device. Lesions that are distal in the SVG also create a significant problem because the catheter shaft length may not be long enough to reach the lesion. This problem is primarily seen in grafts that jump from one territory to another (jump grafts). Patients with jump grafts also experience higher technical risk because the myocardium at risk of a jump graft is larger than that of a graft that only supplies one vascular territory. In addition, it may not be possible to protect both limbs of a jump graft with one embolic protection device.

### No-reflow/Slow Flow

Successful restoration of epicardial coronary artery patency does not guarantee normalization of tissue perfusion. No-reflow is typically defined as failure to restore normal coronary flow despite appropriate treatment of coronary obstruction in the absence of dissection, thrombus formation, or vessel closure. No-reflow during PCI is observed most commonly during SVG intervention, rotational atherectomy, and primary PCI for acute ST-elevation myocardial infarction.[38] The overall prevalence occurs in 0.5%–2% of PCIs.[39,40] This number is higher for patients with acute STEMI (ST segment elevation myocardial infarction) compared with non-infarct patients (11.5 vs 1.5%),[41] although some reports suggest it may be as high as 30%.[42] The incidence is also more frequent during SVG PCI in which it occurs in up to 15% of cases,[43] and during rotational atherectomy, in which the reported incidence is as high as 16%.[44,45] Compared with patients in whom no-reflow is transient, refractory no-reflow is associated with a markedly increased risk of 30-day mortality.[38] Slow flow and no-reflow in SVGs have been observed mostly during percutaneous interventions as a complication from distal embolization and are associated with poor outcome.[46] Patients at the highest risk include those with degenerate vein grafts, ulcerated or thrombotic lesions, and acute coronary syndromes.[47] Spontaneous slow SVG flow is rarely reported and correlation with clinical events not as well documented.[48] The cause of no-reflow is complex and multifactorial but is a result of micro-embolization and occlusion of the microcirculation. Intracoronary vasodilators or embolic protection devices have been shown to prevent or reverse no-reflow (**Table 1**).[46]

## EQUIPMENT REQUIREMENTS FOR COMPLEX PCI TO SVGS OR NATIVE CORONARY ARTERIES

Management of coronary artery disease relies increasingly on percutaneous techniques combined with medical therapy. Although PCI can be

**Table 1**
**Intracoronary vasodilators**

| Drug Category | Medication | Dosage | Side Effects |
|---|---|---|---|
| Purine nucleoside | Adenosine | 12 μg as a single dose to a total of 4 mg | Chest pain, hypotension, bradycardia |
| Calcium channel blockers | Diltiazem | 200 μg as a single dose to a total of 1 mg | Bradycardia, hypotension |
| | Nicardipine | 200 μg as a single dose to a total of 1 mg | Bradycardia, hypotension |
| | Verapamil | 200 μg as a single dose to a total of 5 mg | Bradycardia, transient heart block |
| Vasodilators | Nitroprusside | 100 μg to a total of 1 mg | Bradycardia, hypotension |

*Data from* Kunadian V, Zorkun C, Williams SP, et al. Intracoronary pharmacotherapy in the management of coronary microvascular dysfunction. J Thromb Thrombolysis 2008;26(3):234–42.

performed successfully in most lesions, several difficult lesion subsets continue to present unique technical challenges. These complex lesions may be classified according to anatomic criteria, including extensive calcification, thrombus, and chronic occlusions, bifurcations, and SVGs. PCI of these lesions often requires novel devices, such as drug-eluting stents, hydrophilic guide wires, embolic protection devices, thrombectomy catheters, or rotational atherectomy. An integrated approach that combines these devices with specialized techniques and adjunctive pharmacologic agents has greatly improved PCI success rates for these complex lesions.[49]

## GUIDE CATHETER

Calcified, tortuous, and previously stented coronary anatomy poses an ongoing challenge in the delivery of stents in complex percutaneous coronary intervention. Despite creation of lower-profile intracoronary balloons and stents, technical difficulties with stent deliverability are frequently encountered. Failure to successfully deliver a stent across the target lesion during percutaneous coronary intervention, especially in arteries with calcified tortuous anatomy, is often caused by insufficient backup support from the guiding catheter. Several techniques have been reported as a method to help overcome difficult stent delivery in this setting. These include the use of soft-ended atraumatic catheters for use within standard guide catheters, supportive wires, the anchor balloon technique, deep seating of the guide catheter, and deep inspiration as a method to reduce vascular tortuosity.[50–54] The GuideLiner catheter (Vascular Solutions, Minneapolis, MN) is a modified child guide catheter (GC), which can be delivered through a standard GC, providing an extension for deep seating, added backup support, and coaxial alignment. It contains a highly flexible, super soft rapid exchange section, which facilitates its insertion and allows the use of standard-length guide wires, balloons, or stents through an existing hemostatic valve. The GuideLiner can be used without the need to remove either the GC or the guide wire, which makes it an ideal bail-out device should difficulties be encountered with balloon or stent advancement.[55] A novel technique combining the use of a GuideLiner with a noncompliant balloon, the GuideLiner Anchor Inflated Noncompliant balloon (GAIN) technique, has recently been described.[56] Using this method, a noncompliant balloon is advanced to the lesion and inflated; the 5-in-6 GuideLiner is advanced to the lesion (with or without buddy wire support), using the balloon mandrill as a handle. The balloon is then slowly

deflated and the GuideLiner advanced through the lesion, allowing successful delivery of the stent.

## GUIDE WIRE

The use of a second guide wire, or the so-called buddy wire, may be helpful in several situations during PCI. Compared with other tools used to overcome challenging situations encountered during PCI, the buddy wire has the advantage of being quick and easy to use. Use of 2 wires allows for stabilization of the balloon within the lesion in in-stent restenosis, in which neointima characteristics make it difficult to maintain yield of the lesion, and slippage of the inflated balloon outside the stented segment is undesirable because of the potential risk of edge dissections. Second, they help achieve stabilization of the guiding catheter at the ostium of a vessel, even in the event of suboptimal matching of the catheter and the coronary artery. In the setting of challenging coronary anatomy (eg, tortuosities, sharp bends, calcifications, distal lesions, previously implanted stents) the use of buddy wires helps overcome the anatomic characteristics that impede the steering of devices inside the vessels in addition to facilitating passage of distal protection devices.[57] An extra support wire can be used as a buddy wire to facilitate focal area of plaque modification when a cutting balloon is unable to cross a lesion.[56]

## ROTATIONAL ATHERECTOMY

Techniques used to debulk lesions with extensive calcification include high-speed rotational atherectomy (RotA) and the cutting balloon.[49] RotA devices use a diamond-coated rotating brass burr that pulverizes a portion of the fibrous, calcified, inelastic plaque, modifies the plaque compliance, and leaves a smooth, nonendothelialized surface with intact media. Sequential intravascular ultrasound imaging shows that high-speed rotational atherectomy causes lumen enlargement by selective ablation of hard, especially calcific, atherosclerotic plaque with little tissue disruption and rare arterial expansion.[58]

The true role of RotA is to facilitate stenting, particularly drug eluting stent (DES), in lesions that are not dilatable or to enable stent delivery. Vessel modification with RotA before stenting serves as a valuable strategy in the treatment of heavily calcified lesions. It improves arterial compliance, allowing for the passage of equipment and more uniform and symmetric stent deployment.[59]

The routine use of RotA in SVGs has not been widely accepted. Atherosclerotic plaques in grafts tend to be soft and friable with associated thrombus formation. However, Thomas and colleagues[60] reported that using rotational atherectomy primarily to treat anastomotic sites (aorto-ostial and distal), and restenotic or fibrotic undilatable lesions, situations for which rotablation and debulking may be particularly useful. Moreover, rotational atherectomy may be particularly attractive for smaller vessels with those morphologic features. Case report evidence also suggests the safe and effective use of RotA in the body of SVG.[61] In the appropriate clinical setting, rotational atherectomy may serve as a safe and feasible option for nondilatable, calcified lesions in mature grafts as long as there is no evidence of thrombus or vessel dissection.

## EMBOLIC PROTECTION DEVICES

Clinical experience with various EPDs has shown that the capture and retrieval of potentially embolic debris reduce adverse events in situations in which the amount of debris is largest and in which the end organ is most sensitive (**Table 2**).[62] EPDs were developed in an attempt to reduce distal embolization in the setting of vein graft intervention. They can be categorized according to their mechanism of operation: distal occlusion, distal filter, proximal occlusion, and local plaque trapping. Current guidelines give a class I recommendation for the use of EPD in SVG PCI whenever technically feasible.[63]

## DISTAL OCCLUSION/ASPIRATION SYSTEM

Distal balloon occlusion of the SVG beyond the lesion creates a stagnant column of blood that may prevent plaque embolization into the myocardial bed. After intervention, the blood with contained debris can be removed by an aspiration catheter before occlusion balloon deflation and restoration of antegrade blood flow. Advantages conferred by this technique include achieving a low crossing profile and halting the circulation of serotonin and thromboxane that may have an adverse effect on the distal microvasculature. These advantages may be offset by development of increased ischemia and hemodynamic instability and traumatic injury to the SVG during balloon occlusion. Because a disease-free target zone of approximately 3 cm distal to the lesion is required for placement of the occlusion balloon, distal lesions may not be amenable to distal balloon occlusion devices.[64] The SAFER trial investigators' use of this distal protection device during stenting of stenotic venous grafts was associated with a highly significant reduction in major adverse events compared with stenting over a conventional angioplasty guide wire.[65]

**Table 2**
**Comparison of different embolic protection devices**

| Protection Device | Advantage | Disadvantage |
|---|---|---|
| Distal occlusion | Low crossing profile | Need to cross the lesion before adequate protection |
| | Entrapment of debris of all sizes and neurohumoral mediators | Cessation of antegrade blood flow leading to ischemia |
| | Easy device retrieval | Limited visualization making accurate stent placement difficult |
| | | Balloon-induced injury to SVG |
| Proximal occlusion | Operator can use the guide wire of choice | Inability to use the device in ostial or very proximal lesions |
| | Protection from distal embolization of atheromatous debris | Cessation of antegrade perfusion resulting in myocardial ischemia |
| | Side branches can be protected | Technically challenging to use when compared with distal occlusion devices |
| | No distal landing zone required | |
| Distal filter devices | Ease-of-use | Poor maneuverability |
| | Preservation of antegrade blood flow during intervention | High crossing profile |
| | Ability to inject contrast media to facilitate accurate stent placement | Inability to completely entrap microparticles |
| | | Possible filter occlusion |

*Adapted from* Hindnavis V, Cho SH, Goldberg S. Saphenous vein graft intervention: a review. J Invasive Cardiol 2012;24(2):64–71.

## PROXIMAL OCCLUSION/ASPIRATION SYSTEM

Proximal balloon devices create a stagnant column of blood suspending antegrade blood flow, subsequently preventing debris from embolizing downstream. After completion of the intervention, the blood containing the debris can be aspirated with a suction catheter. Protection from distal embolization of atheromatous debris can be established before crossing the lesion, side branches can be protected, and distal lesions that are not amenable to distal embolic protection because of lack of a landing zone can be treated.[64] The most studied proximal occlusion/flow reversal device is the Proxis system (St. Jude Medical, Maple Groves, MN). This finding was based on the Proximal Protection During Saphenous Vein Graft Intervention Using the Proxis Embolic Protection System (PROXIMAL) trial that showed the Proxis system to be noninferior to distal EPD. Major adverse cardiac events (MACE) at 30 days by intention-to-treat analysis occurred in 10.0% of control and 9.2% of test patients.[66] In addition to offering embolic protection during routine SVG interventions, it can also be used to increase guide support by anchoring the guide catheter by deep intubation and inflation of the Proxis sealing balloon. This device is no longer available in the US market.

## DISTAL FILTRATION SYSTEM

A distal filter system is composed of a tightly wrapped filter attached to a guide wire and sheathed within a delivery catheter for placement distal to the target lesion. It can trap debris that embolize while the intervention is performed over the guide wire. At completion, a retrieval catheter is advanced over the guide wire to collapse the filter and remove it along with retained contents. It may be the preferred system in patients who are undergoing high-risk intervention and are at increased risk for hemodynamic instability in instances of temporary SVG occlusion, such as patients with severe left ventricular dysfunction, last remaining conduit, and need for multiple stents.[64] Distal protection devices require the presence of a landing zone that must be taken into consideration before stent implantation to facilitate stent delivery.

Recent registry data suggest that EPDs are only used in the minority of SVG interventions.[67] This may be because of anatomic difficulties, such as challenging takeoff from the aorta, very large vessel diameter, and the absence of an adequate nondiseased landing zone.[68] EPD use may also be limited because of the higher procedural cost, longer procedural time, and greater radiation exposure.[67] Given the current guidelines regarding EPD use, it is recommended that every effort should be made to use EPDs in SVG interventions whenever technically feasible. The location of the stenosis determines the type of EPD that may be used; ostial lesions require a distal EPD, lesions in the body of the graft can be served either by a proximal or distal device, and distal lesions can only be proximally protected.[68] However, some reports suggest a potential off-label use of these devices for complex SVG interventions in which enhanced backup support is considered crucial.[69]

## CHOICE OF STENT

Percutaneous transluminal coronary angioplasty has proved to be inadequate therapy with unacceptably high rates of restenosis and MACE.[70] Use of stents has helped reduce complications and MACE during SVG PCI. The Saphenous Vein De Novo (SAVED) trial was the first study that compared balloon angioplasty with bare-metal stents (BMS) in SVG lesions. BMS were associated with higher procedural success (92% vs 69%, $P<.001$), a trend toward a reduction in angiographic restenosis (36% vs 47%, $P = .11$), and lower MACE.[71] Observational studies comparing DES with BMS in SVG PCI in terms of death, myocardial infarction, and target vessel revascularization remains inconclusive.[72–78] Randomized prospective studies comparing BMS with DES in SVG PCI are less conclusive because of the small number of studies available and their small sample size.[68] The Reduction in Restenosis in Saphenous Vein Grafts with Cypher (RRISC) trial[79] and the Stenting of Saphenous Vein Graft (SOS) trial[80] compared DES with BMS and found a significant reduction in restenosis and target lesion revascularization (TLR) but no difference in mortality. However, the DELAYED RRISC (Death and Events at Long-Term Follow-Up Analysis: Extended Duration of the Reduction of Restenosis in Saphenous Vein Grafts With Cypher Stent) study reported similar rates of target vessel revascularization at 3 years. Moreover, significantly higher all-cause mortality at 3 years was reported with sirolimus-eluting stents compared with BMS.[81] Several meta-analyses comparing DES with BMS in SVG intervention have demonstrated consistent results of improved efficacy and safety with DES.[82–87]

Covered stents are constructed as 2 coaxial layers of bare metal stents with the polytetrafluoroethylene (PTFE) covering trapped between them. They were created as part of a mechanical strategy to serve as a local filter, trapping plaque against the graft wall to prevent the shower of emboli during stent deployment. They serve as a smooth-muscle cell barrier and, therefore, may theoretically decrease rates of restenosis. Although initial studies suggested that covered stents seemed to be a safe and efficient treatment strategy with a low incidence of restenosis and target-vessel revascularization,[88] prospective, randomized trials failed to show benefit over BMS.[89–91]

## TREATMENT OF OCCLUDED SVGS

The presence of an occluded graft may adversely affect outcomes in patients in whom an acute coronary syndrome develops, because this may affect an even larger myocardial area than the target vessel distribution.[30] Treatment of a native coronary artery chronic total occlusion has been described for acutely thrombosed SVGs that could not be recanalized, but it can be technically challenging.[92] In a small study of patients with chronic total SVG occlusion for which percutaneous revascularization was attempted, successful recanalization with stent implantation was low, and the rates of in-stent restenosis and target vessel revascularization were unacceptably high in patients who underwent successful stenting.[93] Given the poor short- and long-term outcomes of percutaneous revascularization in chronic total occlusion of SVGs, percutaneous revascularization should rarely be considered except for acute occlusion in the setting of myocardial infarction. Instead, attempts to recanalize the native coronary artery are preferred if feasible.[64]

## DECISION TO PERFORM PCI IN PRIOR CABG

The decision regarding whether to intervene in a diseased SVG should be guided by the patient's symptoms, angiographic evidence of a significant stenosis, and noninvasive evidence of myocardial ischemia in the region supplied by the SVG.[64] PCI target vessel and corresponding outcomes in patients with prior CABG are poorly studied. Data from the CathPCI Registry (2004 through 2009) show that (1) most PCIs performed in patients with prior CABG are done in native coronary arteries, (2) most bypass graft PCIs are done in SVGs, and (3) patients undergoing bypass graft PCI have higher-risk clinical characteristics and higher in-hospital mortality. Percutaneous revascularization of SVGs was associated with worse clinical outcomes, including higher rates of in-stent restenosis, target vessel revascularization, myocardial infarction, and death compared with percutaneous coronary intervention of native coronary arteries. PCI in patients with prior CABG represented 17.5% of the total PCI volume. The PCI target vessel in patients with prior CABG was only a native coronary artery in 62.5% and

at least 1 bypass graft in 37.5%. Most of the target grafts were SVGs (34.9%). Compared with patients undergoing native coronary artery PCI, patients undergoing bypass graft PCI had higher rates of postprocedural complications and in-hospital mortality. On multivariable analysis, treatment of a bypass graft was independently associated with higher in-hospital mortality: adjusted odds ratio for SVG was 1.20 (95% confidence interval [CI]: 1.10–1.30; $P<.001$).[30]

Intervening on a native coronary artery instead of an SVG, if feasible, may improve both acute (lower risk of distal embolization) and long-term (as stented native coronary arteries have lower risk for in-stent restenosis than SVGs) results **Fig. 1**.[92] Although the exact factors behind target vessel choice in the CathPCI Registry are not available, the main factors associated with PCI target vessel selection included the severity of SVG disease versus native coronary artery disease. Native coronary artery PCI may be preferred with diffusely degenerated SVGs, whereas SVG PCI may be preferred in the presence of long, tortuous, and calcified native coronary artery lesions or in the presence of chronic total occlusions (**Fig. 2**, **Table 3**).[30]

When attempting to plan a revascularization strategy it is important to answer the following questions before embarking on an unsuccessful procedure:

- Can I predilate?
- Can I deliver a stent? What stent length will I need?
- What type and length guide would I need: 90 versus 100 cm? Supportive versus nonsupportive?
- What is the myocardium at risk? Can I mitigate the risk by treating the native coronary or the SVG?
- Are there any contraindications or special anticoagulation regimens that will favor one approach over another?

The decision to perform angiography and intervention in the setting of prior CABG, should be undertaken with knowledge of the operative report and any previous angiograms. It is imperative to know the number, location, and anatomy of grafts. This reduces contrast load, radiation exposure, and vascular complications that may occur when blindly navigating for graft ostia. Appropriate catheter selection for angiography can also reduce complications and procedural time.[68] Once yield of the lesion is maintained, an EPD is carefully placed in a satisfactory position. Severe stenoses usually require predilation with a small balloon. As opposed to predilation with balloon angioplasty,

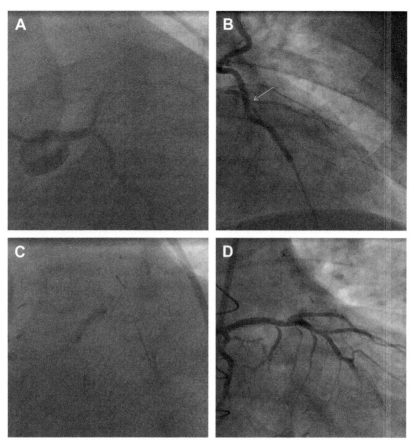

**Fig. 1.** (*A*) Angiogram of a native left coronary artery shows a severe lesion in the proximal segment of the left anterior descending artery in a man presenting with a nonsegment elevation myocardial infarction with antero-lateral ST segment depression. (*B*) Injection of the left internal mammary graft shows good flow distal to the anastomotic segment (*arrow*), with a severe lesion proximal in the native left anterior descending artery proximal to the anastomotic segment of the graft. (*C, D*) Because of the lesion location, the native left anterior descending artery was predilated and stented relieving the culprit obstruction.

direct stenting has the potential benefit of trapping debris and decreasing distal embolization that may occur from repeated balloon inflations.[64] In a registry of unselected patients who underwent SVG intervention, direct stenting was associated with a nearly 50% reduction in CK-MB elevations greater than 4 times normal (13.6% vs 23%, $P$<.12) and fewer non–Q-wave myocardial infarctions (10.7% vs 18.4%, $P$<.02).[94] Currently, there are no prospective randomized trials evaluating whether predilation versus direct stenting is effective in reducing distal embolization.

Stents should be sized one to one, and high-pressure inflation is avoided where possible to reduce the risk of distal embolization. Minimizing poststent manipulation is also important to prevent embolization. Both balloon and stent must be well enough away from the EPD to avoid entanglement. Angiography is then repeated to assess the lesion

intervened on and the flow rates in both the vein grafts and the coronary arteries. The myocardial blush grade should also be carefully assessed. Slow flow may indicate a saturated filter, which should be aspirated and removed. If there is a good angiographic result, the protection balloon is deflated or the filter retrieved. This is a critical step requiring coaxial alignment of the guide to prevent filter entrapment in the stent. A final angiogram is performed to assess the results of the intervention, including the presence of myocardial blush and angiographic flow down the vessel.[68]

If intervention to a lesion in a native coronary artery is not possible via a patent graft for technical reasons, then minimal angioplasty of the native vessel for the purpose of passing interventional hardware and subsequent intervention is an alternative backdoor approach for restoring graft flow to the artery.[95]

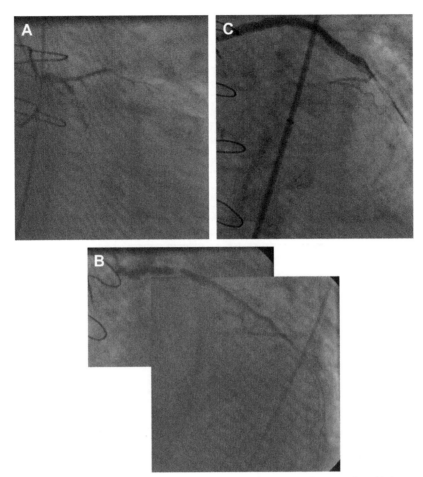

**Fig. 2.** (*A*) Native left coronary artery angiogram shows an occluded circumflex vessel and left anterior descending artery after a large diagonal branch. (*B*) Angiogram of an SVG to the obtuse marginal (OM) branch shows a severely calcified and degenerated vein graft with a critical lesion explaining a lateral non–ST-segment elevation myocardial infarction. (*C*) Because of the presence of a chronic total occlusion in the circumflex territory, PCI of the vein graft was successfully performed after predilatation and placement of an embolic protection device.

**Table 3**
**Factors associated with treatment of native coronary artery lesion**

| Variable | Odds Ratio | Lower 95% CI | Upper 95% CI | P Value |
|---|---|---|---|---|
| Graft stenosis >70% | 0.11 | 0.11 | 0.12 | <0.001 |
| Years from prior CABG (odds ratio for 1 y) | 0.92 | 0.92 | 0.93 | <0.001 |
| Multivessel disease | 2.30 | 2.19 | 2.42 | <0.001 |
| Preprocedure TIMI flow grade | 1.15 | 1.13 | 1.16 | <0.001 |
| Male | 0.82 | 0.81 | 0.84 | <0.001 |
| High-risk lesion | 0.64 | 0.61 | 0.68 | <0.001 |
| Diabetes | 0.93 | 0.92 | 0.94 | <0.001 |
| Right coronary artery stenosis >70% | 0.83 | 0.80 | 0.85 | <0.001 |
| STEMI | 0.75 | 0.72 | 0.79 | <0.001 |
| Left main stenosis >50% | 0.87 | 0.85 | 0.89 | <0.001 |

*Data from* Brilakis ES, Rao SV, Banerjee S, et al. Percutaneous coronary intervention in native arteries versus bypass grafts in prior coronary artery bypass grafting patients a report from the national cardiovascular data registry. JACC Cardiovasc Interv 2011;4(8):844–50.

## OUTCOMES

The risk for subsequent cardiovascular events is high and is thought to be similar between native coronary artery PCI and bypass graft PCI patients. However, when both options are available, native coronary artery PCI seems to be advantageous and serves as the treatment of choice compared with bypass graft PCI in patients with prior CABG requiring coronary revascularization because of lower procedural risk. Previously, the overall outcome in this group was unknown. There is a burgeoning body of evidence reporting on the outcome in this setting. Early registry data from the Mayo Clinic group found that in the setting of acute myocardial infarction, treatment of a vein graft was independently associated with death and adverse cardiac events.[96] Similarly, Varghese and colleagues[97] reported that when compared with bypass graft PCI, native coronary PCI was more likely to be performed and was associated with lower risk of no-reflow. Both groups of patients had similar but high incidence of myocardial infarction, repeat PCI, and death.

## SUMMARY

Complex PCI of native coronary arteries or degenerated SVG are a common scenario in daily practice. The stenting strategy that provides the safest, most complete revascularization with the least risk of restenosis should always be the preferred route. SVG PCI should be performed with an embolic protection device to minimize the risk of periprocedural myocardial infarction. PCI of the native coronary arteries should be considered if the lesion characteristics suggest a favorable outcome because they are associated with the least amount of restenosis with drug eluting stents.

## REFERENCES

1. Alexander JH, Hafley G, Harrington RA, et al. Efficacy and safety of edifoligide, an E2F transcription factor decoy, for prevention of vein graft failure following coronary artery bypass graft surgery: PREVENT IV: a randomized controlled trial. JAMA 2005;294(19):2446–54.
2. Puskas JD, Williams WH, Mahoney EM, et al. Off-pump vs conventional coronary artery bypass grafting: early and 1-year graft patency, cost, and quality-of-life outcomes: a randomized trial. JAMA 2004;291(15):1841–9.
3. Barner HB. Operative treatment of coronary atherosclerosis. Ann Thorac Surg 2008;85(4):1473–82.
4. Widimsky P, Straka Z, Stros P, et al. One-year coronary bypass graft patency: a randomized comparison between off-pump and on-pump surgery angiographic results of the PRAGUE-4 trial. Circulation 2004;110(22):3418–23.
5. Tatoulis J, Buxton BF, Fuller JA. Patencies of 2127 arterial to coronary conduits over 15 years. Ann Thorac Surg 2004;77(1):93–101.
6. Motwani JG, Topol EJ. Aortocoronary saphenous vein graft disease: pathogenesis, predisposition, and prevention. Circulation 1998;97(9):916–31.
7. Loop FD. A 20-year experience in coronary artery re-operation. Eur Heart J 1989;10(Suppl H):78–84.
8. Yap CH, Sposato L, Akowuah E, et al. Contemporary results show repeat coronary artery bypass grafting remains a risk factor for operative mortality. Ann Thorac Surg 2009;87(5):1386–91.
9. Yuan SM, Wang YQ, Shen Y, et al. Transforming growth factor-β in graft vessels: histology and immunohistochemistry. Clinics (Sao Paulo) 2011;66(5):895–901.
10. Shukla N, Jeremy JY. Pathophysiology of saphenous vein graft failure: a brief overview of interventions. Curr Opin Pharmacol 2012;12(2):114–20. http://dx.doi.org/10.1016/j.coph.2012.01.001.
11. Mizuno K, Satomura K, Miyamoto A, et al. Angioscopic evaluation of coronary-artery thrombi in acute coronary syndromes. N Engl J Med 1992;326(5):287–91.
12. Saber RS, Edwards WD, Holmes DR, et al. Balloon angioplasty of aortocoronary saphenous vein bypass grafts: a histopathologic study of six grafts from five patients, with emphasis on restenosis and embolic complications. J Am Coll Cardiol 1988;12(6):1501–9.
13. White CJ, Ramee SR, Collins TJ, et al. Percutaneous angioscopy of saphenous vein coronary bypass grafts. J Am Coll Cardiol 1993;21(5):1181–5.
14. Silva JA, White CJ, Collins TJ, et al. Morphologic comparison of atherosclerotic lesions in native coronary arteries and saphenous vein graphs with intracoronary angioscopy in patients with unstable angina. Am Heart J 1998;136(1):156–63.
15. Mehta RH, Ferguson TB, Lopes RD, et al. Saphenous vein grafts with multiple versus single distal targets in patients undergoing coronary artery bypass surgery: one-year graft failure and five-year outcomes from the Project of Ex-Vivo Vein Graft Engineering via Transfection (PREVENT) IV trial. Circulation 2011;124(3):280–8.
16. Roth JA, Cukingnan RA, Brown BG, et al. Factors influencing patency of saphenous vein grafts. Ann Thorac Surg 1979;28(2):176–83.
17. Cataldo G, Braga M, Pirotta N, et al. Factors influencing 1-year patency of coronary artery saphenous vein grafts. Studio Indobufene nel Bypass Aortocoronarico (SINBA). Circulation 1993;88(5 Pt 2):II93–8.
18. Shah PJ, Gordon I, Fuller J, et al. Factors affecting saphenous vein graft patency: clinical and angiographic study in 1402 symptomatic patients

operated on between 1977 and 1999. J Thorac Cardiovasc Surg 2003;126(6):1972–7.

19. Souza DS, Dashwood MR, Tsui JC, et al. Improved patency in vein grafts harvested with surrounding tissue: results of a randomized study using three harvesting techniques. Ann Thorac Surg 2002; 73(4):1189–95.

20. Björk VO, Ekeström S, Henze A, et al. Early and late patency of aortocoronary vein grafts. Scand J Thorac Cardiovasc Surg 1981;15(1):11–21.

21. Kawaguchi R, Hoshizaki H, Oshima S, et al. Strategy for post coronary artery bypass grafting in patients with bypass graft stenosis: comparison of percutaneous transluminal coronary angioplasty for the native coronary artery, internal mammary artery and saphenous vein graft. J Cardiol 2001;38(5): 239–44.

22. Gyöngyösi M, Yang P, Khorsand A, et al. Longitudinal straightening effect of stents is an additional predictor for major adverse cardiac events. Austrian Wiktor Stent Study Group and European Paragon Stent Investigators. J Am Coll Cardiol 2000;35(6): 1580–9.

23. Gyöngyösi M, Posa A, Pavo N, et al. Differential effect of ischaemic preconditioning on mobilisation and recruitment of haematopoietic and mesenchymal stem cells in porcine myocardial ischaemia-reperfusion. Thromb Haemost 2010;104(2):376–84.

24. Gerszten RE, Lim YC, Ding HT, et al. Adhesion of monocytes to vascular cell adhesion molecule-1-transduced human endothelial cells: implications for atherogenesis. Circ Res 1998;82(8):871–8.

25. Barth KH, Virmani R, Froelich J, et al. Paired comparison of vascular wall reactions to Palmaz stents, Strecker tantalum stents, and Wallstents in canine iliac and femoral arteries. Circulation 1996; 93(12):2161–9.

26. Wentzel JJ, Krams R, Schuurbiers JC, et al. Relationship between neointimal thickness and shear stress after Wallstent implantation in human coronary arteries. Circulation 2001;103(13):1740–5.

27. Hirshfeld JW, Schwartz JS, Jugo R, et al. Restenosis after coronary angioplasty: a multivariate statistical model to relate lesion and procedure variables to restenosis. The M-HEART Investigators. J Am Coll Cardiol 1991;18(3):647–56.

28. Bourassa MG, Lespérance J, Eastwood C, et al. Clinical, physiologic, anatomic and procedural factors predictive of restenosis after percutaneous transluminal coronary angioplasty. J Am Coll Cardiol 1991;18(2):368–76.

29. Elezi S, Kastrati A, Neumann FJ, et al. Vessel size and long-term outcome after coronary stent placement. Circulation 1998;98(18):1875–80.

30. Brilakis ES, Rao SV, Banerjee S, et al. Percutaneous coronary intervention in native arteries versus bypass grafts in prior coronary artery bypass grafting patients a report from the national cardiovascular data registry. JACC Cardiovasc Interv 2011;4(8): 844–50.

31. Moussa I, Ellis SG, Jones M, et al. Impact of coronary culprit lesion calcium in patients undergoing paclitaxel-eluting stent implantation (a TAXUS-IV sub study). Am J Cardiol 2005;96(9):1242–7.

32. Dardas P, Mezilis N, Ninios V, et al. The use of rotational atherectomy and drug-eluting stents in the treatment of heavily calcified coronary lesions. Hellenic J Cardiol 2011;52(5):399–406.

33. Hoffmann R, Mintz GS, Popma JJ, et al. Treatment of calcified coronary lesions with Palmaz-Schatz stents. An intravascular ultrasound study. Eur Heart J 1998;19(8):1224–31.

34. Kaplan BM, Benzuly KH, Kinn JW, et al. Treatment of no-reflow in degenerated saphenous vein graft interventions: comparison of intracoronary verapamil and nitroglycerin. Cathet Cardiovasc Diagn 1996; 39(2):113–8.

35. Hong MK, Mehran R, Dangas G, et al. Creatine kinase-MB enzyme elevation following successful saphenous vein graft intervention is associated with late mortality. Circulation 1999;100(24):2400–5.

36. Sano K, Mintz GS, Carlier SG, et al. Intravascular ultrasonic differences between aorto-ostial and shaft narrowing in saphenous veins used as aortocoronary bypass grafts. Am J Cardiol 2006;97(10): 1463–6.

37. Hong YJ, Jeong MH, Ahn Y, et al. Impact of lesion location on intravascular ultrasound findings and short-term and five-year long-term clinical outcome after percutaneous coronary intervention for saphenous vein graft lesions. Int J Cardiol, in press.

38. van Gaal WJ, Banning AP. Percutaneous coronary intervention and the no-reflow phenomenon. Expert Rev Cardiovasc Ther 2007;5(4):715–31.

39. Piana RN, Paik GY, Moscucci M, et al. Incidence and treatment of "no-reflow" after percutaneous coronary intervention. Circulation 1994;89(6):2514–8.

40. Abbo KM, Dooris M, Glazier S, et al. Features and outcome of no-reflow after percutaneous coronary intervention. Am J Cardiol 1995;75(12):778–82.

41. Ito H, Tomooka T, Sakai N, et al. Lack of myocardial perfusion immediately after successful thrombolysis. A predictor of poor recovery of left ventricular function in anterior myocardial infarction. Circulation 1992;85(5):1699–705.

42. Ito H, Maruyama A, Iwakura K, et al. Clinical implications of the "no reflow" phenomenon. A predictor of complications and left ventricular remodeling in reperfused anterior wall myocardial infarction. Circulation 1996;93(2):223–8.

43. Resnic FS, Wainstein M, Lee MK, et al. No-reflow is an independent predictor of death and myocardial infarction after percutaneous coronary intervention. Am Heart J 2003;145(1):42–6.

44. Ellis SG, Popma JJ, Buchbinder M, et al. Relation of clinical presentation, stenosis morphology, and operator technique to the procedural results of rotational atherectomy and rotational atherectomy-facilitated angioplasty. Circulation 1994;89(2):882–92.

45. Hanna GP, Yhip P, Fujise K, et al. Intracoronary adenosine administered during rotational atherectomy of complex lesions in native coronary arteries reduces the incidence of no-reflow phenomenon. Catheter Cardiovasc Interv 1999;48(3):275–8.

46. Habibzadeh MR, Thai H, Movahed MR. Prophylactic intragraft injection of nicardipine prior to saphenous vein graft percutaneous intervention for the prevention of no-reflow: a review and comparison to protection devices. J Invasive Cardiol 2011;23(5):202–6.

47. Sdringola S, Assali AR, Ghani M, et al. Risk assessment of slow or no-reflow phenomenon in aortocoronary vein graft percutaneous intervention. Catheter Cardiovasc Interv 2001;54(3):318–24.

48. Ho PC. Spontaneous slow flow in the saphenous vein graft: a relevant distinction of macrovascular endothelial dysfunction. Heart Vessels 2007;22(4): 274–7.

49. Baber U, Kini AS, Sharma SK. Stenting of complex lesions: an overview. Nat Rev Cardiol 2010;7(9): 485–96.

50. Feldman T. Tricks for overcoming difficult stent delivery. Catheter Cardiovasc Interv 1999;48(3): 285–6.

51. Kumar S, Gorog DA, Secco GG, et al. The Guide-Liner "child" catheter for percutaneous coronary intervention—early clinical experience. J Invasive Cardiol 2010;22(10):495–8.

52. Saucedo JF, Muller DW, Moscucci M. Facilitated advancement of the Palmaz-Schatz stent delivery system with the use of an adjacent 0.018″ stiff wire. Cathet Cardiovasc Diagn 1996;39(1):106–10.

53. Bartorelli AL, Lavarra F, Trabattoni D, et al. Successful stent delivery with deep seating of 6 French guiding catheters in difficult coronary anatomy. Catheter Cardiovasc Interv 1999;48(3):279–84.

54. Attaran RR, Butman S, Movahed MR. Going around the bend: deep inspiration facilitates difficult stent delivery in the native coronary arteries. Tex Heart Inst J 2011;38(3):270–4.

55. Wiper A, Mamas M, El-Omar M. Use of the Guide-Liner catheter in facilitating coronary and graft intervention. Cardiovasc Revasc Med 2011;12(1): 68.e5–7.

56. Lin CH, Kurz H, Lasala J, et al. Delivery of stent in prohibitive coronary anatomy using the Guideliner Anchor Inflated Noncompliant Balloon (GAIN) technique, a case series [abstract]. In: Abstracts of the society for cardiovascular angiography and interventions 34th annual scientific sessions. May 4–7, 2011. Baltimore (MD): Catheter Cardiovasc Interv; 2011. p. S40 Abstract nr B-007.

57. Goldberg A, Klein R, Marmor A. Buddy wire, buddy balloon or better together! J Invasive Cardiol 2007; 19(12):E363–5.

58. Kovach JA, Mintz GS, Pichard AD, et al. Sequential intravascular ultrasound characterization of the mechanisms of rotational atherectomy and adjunct balloon angioplasty. J Am Coll Cardiol 1993;22(4): 1024–32.

59. Tran T, Brown M, Lasala J. An evidence-based approach to the use of rotational and directional coronary atherectomy in the era of drug-eluting stents: when does it make sense? Catheter Cardiovasc Interv 2008;72(5):650–62.

60. Thomas WJ, Cowley MJ, Vetrovec GW, et al. Effectiveness of rotational atherectomy in aortocoronary saphenous vein grafts. Am J Cardiol 2000;86(1): 88–91.

61. Don CW, Palacios I, Rosenfield K. Use of rotational atherectomy in the body of a saphenous vein coronary graft. J Invasive Cardiol 2009;21(9): E168–70.

62. Mauri L, Rogers C, Baim DS. Devices for distal protection during percutaneous coronary revascularization. Circulation 2006;113(22):2651–6.

63. Levine GN, Bates ER, Blankenship JC, et al. 2011 ACCF/AHA/SCAI guideline for percutaneous coronary intervention: Executive Summary: A Report of the American College of Cardiology Foundation/ American Heart Association Task Force on Practice Guidelines and the Society for Cardiovascular Angiography a. Catheterization and cardiovascular interventions. Catheter Cardiovasc Interv 2012;79(3): 453–95.

64. Lee MS, Park SJ, Kandzari DE, et al. Saphenous vein graft intervention. JACC Cardiovasc Interv 2011;4(8):831–43.

65. Baim DS, Wahr D, George B, et al. Randomized trial of a distal embolic protection device during percutaneous intervention of saphenous vein aorto-coronary bypass grafts. Circulation 2002;105(11):1285–90.

66. Mauri L, Cox D, Hermiller J, et al. The PROXIMAL trial: proximal protection during saphenous vein graft intervention using the Proxis Embolic Protection System: a randomized, prospective, multicenter clinical trial. J Am Coll Cardiol 2007;50(15):1442–9.

67. Mehta SK, Frutkin AD, Milford-Beland S, et al. Utilization of distal embolic protection in saphenous vein graft interventions (an analysis of 19,546 patients in the American College of Cardiology-National Cardiovascular Data Registry). Am J Cardiol 2007;100(7):1114–8.

68. Hindnavis V, Cho SH, Goldberg S. Saphenous vein graft intervention: a review. J Invasive Cardiol 2012;24(2):64–71.

69. Banerjee S, Brilakis ES. Use of the Proxis embolic protection device for guide anchoring and stent delivery during complex saphenous vein graft

interventions. Cardiovasc Revasc Med 2009;10(3): 183–7.

70. de Feyter PJ, van Suylen RJ, de Jaegere PP, et al. Balloon angioplasty for the treatment of lesions in saphenous vein bypass grafts. J Am Coll Cardiol 1993;21(7):1539–49.

71. Savage MP, Douglas JS, Fischman DL, et al. Stent placement compared with balloon angioplasty for obstructed coronary bypass grafts. Saphenous Vein De Novo Trial Investigators. N Engl J Med 1997;337(11):740–7.

72. Ge L, Iakovou I, Sangiorgi GM, et al. Treatment of saphenous vein graft lesions with drug-eluting stents: immediate and midterm outcome. J Am Coll Cardiol 2005;45(7):989–94.

73. Lee MS, Shah AP, Aragon J, et al. Drug-eluting stenting is superior to bare metal stenting in saphenous vein grafts. Catheter Cardiovasc Interv 2005;66(4): 507–11.

74. Ramana RK, Ronan A, Cohoon K, et al. Long-term clinical outcomes of real-world experience using sirolimus-eluting stents in saphenous vein graft disease. Catheter Cardiovasc Interv 2008;71(7): 886–93.

75. Assali A, Raz Y, Vaknin-Assa H, et al. Beneficial 2-years results of drug-eluting stents in saphenous vein graft lesions. EuroIntervention 2008; 4(1):108–14.

76. Chu WW, Rha SW, Kuchulakanti PK, et al. Efficacy of sirolimus-eluting stents compared with bare metal stents for saphenous vein graft intervention. Am J Cardiol 2006;97(1):34–7.

77. Baldwin DE, Abbott JD, Trost JC, et al. Comparison of drug-eluting and bare metal stents for saphenous vein graft lesions (from the National Heart, Lung, and Blood Institute Dynamic Registry). Am J Cardiol 2010;106(7):946–51.

78. Shishehbor MH, Hawi R, Singh IM, et al. Drug-eluting versus bare-metal stents for treating saphenous vein grafts. Am Heart J 2009;158(4): 637–43.

79. Vermeersch P, Agostoni P, Verheye S, et al. Randomized double-blind comparison of sirolimus-eluting stent versus bare-metal stent implantation in diseased saphenous vein grafts: six-month angiographic, intravascular ultrasound, and clinical follow-up of the RRISC Trial. J Am Coll Cardiol 2006;48(12):2423–31.

80. Brilakis ES, Lichtenwalter C, Abdel-karim AR, et al. Continued benefit from paclitaxel-eluting compared with bare-metal stent implantation in saphenous vein graft lesions during long-term follow-up of the SOS (Stenting of Saphenous Vein Grafts) trial. JACC Cardiovasc Interv 2011;4(2):176–82.

81. Vermeersch P, Agostoni P, Verheye S, et al. Increased late mortality after sirolimus-eluting stents versus bare-metal stents in diseased saphenous

vein grafts: results from the randomized DELAYED RRISC Trial. J Am Coll Cardiol 2007;50(3):261–7.

82. Wiisanen ME, Abdel-Latif A, Mukherjee D, et al. Drug-eluting stents versus bare-metal stents in saphenous vein graft interventions: a systematic review and meta-analysis. JACC Cardiovasc Interv 2010;3(12):1262–73.

83. Lee MS, Yang T, Kandzari DE, et al. Comparison by meta-analysis of drug-eluting stents and bare metal stents for saphenous vein graft intervention. Am J Cardiol 2010;105(8):1076–82.

84. Meier P, Brilakis ES, Corti R, et al. Drug-eluting versus bare-metal stent for treatment of saphenous vein grafts: a meta-analysis. PLoS One 2010;5(6): e11040.

85. Joyal D, Filion KB, Eisenberg MJ. Effectiveness and safety of drug-eluting stents in vein grafts: a meta-analysis. Am Heart J 2010;159(2):159–169.e4.

86. Paradis JM, Bélisle P, Joseph L, et al. Drug-eluting or bare metal stents for the treatment of saphenous vein graft disease: a Bayesian meta-analysis. Circ Cardiovasc Interv 2010;3(6):565–76.

87. Hakeem A, Helmy T, Munsif S, et al. Safety and efficacy of drug eluting stents compared with bare metal stents for saphenous vein graft interventions: a comprehensive meta-analysis of randomized trials and observational studies comprising 7,994 patients. Catheter Cardiovasc Interv 2011;77(3): 343–55.

88. Baldus S, Köster R, Elsner M, et al. Treatment of aortocoronary vein graft lesions with membrane-covered stents: A multicenter surveillance trial. Circulation 2000;102(17):2024–7.

89. Turco MA, Buchbinder M, Popma JJ, et al. Pivotal, randomized U.S. study of the Symbiottrade mark covered stent system in patients with saphenous vein graft disease: eight-month angiographic and clinical results from the Symbiot III trial. Catheter Cardiovasc Interv 2006;68(3):379–88.

90. Stankovic G, Colombo A, Presbitero P, et al. Randomized evaluation of polytetrafluoroethylene-covered stent in saphenous vein grafts: the Randomized Evaluation of polytetrafluoroethylene COVERed stent in Saphenous vein grafts (RECOVERS) Trial. Circulation 2003;108(1):37–42.

91. Stone GW, Goldberg S, O'Shaughnessy C, et al. 5-year follow-up of polytetrafluoroethylene-covered stents compared with bare-metal stents in aortocoronary saphenous vein grafts the randomized BARRICADE (barrier approach to restenosis: restrict intima to curtail adverse events) trial. JACC Cardiovasc Interv 2011;4(3):300–9.

92. Brilakis ES, Banerjee S. What can we do for patients undergoing saphenous vein graft interventions? Catheter Cardiovasc Interv 2011;78(1):30–1.

93. Al-Lamee R, Ielasi A, Latib A, et al. Clinical and angiographic outcomes after percutaneous

recanalization of chronic total saphenous vein graft occlusion using modern techniques. Am J Cardiol 2010;106(12):1721–7.

94. Leborgne L, Cheneau E, Pichard A, et al. Effect of direct stenting on clinical outcome in patients treated with percutaneous coronary intervention on saphenous vein graft. Am Heart J 2003;146(3): 501–6.

95. Chan RY, Gunalingam B. "Backdoor" alternative approach to stenting of a post-anastomotic coronary artery lesion via a chronically obstructed right coronary artery after failure to stent through a tortuous free internal mammary graft. J Interv Cardiol 2007; 20(4):243–7.

96. Al Suwaidi J, Velianou JL, Berger PB, et al. Primary percutaneous coronary interventions in patients with acute myocardial infarction and prior coronary artery bypass grafting. Am Heart J 2001;142(3): 452–9.

97. Varghese I, Samuel J, Banerjee S, et al. Comparison of percutaneous coronary intervention in native coronary arteries vs. bypass grafts in patients with prior coronary artery bypass graft surgery. Cardiovasc Revasc Med 2009;10(2):103–9.

# Management of Complications During Saphenous Vein Graft Interventions

Satya Shreenivas, MD, Saif Anwaruddin, MD*

## KEYWORDS

• Saphenous vein grafts • Complications • Embolic protection devices

## KEY POINTS

• The approach to saphenous vein graft (SVG) interventions is different in many regards from native coronary interventions, including different risks and complications that occur.
• Immediate recognition and timely management of mechanical complications during intervention on SVGs can help ensure optimal patient outcomes.
• Several strategies exist to reduce the risk of periprocedural complications related to SVG interventions.

## INTRODUCTION

Despite the ongoing use of percutaneous coronary revascularization, coronary artery bypass grafting (CABG) remains the standard of care for patients with significant multivessel and left main coronary atherosclerosis. SVGs make up the vast majority of conduits used to bypass diseased native vessels. Unlike arterial grafts, SVGs have higher rates of degeneration, and it is estimated that up to 5% of SVGs fail each year.[1] As an increasing number of SVGs age, they eventually require replacement or percutaneous repair. In a recent review of the National Cardiovascular Data Registry (NCDR), 17.5% of all percutaneous interventions (PCIs) were done on patients with prior CABG and in these cases approximately 40% of the interventions were performed on diseased SVGs.[2]

SVG PCI carries a higher risk of periprocedural complications.[2,3] In the aforementioned NCDR review, patients undergoing PCI of an SVG had an in-hospital mortality rate of 1.5% versus an in-hospital mortality rate of 0.9% for those patients undergoing PCI of native vessels only ($P$ <.001).

Increased intraprocedural complications, transfusion requirements, risk of no-reflow, and higher 90-day mortality have all been previously reported with SVG interventions.[4,5] Part of this increased risk is attributable to the older age and increased comorbidities of patients presenting with SVG disease.[6] The challenge of SVG PCI cannot be underestimated, however, in this population as well.

Some of the challenges with SVG PCI include the use of proper guide support, use of adequate distal or proximal embolic protection devices, controversies in the use of bare metal stents versus drug-eluting stents, and characteristics unique to SVGs that make intervention challenging, such as the risk of no-reflow and the risk of perforation. SVGs do not behave in a fashion similar to native coronary arteries, and any approach to percutaneous procedures involving SVGs should account for these differences.

## HISTORY

Over the years, many different surgical approaches have been attempted to relieve angina.[7]

Division of Cardiovascular Medicine, Hospital of the University of Pennsylvania, 3400 Spruce Street, Philadelphia, PA 19104, USA
* Corresponding author. Hospital of the University of Pennsylvania, 3400 Spruce Street, 9 Gates, Philadelphia, PA 19104.
E-mail address: saif.anwaruddin@uphs.upenn.edu

Intervent Cardiol Clin 2 (2013) 339–346
http://dx.doi.org/10.1016/j.iccl.2012.12.003
2211-7458/13/$ – see front matter © 2013 Published by Elsevier Inc.

Extracardiac operations, such as sympathetic denervation and thyroidectomy, were reported to elicit chest pain relief.[8] Attempts to both decrease collateral flow to the coronaries and increase collateral flow to coronaries were attempted. Bilateral internal mammary arteries were ligated to prevent coronary steal and thus relieve angina but in one of the first randomized trials on coronary artery disease, this operation was shown ineffective.[9] Attempts to increase collateral flow to the coronaries from the pericardium led Beck[10] and O'Shaughnessy[11] to try pericardial poudrage (mechanical irritation instilled in the pericardium to cause adhesions and presumably new vessel growth).[10,11] On discovering the existence of subendocardial vessels that provide myocardial perfusion, internal mammary artery grafts sewn directly to the myocardium (Vineberg procedure) were used to relive angina with mixed results.[12] It was not until the chance direct engagement of coronary arteries by Sones and Shirey[13] at the Cleveland Clinic, however, that the possibility arose of directly diagnosing and then bypassing a critical coronary stenosis.

The first SVG used to bypass native coronary artery disease was performed in 1962 by David Sabiston and the surgical group at Johns Hopkins Hospital.[14,15] In this case, the right coronary artery was bypassed with an SVG but the patient died 3 days postsurgery.[16] In 1964, Kolesov (Russia) also performed a successful coronary artery bypass surgery using an SVG and continued to perform selective bypass surgeries over the next few years.[17] The procedure was further refined by DeBakey and others, but it was Favaloro and the group at the Cleveland Clinic who popularized the routine use of SVGs for CABG.[18,19]

## CAUSES OF SAPHENOUS VEIN GRAFT FAILURE

The causes of SVG failure vary and include vein trauma during harvest, mechanical complications with the anastomotic site, and eventual vein degeneration due to atherosclerotic disease. Graft failure immediately after CABG is usually due to acute thrombosis, graft damage due to misplacement, suture line stenosis, or bypassing an incorrect vessel. In addition to the mechanical complications, acute thrombosis of the graft is likely due to the endothelial dysfunction directly related to vein graft harvest and manipulation.[20] A recent study of 366 patients who underwent immediate postoperative angiography revealed that 12% of grafts had clinically significant problems that were only identified with the use of angiography but otherwise would have gone

unrecognized.[21] Due to the presence of chest pain from other causes, such as the sternotomy site and the patient's sedation, immediate mild ischemia can be missed. Immediate ischemia post CABG is either dealt with conservatively (medical management) or with a redo sternotomy and surgical repair if a patient is unstable. Ischemia after the first month from CABG out to the first year can be the result of perianastamotic stenosis or from accelerated intimal hyperplasia within the graft and can be successfully treated with balloon angioplasty.

Most of the patients who present to a catheterization laboratory after CABG do so several years after the initial surgery, and any identifiable ischemia is usually due to progressive SVG atherosclerotic disease. In 70% to 85% of patients presenting with an acute coronary syndrome 1 year or more removed from CABG, the identified culprit vessel was an SVG.[22,23] The risk of clinically significant graft atherosclerosis increases markedly after 5 to 7 years.[24–26] Unlike native coronary artery atherosclerosis, progressive SVG dysfunction has a different pathogenesis and appears histologically different. Just a few weeks after exposure to arterial pressure, SVGs develop intimal hyperplasia, a finding that has been associated with the atherosclerosis progression.[24,27] With the influx of smooth muscle cells and the loss of normal endothelial function, SVGs develop prothrombotic regions that result in fibrin deposition and further proinflammatory changes.[28] Histologically, SVG lesions are more friable, less calcified, and more diffuse than native coronary artery lesions. Procedurally, this becomes important because device manipulation and balloon or stent inflation across the lesion can result in distal embolization and eventual poor reflow in the vessel.

## PERCUTANEOUS INTERVENTION OF SAPHENOUS VEIN GRAFTS AND COMPLICATIONS

Although PCI of native coronary vessels is well established, the use of percutaneous revascularization techniques for SVGs has remained a challenge. The equipment used and the complications encountered are different; hence, the approach to SVG intervention must be as well. Patient outcomes are also different, as evidenced by pooled data suggesting higher mortality in patients undergoing SVG intervention versus native vessel PCI in the pre-embolic filter experience.[29]

The Saphenous Vein de Novo Trial trial demonstrated the superiority of stenting over angioplasty in SVG intervention.[30] In the modern era of PCI, several issues remain. The use of bare metal stents versus drug-eluting stents in SVG PCI has been debated. With drug-eluting stents, there is less target vessel revascularization early on; it remains questionable as to whether this advantage remains over the long term.[31,32] In addition to selecting the proper equipment, recognition and management of complications of SVG intervention are vitally important to ensuring excellent patient outcomes.

Although several of the complications encountered in SVG intervention are not unique to SVG intervention, they occur more commonly with SVG interventions, and they must be recognized and managed slightly differently than in the native coronary PCI. As such, a well thought-out preprocedural strategy and intraprocedural management of both the procedural aspects and any encountered complications are necessary. This article discusses some of the common complications associated with SVG interventions and how to deal with these issues and challenges.

## DISTAL EMBOLIZATION

As discussed previously, atherosclerotic plaque in SVGs versus native coronary arteries is larger, more friable, and less calcified. As such, the potential for periprocedural embolization during PCI remains a problem. Several trials have shown a higher risk of periprocedural complications, notably periprocedural myocardial infarction and poor reflow after balloon and/or stent deployment.[33,34] Clinically, this is significant and, in pooled analysis of several randomized studies, there was a doubling of 30-day mortality in SVG intervention versus native coronary vessel PCI where revascularization of an SVG was identified as an independent predictor of mortality.[29] This is not to say that that distal embolization does not occur in native coronary circulation PCI, because this phenomenon has been well established in native vessel PCI.[35]

The incidence of poor reflow or no-reflow after SVG intervention without the use of distal vessel protection is as high as 15%.[36] It is hypothesized that the increased risk of no-reflow and subsequent increased risk of periprocedural myocardial infarction is related to distal microembolization, poor microvascular circulation, and vasospasm of the micovasculature due, in part, to the release of various neurohormonal factors.[37]

Clinically, distal embolization and no-reflow resulting in periprocedural myocardial infarction have important prognostic implications. With periprocedural myocardial infarction after SVG interventions in the pre-embolic protection filter era, 30-day mortality was significantly higher.[38] Significant periprocedural biomarker elevation after SVG intervention was observed the most important predictor of 1-year mortality as well.[39]

Several strategies have been tried in preventing distal microemboli and include direct stenting versus pre–balloon dilation, covered stents, proximal occlusion devices, distal occlusion devices, and filter devices. Prevention of distal microemboli decreases the risk of no-reflow and the risk of periprocedural myocardial infarction and the use of embolic protection devices in SVG interventions is currently an American College of Cardiology/American Heart Association class I indication.[40]

Two early methods used to prevent distal microemboli included direct stenting and using covered stents. Direct stenting has the theoretic benefit of minimizing distal embolization by theoretically capturing the debris between stent struts and the vessel wall. There are biomarker data that show that SVG interventions that were done with a direct stent approach resulted in a lower rise in creatine kinase–MB (9.5 vs 19.6, P<.001).[41] A similar rationale led to several trials examining the benefits of covered stents (Jostent [Abbott Vascular, Abbott Park, Illinois] and Symbiot [Boston Scientific, Natick, Massachusetts] stents) in SVG interventions. Three multicenter randomized trials compared covered stents with bare metal stents and showed a slightly higher incidence of major adverse cardiovascular events and a higher incidence of long-term (5-year) vessel failure with the use of covered stents.[42–44]

Other methods to prevent distal microembolization include proximal and distal occlusion devices and filter devices (**Table 1**). Distal occlusion devices involve crossing the lesion and then inflating a balloon distal to the lesion. This physical barrier prevents embolization during intervention. Before deflating the distal balloon, debris is aspirated. The disadvantages to this include distal vessel ischemia with prolonged balloon inflation, the possibility of distal vessel injury during balloon inflation, and the difficulty visualizing the extent of the lesion in a thrombotic occlusion. Despite its limitations, several trials with both the PercuSurge GuardWire (Medtronic, Minneapolis, Minnesota) and TriActiv (Kensey Nash, Exton, Pennsylvania) systems showed decreased incidence of no-reflow with the use of these devices.[45,46] The Saphenous Vein Graft Angioplasty Free of Emboli Randomized trial examined the use of the PercuSurge GuardWire in SVG intervention.[45] In total, 801 patients were randomized to either stenting of SVG lesions with or without the use of the PercuSurge device.

**Table 1**
**Embolization protection devices**

| Study Name | No. of Patients | Device(s) | MACE (%) | MI (%) | Summary |
|---|---|---|---|---|---|
| SAFER[45] | 801 | GuardWire | 9.6 | 8.6 | Embolic protection superior to no |
|  |  | Control | 16.5 | 14.7 | embolic protection |
| FIRE[48] | 651 | GuardWire | 11.6 | 10 | FilterWire EX noninferior to GuardWire |
|  |  | FilterWire EX | 9.9 | 9 | (distal occlusion) |
| PRIDE | 631 | TriActiv | 11.2 | 9.9 | TriActiv aspiration noninferior to |
|  |  | FilterWire/guard wire | 10.1 | 8.8 | established distal embolic protection |
| PROXIMAL[47] | 594 | Proxis | 9.2 | 6.4 | Proximal protection noninferior |
|  |  | Control | 10 | 7.9 |  |

*Abbreviations:* FIRE, FilterWire EX During Transluminal Intervention of Saphenous Vein Grafts; MACE, major adverse cardiac events; MI, myocardial infarction; PRIDE, Protection During Saphenous Vein Graft Intervention to Prevent Distal Embolization; PROXIMAL, Proximal Protection During Saphenous Vein Graft Intervention Using the Proxis Embolic Protection System: A Randomized, Prospective, Multicenter Trial; SAFER, Saphenous Vein Graft Angioplasty Free of Emboli Randomized trial.

The primary endpoint, a composite of death, myocardial infarction, emergency bypass, or target vessel revascularization at 30 days, was observed to occur in 9.6% of patients randomized to the PercuSurge device and 16.5% of patients in the control group ($P = .004$), primarily driven by a reduction in no-flow. The TriActiv distal occlusion device uses an active flush and aspiration component and has been shown to be similar to other distal embolic protection devices.

Proximal vessel occlusion with the Proxis device (St. Jude Medical, St. Paul, Minnesota) creates a brief lack of blood flow and thus prevents microemboli from reaching the distal vasculature. A balloon is inflated proximal to the lesion, creating an area distal to the balloon that has no blood flow. After stenting the lesion, an aspiration catheter is used for debris removal before balloon disengagement. The advantage of using this approach over the distal occlusion devices is that it allows establishment of distal embolic protection before delivering a guide wire and it allows for distal vessel protection even when the culprit lesion is very distal or in a tortuous segment. The disadvantages to the proximal occlusion device are the possibility of both vessel injury with proximal balloon inflation and ischemia due to lack of blood flow during a prolonged intervention. In the Proximal Protection During Saphenous Vein Graft Intervention Using the Proxis Embolic Protection System trial, 594 patients were randomized to proximal versus distal emboli protection in a noninferiority design.[47] Investigators reported similar outcomes with proximal protection versus distal embolic protection.

The use of distal embolic protection in the form of a filter wire is another widely used device (**Fig. 1**). The filter wire system is composed of a filter basket attached to a guide wire that is deployed distal to the lesion. During intervention, any debris that embolize are theoretically caught by the filter and then retrieved after the intervention using a separate retrieval catheter. There are several technical challenges to using such a device, including incomplete apposition in some cases, delivery of a bulky filter device across a severe stenosis, inability to ensure complete particle capture, and inability to use in distal SVG lesions. In a randomized study of 651 patients using either the FilterWire EX system or the PercuSurge GuardWire balloon system, both systems allowed for similar procedural success and there was a similar rate of major adverse cardiac events with the devices, including death, myocardial infarction, and target vessel revascularization at 30 days.[48]

Difficulties with using distal vessel protection devices include crossing the lesion, positioning the device accurately in the distal vessel (with no distal flow it can be difficult to determine the extent

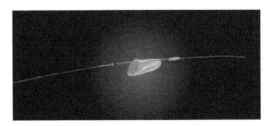

**Fig. 1.** FilterWire EZ system. (*Courtesy of* Boston Scientific Corporation; with permission.)

of the lesion and distal vessel size), and protection of side branches. It is likely that these limitations are part of the reason that despite a class IA indication for distal embolic protection, a recent NCDR review revealed that only 23% of SVG PCIs used distal embolic protection.[49]

In addition to device-based strategies to reduce the distal embolization of particulate matter, pharmacologic therapies have been examined in this regard. Several analyses have suggested a lack of benefit of glycoprotein IIb/IIIa inhibitors in SVG intervention. In an analysis of patients from the Evaluation of 7E3 for the Prevention of Ischemic Complications and Evaluation of PTCA To Improve Long-Term Outcome with Abciximab GP IIb/IIIa Blockade studies, there was a benefit to abciximab in all lesion morphologies with the exception of degenerated SVGs.[50] The lack of benefit of glycoprotein IIb/IIIa inhibitors in SVG intervention in these studies was likely due to the face that these studies were conducted before the widespread use of distal embolic protection. In a separate propensity analysis of the FilterWire EX During Transluminal Intervention of Saphenous Vein Grafts trial (discussed previously), comparing the FilterWire EX to the GuardWire, examining the use of glycoprotein IIb/IIIa inhibitors with the FilterWire system, there was reduction in major adverse cardiac events using the combination of the FilterWire and glycoprotein IIb/IIIa inhibitors despite that those patients receiving adjunctive pharmacotherapy were at higher risk.[51]

Other adjunctive pharmacotherapies have been examined. In addition to distal embolization of particulate matter, vasospasm resulting from release of soluble vasoconstrictive factors can contribute to microvascular dysfunction after stenting. Several agents, such as adenosine, nitroprusside, and calcium channel blockers, have been used to reduce or treat no-reflow in addition to embolic protection devices.

## MECHANICAL COMPLICATIONS

Mechanical complications during graft interventions occur rarely but at an increased rate compared with interventions on native coronary arteries.[52] Mechanical complications include dissections, perforations, aneurysms, and fistulas to other cardiac structures.

## PERFORATION

SVG perforation can occur from guide wire perforation, use of atherectomy devices, or oversizing of either balloon or stent during treatment of the lesion. The incidence of perforations during SVG interventions has been reported to be approximately 0.5%.[52] SVG perforation can cause loss of vessel patency, aneurysm formation, severe hemorrhage and shock, tamponade, and even death. Isolated case reports of pulmonary artery compression and severe right heart failure have also been described.[53] In contrast to the aforementioned grave clinical consequences, however, SVG perforations can also be subclinical and treated conservatively. Other than the size of the initial perforation, it is unclear why some perforations resolve with conservative treatment. One theory is that there is significant mediastinal scarring from the initial sternotomy and bypass surgery that helps contain any perforation.[54]

In some cases, conservative treatment of a promptly recognized SVG perforation includes cessation and/or reversal of anticoagulants and prolonged balloon inflation. If this does not stop, then a covered stent (Jostent) should be used to contain extravascular bleeding and retain vessel patency.[55] The difficulty with covered stents includes challenges with deliverability of a noncompliant stent to a tortuous segment, especially if the segment is very distal and long-term restenosis concerns. Despite these limitations, a covered stent and rapid reversal of anticoagulation are indicated to treat rapid clinical deterioration.

## ANEURYSM AND FISTULA

Aneurysm formation in an SVG is a rare complication that usually occurs greater than 10 years after bypass.[56] Aneurysms can also form after focal dissection of the SVG during a PCI. Depending on the size and location of the aneurysm (**Fig. 2**), patients can be asymptomatic and the aneurysm discovered incidentally (occasionally large enough to be seen on a chest radiograph as a mediastinal mass), or they can present with shortness of breath due to local compression of the pulmonary artery, vein, or atria.[57] Infrequently, the entire aneurysm can thrombose and patients can present with chest pain and an acute coronary syndrome.

Data behind the appropriate management of SVG aneurysms are lacking. Incidentally discovered aneurysms can be treated with a conservative approach that involves frequent monitoring, usually by cardiac CT. Triggers for intervening on coronary aneurysms include a rapidly enlarging aneurysm, an aneurysm that is causing local compression on cardiac structures, and an aneurysm that has ruptured (possibly leading to fistula formation to another cardiac structure). Treatment of SVG aneurysms includes wire coiling/embolization, the use of a covered stent, and surgical excision.

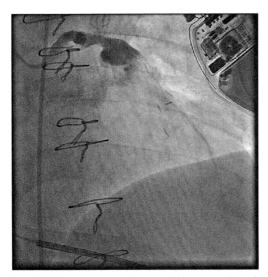

**Fig. 2.** SVG aneurysm: 55-year-old man with past medical history significant for coronary artery bypass surgery in 2004 who presents with chest pain and is noted by CT scan to have an enlarging SVG aneurysm compared over the prior year. Left heart catheterization revealed a large SVG aneurysm to the first diagonal branch with very slow flow to the distal vessel.

Infrequently, an aneurysm can expand and eventually rupture, sometimes leading to a fistula between the vein graft and native cardiac structures, such as the right atrium or pulmonary artery. Most of the case reports of SVG fistula formation involve an SVG to the right coronary artery with the fistula communicating between the vein graft and the right atrium.[58,59] Data behind the appropriate management of an SVG fistula are scarce. The few case reports of SVG fistulas that are cited all involved surgical fixes for the fistula.

## SUMMARY

Due to greater patient comorbidities, more diffusely diseased vessels, and the greater possibility of mechanical complications due to the thin-walled and friable nature of a diseased vein graft, SVG interventions are fraught with complications. The greatest risk with SVG interventions is the higher risk of periprocedural myocardial infarction due to distal embolization of microemboli. The risk for no-reflow in patients with concomitant native critical vessel disease can have grave consequences. Minimizing the risk of periprocedural myocardial infarction with the use of distal embolic protection, understanding the role of adjunctive pharmacotherapy, and learning how to manage less common but serious mechanical complications during SVG intervention are important to ensuring optimal patient outcomes.

## REFERENCES

1. Fitzgibbon GM, Kafka HP, Leach AJ, et al. Coronary bypass graft fate and patient outcome: angiographic follow-up of 5,065 grafts related to survival and reoperation in 1,388 patients during 25 years. J Am Coll Cardiol 1996;28:616–26.
2. Brilakis ES, Rao SV, Banerjee S, et al. Percutaneous coronary intervention in native arteries versus bypass grafts in prior coronary artery bypass grafting patients. JACC Cardiovasc Interv 2011;4:844–50.
3. Pucelikova T, Mehran R, Kirtane AJ, et al. Short and long-term outcomes after stent-assisted percutaneous treatment of saphenous vein grafts in the drug-eluting stent era. Am J Cardiol 2008;101:63–8.
4. Varghese I, Samuel J, Banerjee S, et al. Comparison of percutaneous coronary intervention in native coronary arteries vs. bypass grafts in patients with prior coronary artery bypass graft surgery. Cardiovasc Revasc Med 2009;10:103–9.
5. Welsh RC, Granger CB, Westerhout CM, et al. Prior coronary artery bypass graft patients with ST-segment elevation myocardial infarction treated with primary percutaneous coronary intervention. JACC Cardiovasc Interv 2010;3:343–51.
6. Stone GW, Brodie BR, Griffin JJ, et al. Clinical and angiographic outcomes in patients with previous coronary artery bypass graft surgery treated with primary balloon angioplasty for acute myocardial infarction. Second primary angiopalsty in myocardial infarction trial (PAMI-s) investigators. J Am Coll Cardiol 2000;35:605–11.
7. Greason KL, Schaff HV. Myocardial revascularization by coronary arterial bypass graft: past, present, and future. Curr Probl Cardiol 2011;36:325–68.
8. Mueller RL, Rosengart TK, Isom OW. The history of surgery forischemic heart disease. Ann Thorac Surg 1997;63:869–78.
9. Cobb LA, Thomas GI, Dillard DH, et al. An evaluation of internal-mammary-artery ligation by a double-blind technic. N Engl J Med 1959;260:1115–8.
10. Beck CS. The development of a new blood supply to the heart by operation. Ann Surg 1935;102:801–13.
11. O'Shaughnessy L. Angina pectoris treated by cardio-pneumonopexy. Proc R Soc Med 1939;32:437.
12. Vineberg A, Miller G. Treatment of coronary insufficiency. CMAJ 1951;64:204–10.
13. Sones FM Jr, Shirey EK. Cine coronary arteriography. Mod Concepts Cardiovasc Dis 1962;31:735–8.
14. Cheng TO. History of coronary artery bypass surgery—half of a century of progress. Int J Cardiol 2012;157(1):1–2.
15. Buxton B, Frazier OH, Westaby S. Ischemic heart disease surgical management. London: Mosby International; 1999. p. 3.

16. Sabiston DC. The William F Reinhoff Jr. lecture. The coronary circulation. Johns Hopkins Med J 1974; 134:314–29.

17. Konstantinov IE. The first coronary artery bypass operation and forgotten pioneers. Ann Thorac Surg 1997;64:1522–3.

18. Favaloro RG. Saphenous vein autograft replacement of severe segmental coronary artery occlusion. Operative technique. Ann Thorac Surg 1968;5:334–9.

19. Garrett HE, Dennis EW, DeBakey ME. Aortocoronary bypass with saphenous vein graft. Seven-year follow-up. JAMA 1973;223:792–4.

20. Roubos N, Rosenfeldt FL, Richards SM, et al. Improved preservation of saphenous vein grafts by the use of glyceryl trinitrate - verapamil solution during harvesting. Circulation 1995;92(Suppl II): II-31–6.

21. Zhao DX, Leacche M, Balaguer JM, et al. Routine intraoperative completion angiography after coronary artery bypass grafting and 1-stop hybrid revascularization. Results from a fully integrated hybrid catheterization laboratory/operating room. J Am Coll Cardiol 2009;53:232–41.

22. Chen L, Theroux P, Lesperance J, et al. Angiographic features of vein grafts versus ungrafted coronary arteries in patients with unstable angina and previous bypass surgery. J Am Coll Cardiol 1996;28:1493–9.

23. Douglas JS. Percutaneous approaches to recurrent myocardial ischemia in patients with prior surgical revascularization. Semin Thorac Cardiovasc Surg 1994;6:98–108.

24. Motwani JG, Topol EJ. Aortocoronary saphenous vein graft disease: pathogenesis, predisposition, and prevention. Circulation 1998;97:916–31.

25. Kalan JM, Roberts WC. Morphologic findings in saphenous veins used as coronary arterial bypass conduits for longer than 1 year: necropsy analysis of 53 patients, 123 saphenous veins, and 1865 five-millimeter segments of veins. Am Heart J 1990;119: 1164–84.

26. Neitzel GF, Barboriak JJ, Pintar K, et al. Atherosclerosis in aortocoronary bypass grafts: morphologic study and risk factor analysis 6 to 12 years after surgery. Arteriosclerosis 1986;6:594–600.

27. Chesebro JM, Fuster V. Platelet-inhibitor drugs before and after coronary artery bypass surgery and coronary angioplasty: the basis of their use, data from animal studies, clinical trial data, and current recommendations. Cardiology 1986;73:292–305.

28. Ratliff NB, Myles JL. Rapidly progressive atherosclerosis in aortocoronary saphenous vein grafts: possible immune-mediated disease. Arch Pathol Lab Med 1989;113:772–6.

29. Roffi M, Mukherjee D, Chew DP, et al. Lack of benefit from intravenous platelet glycoprotein IIb/IIIa receptor inhibition as adjunctive treatment for percutaneous interventions of aortocoronary bypass grafts: a pooled analysis of five randomized clinical trials. Circulation 2002;106(24):3063–7.

30. Savage MP, Douglas JS, Fischman DL, et al. Stent placement compared with balloon angioplasty for obstructed coronary bypass grafts. Saphenous Vein De Novo Trial Investigators. N Engl J Med 1997;337(11):740–7.

31. Brodie BR, Stuckey T, Downey W, et al. Outcomes and complications with off-label use of drug-eluting stents: results from the STENT (strategic transcatheter evaluvation of new therapies) group. JACC Cardiovasc Interv 2008;1:405–14.

32. Meier P, Brilakis ES, Corti R, et al. Dug-eluting ersus bare-metal stent for treatment of saphenous vein grafts: a meta-analysis. PLoS One 2010;5:e11040.

33. Gorog DA, Foale RA, Malik I. Distal myocardial protection during percutaneous coronary intervention: when and where. J Am Coll Cardiol 2005;46: 1434–45.

34. Piana RN, Paik GY, Moscucci M, et al. Incidence and treatment of 'no-reflow' after percutaneous coronary intervention. Circulation 1994;89:2514–8.

35. Angelini A, Rubartelli P, Mistrorigo F, et al. Distal protection with a filter device during coronary stenting in patients with stable and unstable angina. Circulation 2004;110(5):515–21.

36. Sdringola S, Assali AR, Ghani M, et al. Risk assessment of slow or no-reflow phenomenon in aortocoronary vein graft percutaneous intervention. Catheter Cardiovasc Interv 2001;54:318–24.

37. Lee MS, Park SJ, Kandzari DE. Saphenous vein graft intervention. JACC Cardiovasc Interv 2011;4: 831–43.

38. Giugliano GR, Kuntz RE, Popma JJ, et al. Determinants of 30-day adverse events following saphenous ein graft intervention with an without a distal occlusion embolic protection device. Am J Cardiol 2005; 95(2):173–7.

39. Hong MK, Mehran R, Dangas G, et al. Creatine kinase-MB enzyme elevation following successful saphenous vein graft intervention is associated with late mortality. Circulation 1999;100(24):2400–5.

40. ACC/AHA PCI Guidelines reference. Distal protection is a class I indication.

41. Leborgne L, Cheneau E, Pichard A, et al. Effect of direct stenting on clinical outcome in patients treated with percutaneous coronary intervention on saphenous vein graft. Am Heart J 2003;146:501–6.

42. Turco MA, Buchbinder M, Popma JJ, et al. Pivotal, randomized U.S. study of the Symbiot covered stent system in patients with saphenous vein graft disease: eight-month angiographic and clinical results from the Symbiot III trial. Catheter Cardiovasc Interv 2006;68:379–88.

43. Stankovic G, Colombo A, Presbitero P, et al, for the RECOVERS Trial Investigators. Randomized

evaluation of polytetrafluoroethylenecovered stent in saphenous vein grafts: the Randomized Evaluation of polytetrafluoroethylene COVERed stent in Saphenous vein grafts (RECOVERS) trial. Circulation 2003; 108:37–42.

44. Stone GW, Goldberg S, O'Shaughnessy C, et al. Five-year follow-up of polytetrafluoroethylene-covered stents compared with bare-metal stents in aortocoronary saphenous vein graft: the randomized BARRICADE (Barrier Approach to Restenosis: restrict Intima to Curtail Adverse Events) Trial. JACC Cardiovasc Interv 2011;4:300–9.

45. Baim DS, Wahr D, George B, et al, for the SAFER Trial Investigators. Randomized trial of a distal embolic protection device during percutaneous intervention of saphenous vein aorto-coronary bypass grafts. Circulation 2002;105(11):1285–90.

46. Carrozza JP, Mumma M, Breall JA, et al, for the PRIDE Study Investigators. Randomized evaluation of the TriActiv balloon protection flush and extraction system for the treatment of saphenous vein graft disease. J Am Coll Cardiol 2005;46:1677–83.

47. Mauri L, Cox D, Hermiller J, et al. The PROXIMAL trial: proximal protection during saphenous vein graft intervention using the Proxis Embolic Protection System: a randomized, prospective, multicenter clinical trial. J Am Coll Cardiol 2007;50:1442–9.

48. Stone GW, Rogers C, Hermiller J, et al, for the Filter-Wire EX Randomized Evaluation Investigators. Randomized comparison of distal protection with a filter-based catheter and a balloon occlusion and aspiration system during percutaneous intervention of diseased saphenous vein aortocoronary bypass grafts. Circulation 2003;108:548–53.

49. Brilakis ES, Wang TY, Rao SV, et al. Frequency and predictors of drug-eluting stent use in saphenous vein bypass graft percutaneous coronary interventions: a report from the American College of Cardiology National Cardiovascular Data CathPCI Registry. JACC Cardiovasc Interv 2010;3:1068–73.

50. Ellis SG, Lincoff AM, Miller D, et al. Reduction in ocmplications of angioplasty with abciximab occurs largely independently of baseline lesion morphology. EPIC and EPILOG investigators. Evaluation of 7E3 for the prevention of ischemic complications. Evaluation of PTCA to improve long-term outcome with abciximab GP IIb/IIIa receptor blockade. J Am Coll Cardiol 1998;32(6):1619–23.

51. Jonas M, Stone GW, Mehran R, et al. Platelet glycoprotein IIb/IIIa receptor inhibition as adjunctive treatment during saphenous vein graft stenting: differential deffecs after randomization to occlusion or filter-based embolic protection. Eur Heart J 2006; 27(8):920–8.

52. Douglas J, Robinson K, Schlumpf M. Percutaneous transluminal angioplasty in aortocoronary venous graft stenoses: immediate results and complications. Circulation 1986;74(Suppl II):I1–281.

53. Poulter RS, Dorris M. Localized pulmonary artery compression due to saphenous vein graft perforation during percutaneous coronary intervention. Can J Cardiol 2011;27(389):e25–8.

54. Teirstein PS, Hartzler GO. Nonoperative mamagement of aorto-coronary saphenous vein graft rupture during percutaneous transluminal coronary angioplasty. Am J Cardiol 1987;60:377–8.

55. Hernandez-Antolin R, Banuelos C, Alfonso F, et al. Successful sealing of an angioplasty related saphenous vein graft rupture with a PTFE-covered stent. J Invasive Cardiol 2000;12:589–93.

56. Gruberg L, Satler LF, Pfister AJ, et al. A large coronary artery saphenous vein bypass graft aneurysm with a fistula: case report and review of the literature. Catheter Cardiovasc Interv 1999;48:214–6.

57. Austin D, Asopa S, Owens WA, et al. Compression of main pulmonary artery by giant saphenous vein graft aneurysm. Ann Thorac Surg 2011;92:742.

58. Le Breton H, Langanay T, Roland Y, et al. Aneurysms and pseudoaneurysms of saphenous vein coronary artery bypass grafts. Heart 1998;79:505–8.

59. Jukema JW, Van Dickman PR, Van Der Wall EE. Pseudoaneurysm of a saphenous vein coronary artery bypass graft with a fistula draining into the right atrium. Am Heart J 1992;124:1397–9.

# Thrombectomy Devices in Coronary Intervention

Aaron Horne Jr, MD, Matthews Chacko, MD*

## KEYWORDS

- Thrombectomy • Percutaneous coronary intervention • ST-elevation myocardial infarction
- Rheolysis

## KEY POINTS

- TAPAS was the first multicenter randomized controlled trial to find that manual thrombus aspiration could be performed in most patients with STEMI, irrespective of their clinical or angiographic features (eg, a visible thrombus on angiography) resulting in improved myocardial reperfusion and clinical outcome compared with conventional PCI.
- INFUSE-AMI demonstrated that in patients with large anterior STEMI undergoing primary PCI with bivalirudin for anticoagulation, infarct size at 30 days was significantly reduced by bolus intracoronary abciximab delivered to the infarct lesion site through an infusion catheter but not by manual aspiration thrombectomy.
- The results of the TOTAL, TASTE, and SMART PCI trials will provide additional insight concerning optimal management of this vulnerable patient population.

## BACKGROUND AND INTRODUCTION

Ruptured atherosclerotic plaque causing thrombosis and occlusion of the infarct-related coronary artery was identified as the cause of acute myocardial infarction in the 1970s.[1] Improvements in adjunctive pharmacotherapy and the recognition that prompt restoration of coronary blood flow salvages myocardium, reduces infarct size, and prolongs life ultimately led to coupling antithrombotic therapy with percutaneous coronary intervention (PCI).[2] Because of improvements in PCI technique and adjunctive pharmacotherapy, timely PCI is the preferred reperfusion strategy in patients with ST-elevation myocardial infarction (STEMI).[2]

Early studies demonstrated that patent epicardial vessels did not guarantee optimal myocardial perfusion.[3] The "no-reflow" phenomenon, an open epicardial artery without flow into the myocardium, is a well-known complication of reperfusion therapy with PCI and its presence is predictive of downstream complications and left ventricular dilation.[4,5] No-reflow is thought to be secondary to distal embolization of platelet-rich thrombus and atherosclerotic debris from ruptured plaque leading to microvascular obstruction. This insight led to the development of devices to minimize distal thromboembolization during PCI for STEMI.

Thrombectomy catheters generally use one of two mechanisms to extract thrombus: manual aspiration or rheolysis, with the primary difference being that the rheolytic devices fragment the thrombus before extraction. The latest American College of Cardiology/American Heart Association guidelines[6] give thrombectomy a class IIa recommendation; however, this recommendation may need to be revisited depending on the results of recent and ongoing multicenter clinical trials. This article provides a comprehensive overview of key trials of mechanical and rheolytic thrombectomy in the management of STEMI.

Division of Cardiology, Johns Hopkins Hospital, Johns Hopkins University, 1800 Orleans Street, Baltimore, MD 21287, USA
* Corresponding author. Sheikh Zayed Tower 7125V, Carnegie 568, Baltimore, MD 21287.
E-mail address: mchacko@jhmi.edu

Intervent Cardiol Clin 2 (2013) 347–359
http://dx.doi.org/10.1016/j.iccl.2012.12.001
2211-7458/13/$ – see front matter © 2013 Elsevier Inc. All rights reserved.

## RHEOLYTIC THROMBECTOMY

Two rheolytic thrombectomy devices have been investigated in randomized controlled trials, the X-sizer (Covidien, Mansfield, MA), which is no longer available, and the Angiojet (Medrad, Indianola, PA). The first thrombectomy trial was a single-center prospective randomized controlled trial published by Beran and colleagues[7] in 2002 comparing conventional PCI with thrombectomy using the X-sizer thrombectomy device in 66 patients with acute coronary syndromes. Thrombolysis in myocardial infarction (TIMI) flow grade 3 was obtained in 90% of X-sizer–treated patients and in 84% of control subjects; however, corrected TIMI frame count was lower in X-sizer–treated patients and there were no significant differences between the intervention and control groups observed in final coronary flow reserve, myocardial blush grade (MBG), and myocardial dye intensity. However, in patients with STEMI (representing 49 of the 66 patients enrolled in the study) the sum of ST elevation was significantly lower with X-sizer immediately and 6 hours after intervention. ST resolution (>50%) was observed in 83% of X-sizer–treated patients and in 52% of control subjects ($P<.03$). Multivariate analysis identified X-sizer treatment as the single independent predictor of ST resolution. The results of this trial were inconclusive but the improvement of surrogate end points in the X-sizer arm of patients with STEMI undoubtedly spurred cautious optimism regarding the potential use of thrombectomy in this subgroup of patients with subsequent studies structured to better assess clinical outcomes in patients with STEMI.

After this, additional rheolytic thrombectomy devices were evaluated with more rigor and emphasis on hard clinical end points. In 2005, Lefevre and colleagues[8] published the X-AMINE ST trial, which was a prospective randomized multicenter study of 201 patients with STEMI and TIMI flow grade 0 to 1 randomized to thrombectomy using the X-Sizer plus PCI versus conventional PCI with a primary end point of ST resolution 1 hour after PCI. The magnitude of ST resolution was greater in the X-Sizer group compared with the conventional group (7.5 vs 4.9 mm, respectively; $P = .033$) and ST resolution greater than 50% (68% vs 53%; $P = .037$). Furthermore, the occurrence of distal embolization was reduced (2% vs 10%; $P = .033$) and TIMI flow grade 3 was obtained in 96% versus 89% in the X-sizer and conventional groups, respectively ($P = .105$). Although the ST resolution and distal embolization surrogate end points were encouraging, the comparable MBGs and 6-month clinical

outcomes between the intervention and control arms left many with lingering uncertainty. Criticisms of the study were that it was limited to patients with TIMI flow grade 0 or 1, did not include the entire STEMI population, and that the possible treatment benefit of adjunctive pharmacologic therapy was not evaluated.

The enthusiasm for thrombectomy in patients with STEMI was further diminished with the AIMI trial, published by Ali and colleagues[9] in 2006, which was a trial of 480 patients with STEMI that showed no benefit of the Angiojet device in terms of TIMI flow, MBG, or ST resolution and actually showed higher 30-day Major Adverse Cardiac Event (MACE) rates ($P = .01$) and infarct sizes by nuclear imaging.

The JETSTENT trial,[10] published in 2010, restored some faith in thrombectomy showing that despite comparable TIMI flow, MBG, and infarct sizes (by nuclear imaging), there was more ST resolution (85.8% vs 78.8%; $P = .043$), a reduction in 6-month MACE rates (11.2% vs 19.4%; $P = .011$), and better 1-year event-free survival rates (85.2% vs 75.0%; $P = .009$) with the Angiojet device compared with direct stenting in 501 patients presenting with STEMI. JETSTENT included all patients with STEMI without restriction based on age or clinical status on presentation. Additionally, patients with angiographic evidence of thrombus were included, which is not an attribute that is replicated across all thrombectomy randomized controlled trials, and potentially resulted in the different outcomes seen in AIMI. Of note, all of the patients received abciximab unless contraindicated, which was an important component of this trial because investigators continued to clarify the potential synergistic role that adjunctive devices and pharmacotherapy play in the management of patients with STEMI.

## MANUAL ASPIRATION THROMBECTOMY

The first study examining manual aspiration thrombectomy in patients with STEMI was published in 2004 by Dudek and colleagues[11] using the Rescue catheter (Boston Scientific, Natick, MA). The investigators prospectively randomized 100 consecutive patients with STEMI to PCI with or without manual thrombus aspiration. The results favored thrombectomy, with the higher rates of postprocedural MBG greater than or equal to 2 (68% vs 58%) and ST resolution greater than 70% (44.9% vs 36.7%) in the thrombus-aspiration group versus the standard PCI group. In multivariate analysis, thrombus-aspiration was a significant independent predictor of MBG greater than or equal to 2 and ST resolution greater than 70% ($P = .013$). The results showed that aspiration thrombectomy in unselected patients with STEMI undergoing primary or rescue PCI was clinically feasible and resulted in better angiographic and electrocardiogram myocardial reperfusion compared with those achieved by standard PCI, although clinical end points were not assessed.

After this, multiple trials[12–16] of aspiration thrombectomy showed variable and disparate results with a consistent theme being the lack of decreased mortality or MACE associated with the use of these devices. In 2008, Svilaas and colleagues[17] published the results of the pivotal TAPAS trial, which was a prospective single-center trial of 1071 patients with STEMI undergoing primary PCI randomly assigned (before angiography) to aspiration thrombectomy with the Export catheter (Medtronic, Minneapolis, MN) or to conventional PCI. An MBG of 0 or 1 occurred in 17.1% of the patients in the thrombus-aspiration group and 26.3% of those in the conventional PCI group (P<.001). Complete resolution of ST elevation occurred in 56.6% and 44.2% of patients, respectively (P<.001). Additionally, there was a trend toward better short-term MACE rates and reinfarction with a statistically significant reduction in cardiac death at 1 year (3.6% vs 6.7%; P = .02) in favor of aspiration thrombectomy.[18] Criticisms of the trial included that it was a single-center experience using surrogate end points, randomization occurred before coronary angiography resulting in some patients not undergoing PCI or receiving the alternative therapy, and the use of balloon predilation before stenting. An important observation from the TAPAS trial was that the benefit of aspiration thrombectomy was seen regardless of baseline features, such as infarct-related artery, preprocedural TIMI flow, or visible thrombus at angiography. Furthermore, atherothrombotic debris was retrieved in 72.9% of the patients who underwent thrombus aspiration with the main constituent of the aspirate being platelet-rich thrombi, even if no visible thrombus was seen on initial angiography. This underscores the importance of platelets and antiplatelet therapy in combating no-reflow.

Studies subsequent to TAPAS have reproduced the findings that manual aspiration thrombectomy devices can improve clinical outcomes in patients with STEMI. Among them was the EXPIRA trial,[19] which randomized 175 patients with STEMI at a single center to standard PCI (n = 87) or manual thrombectomy with the Export catheter in a subset of patients with anterior STEMI (n = 88). MBG greater than or equal to 2 (88% vs 60%; P = .001) and ST resolution (64% vs 39%; P = .001) occurred more frequently in the thrombectomy group with a lower incidence of cardiac death in the thrombectomy group (4.6% vs 0%; P = .02) at 9 months.

To assess the possible synergy between antithrombotic pharmacotherapy and aspiration thrombectomy, the INFUSE AMI trial,[20] published in 2012, was a multicenter study of 452 patients presenting within 4 hours of STEMI caused by proximal or mid-left anterior descending (LAD) artery occlusion undergoing PCI with bivalirudin. The trial compared bolus intracoronary abciximab delivered locally through an infusion catheter (Clearway Rx; Atrium Medical, Hudson, NH) and aspiration thrombectomy (Export catheter). Patients were randomized to one of four groups: (1) thrombectomy followed by intracoronary bolus abciximab, (2) thrombectomy without abciximab, (3) intracoronary bolus abciximab without thrombectomy, or (4) no abciximab and no thrombectomy. The primary end point was 30-day infarct size assessed by cardiac magnetic resonance imaging. Patients randomized to intracoronary abciximab (n = 181) compared with no abciximab (n = 172) had a significant reduction in 30-day infarct size (15.1% vs 17.9%; P = .03). Patients randomized to thrombectomy (n = 174) compared with no thrombectomy (n = 179) had no significant difference in 30-day infarct size (17% vs 17.3%; P = .51). The thrombectomy plus abciximab group showed the lowest median 30-day infarct size of 14.7% compared with 17.6% for the other three groups combined. The study was limited by several factors: (1) being single-blinded; (2) containing a highly selected population of primarily Killip class I patients with STEMI with only 7.2% of the 6318 screened patients with STEMI enrolled; (3) the confounding issue of unavoidable mechanical disruption of thrombus with the infusion catheter perhaps contributing to the lowest 30-day infarct sizes in the combined thrombectomy plus abciximab group; and (4) incomplete follow-up relevant to the primary end point with infarct size assessment by cardiac magnetic resonance imaging available in only 353 of 452 (78%) of patients. Nevertheless, the authors concluded that in patients with anterior STEMI presenting early and undergoing primary PCI with bivalirudin for anticoagulation, 30-day infarct size was significantly reduced by bolus intracoronary abciximab delivered to the infarct lesion site through an infusion catheter but not by thrombectomy.

## FUTURE DIRECTIONS

The results of the INFUSE-AMI trial have reinfused controversy into the discussion about the optimal management strategy for patients with STEMI in light of the lack of benefit demonstrated in the adjunctive thrombectomy arm of the INFUSE-AMI trial in contrast to the findings of the TAPAS

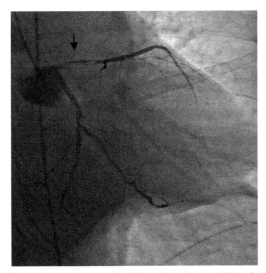

Fig. 1. Angiogram of visible thrombus within the proximal LAD.

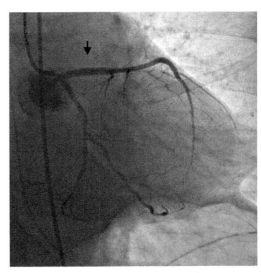

Fig. 3. Angiogram of the stented LAD after aspiration thrombectomy.

trial. Given this, there is heightened interest in the forthcoming TOTAL and TASTE trials. The TOTAL trial[21] is a randomized trial of aspiration thrombectomy (Export catheter) versus no thrombectomy in patients with STEMI undergoing primary PCI. End points include cardiovascular death, recurrent myocardial infarction, cardiogenic shock, and new or worsening New York Heart Association Class IV heart failure at 180 days.

Similar to TOTAL but larger in scale and potential long-term impact is the TASTE trial,[22] which is a multicenter, prospective, randomized, controlled, open-label trial of 5000 patients with

STEMI assigned to conventional PCI or to thrombectomy with PCI and subsequently followed in the Swedish Coronary Angiography and Angioplasty Registry platform with blinded evaluation of end points. This design allows a broad population of all-comers in the registry network to be enrolled to assess the primary end point of all-cause death at 30 days. Notably, a variety of aspiration thrombectomy catheters will be used in the TASTE trial including the Export, OXT (Vascular Solutions, Minneapolis, MN), and Pronto catheters (Vascular Solutions). Furthermore, the use of a glycoprotein IIb/IIIa inhibitor will be left to the discretion of the operator. The TASTE trial will be the largest trial to date to evaluate the impact of aspiration thrombectomy on death in patients with STEMI undergoing PCI.

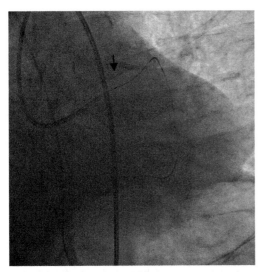

Fig. 2. Angiogram of aspiration thrombectomy being performed (Export catheter; Medtronic, Minneapolis, MN).

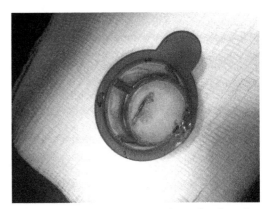

Fig. 4. Contents of the aspirate from the thrombectomized LAD.

**Table 1**
**Thrombectomy devices in randomized trials**

| Device | Mechanism of Action | Picture of Device | Manufacturer |
|--------|---------------------|-------------------|--------------|
| *Aspiration Thrombectomy* | | | |
| Diver C.E. | Rapid-exchange, 6F catheter compatible, thrombus-aspirating catheter with central aspiration lumen and soft, flexible, 0.026-in, nontraumatic tip with multiple holes (one large anterior and three smaller lateral holes) communicating with the central lumen; 30-mL Luer-lock syringe connected to proximal hub of central lumen for thrombus aspiration | | Medtronic, Inc (Photo courtesy of Medtronic Inc., Minneapolis MN; with permission.) |

*(continued on next page)*

**Table 1**
*(continued)*

| Device | Mechanism of Action | Picture of Device | Manufacturer |
|---|---|---|---|
| Export | 6F catheter with an obilque tip and a 0.041-in aspiration lumen with a 0.068-in crossing profile; aspiration is provided by hand with a lockable 20-mL syringe, which allows a suction rate of 1 mL/s | 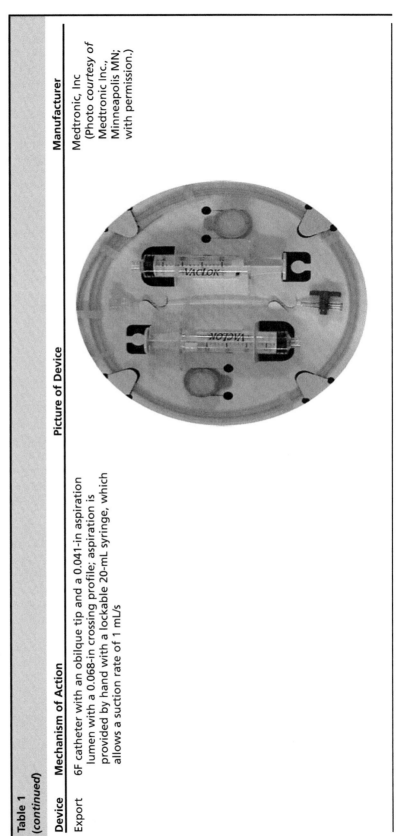 | Medtronic, Inc (Photo courtesy of Medtronic Inc., Minneapolis MN; with permission.) |

| | | |
|---|---|---|
| Pronto | 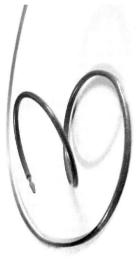 | Vascular Solutions, Inc (Photo courtesy of Vascular Solutions, Inc., Minneapolis MN; with permission.) |
| | Dual-lumen monorail design with 6F catheter compatible catheter, the smaller lumen accommodates a 0.014-in guidewire, and the larger extraction lumen allows thrombus removal, which is aspirated with a 30-mL locking-vacuum syringe, the catheter has a round distal tip designed to maximize thrombus aspiration and protect the vessel wall while advancing and during aspiration. | |
| Rescue | | Boston Scientific Corporation (Photo courtesy of Boston Scientific, Natick, MA; with permission.) |
| | 4.5F catheter advanced over a guidewire through a 7F guiding catheter, the proximal end of the catheter has an extension tube connected to a vacuum pump (0.8 bar) with a collection bottle, a continuous suction is applied while the catheter is advanced and pulled through the thrombus. | Aspiration regulation system; Aspiration tube extension; Aspiration catheter; Connection to vacuum console; Distal end of the catheter; Vacuum bottle; Intracoronary guide exit opening (monorail); B |
| TVAC | Picture not available | Nipro |
| | Single-lumen, rapid-exchange aspiration shaft compatible with a 7F guiding catheter and has a dedicated vacuum pump; the catheter has a block-shaped distal tip and a shaft with spring support. | |

(continued on next page)

**Table 1**
*(continued)*

| Device | Mechanism of Action | Picture of Device | Manufacturer |
|---|---|---|---|
| *Rheolytic Thrombectomy* | | | |
| Angiojet | Rheolytic thrombectomy system comprising a drive unit console, disposable pump set, and 4F catheter, high-velocity saline jets contained within the distal catheter tip, creating a strong negative pressure (Bernoulli effect) that entrains the thrombus to the catheter inflow windows where it is captured, fragmented, and evacuated through the outflow lumen. | | Medrad Interventional (Photo courtesy of Bayer HealthCare LLC, Wayne, NJ; with permission.) |
| X-Sizer | Two-lumen, over-the-wire system with a helical shape cutter at its distal tip; the cutter rotates at 2100 rpm driven by a hand-held battery motor, one catheter lumen is connected to a 250-mL vacuum bottle, and aspirated debris is collected in an inline filter. | Picture not available | Covidien |

*Adapted from* Yetgin T, Magro M, van Geuns RJ, et al. Utilizing thrombectomy during PCI for STEMI. Current evidence, unresolved questions, and future trials. Cardiac Interventions Today 2012; with permission.

**Table 2**
**Randomized clinical trials investigating thrombectomy in STEMI**

| Study | Study Acronym | Number of Centers | N | Device | Primary End Point and Outcome | Clinical End point and Outcome |
|---|---|---|---|---|---|---|
| *Single-Center Rheolytic Thrombectomy Trials* | | | | | | |
| Beran et al,[7] 2002 | N/A | Single | 46 | X-Sizer | (+) STR | ($\neq$) 30-d MACE |
| Napodano et al,[28] 2003 | N/A | Single | 92 | X-Sizer | (+) MBG-3 | ($\neq$) 30-d MACE |
| Antoniucci et al,[29] 2004 | N/A | Single | 100 | Angiojet | (+) STR | ($\neq$) 30-d MACE |
| Lefevre et al,[8] 2005 | X-AMINE ST | Single | 201 | X-Sizer | (+) STR | ($\neq$) 60-d MACE ($\neq$) 60-d MACE |
| *Multicenter Rheolytic Thrombectomy Trials* | | | | | | |
| Ali et al,[9] 2006 | AIMI | Thirty-one | 480 | Angiojet | (−) IS | (−) 30-d MACE ($P = .01$) |
| Migliorini et al,[10] 2010 | JETSTENT | Eight | 501 | Angiojet | (+) STR, (−) IS | (−) 30-d MACE ($P = .04$) |
| *Single-Center Manual Aspiration Thrombectomy Trials* | | | | | | |
| Dudek et al,[11] 2004 | N/A | Single | 72 | Rescue | $\neq$ TIMI3, cTFC, tMPG (+) STR | N/A |
| Burzotta et al,[30] 2005 | REMEDIA | Single | 99 | Diver C.E. | (+) MBG $\geq$2, STR | $\neq$ 30-d MACE |
| De Luca et al,[12] 2005 | N/A | Single | 76 | Diver C.E. | (+) MBG3, STR | $\neq$ 6-mo MACE |
| Silva-Orrego et al,[13] 2006 | DEAR-MI | Single | 148 | Pronto | (+) MBG3, STR | $\neq$ in-hospital MACE |
| Kaltoft et al,[14] 2006 | N/A | Single | 215 | Rescue | $\neq$ Myocardial Salvage | $\neq$ 30-d MACE |
| Andersen et al,[31] 2007 | N/A | Single | 122 | Rescue | $\neq$ Left ventricular function | N/A |
| Chao et al,[16] 2008 | N/A | Single | 74 | Export | (+) Post-TIMI flow, MBG | N/A |
| Silvaas et al,[17] 2008 | TAPAS | Single | 1071 | Export | (+) MBG 0/1 | (+) 1-y mortality ($P = .04$) (+) 1-y cardiac death ($P = .02$) |
| Lipiecki et al,[32] 2009 | N/A | Single | 44 | Export | $\neq$ IS | N/A |
| Liistro et al,[33] 2009 | N/A | Single | 111 | Export | (+) STR | $\neq$ 6-mo MACE |
| Sardella et al,[19] 2009 | EXPIRA | Single | 175 | Export | (+) MBG $\geq$2, STR | (+) 2-y cardiac death ($P = .0001$) (+) 2-y MACE ($P = .04$) |
| Ciszewski et al,[34] 2011 | N/A | Single | 137 | Rescue/ Diver C.E. | (+) Myocardial salvage | $\neq$ In-hospital mortality |
| *Multicenter Manual Aspiration Thrombectomy Trials* | | | | | | |
| Dudek et al,[15] 2010 | PIHRATE | Ten | 196 | Diver CE | $\neq$ STR | $\neq$ 6-mo mortality |
| Ikari et al,[35] 2008 | VAMPIRE | Twenty-three | 355 | TVAC | (+trend) SRNR (TTMI <3) | (+) 8-mo MACE ($P<.05$) |

*(continued on next page)*

**Table 2**
*(continued)*

| Study | Study Acronym | Number of Centers | N | Device | Primary End Point and Outcome | Clinical End point and Outcome |
|---|---|---|---|---|---|---|
| Chevalier et al,[36] 2008 | EXPORT | Twenty-four | 249 | Export | (+) MBG3, STR | ≠ 30-d MACCE |
| Frobert et al,[22] rationale published in 2010 | TASTE | Twenty-nine | 5000 | Export/OXT/Pronto | | Time to all-cause death at 30 d |
| Stone et al,[20] 2012 | INFUSE-AMI | Thirty-seven | 452 | Export | (+) IS in abciximab but not manual aspiration group | ≠ 30 d clinical events |
| Jolly et al,[21] June 2014 is the final data collection date for primary outcome | TOTAL | Twenty-nine | 4000 | Export | | First occurrence of CV death, recurrent MI, cardiogenic shock or new or worsening New York Heart Association class IV heart failure |
| *Intramanual Aspiration Thrombectomy Trial* | | | | | | |
| Sardella et al,[26] 2008 | RETAMI | Single-center | 103 | Diver-Invatec1 (DI) vs Export Medtronic (EM) | (+) TS ≤2, TIMI flow grade ≥2, MBG ≥2 in the EM compared with the DI group | ≠ MACE at 1 and 12 mo |
| *Manual Aspiration vs Rheolytic Thrombectomy Trial* | | | | | | |
| Antoniucci[25] March 2012 is estimate study completion date | SMART-PCI | Single-center | 80 | Export vs Angiojet | Postthrombectomy thrombus burden assessed by coronary OCT | 6- and 12-mo MACE |

*Abbreviations:* (+), improved end point; (≠), neutral effect on end point; (−), worsened end point; AIMI, AngioJet Rheolytic Thrombectomy in Patients Undergoing Primary Angioplasty for Acute Myocardial Infarction; cTFC, corrected TIMI frame count; DEAR-MI, Dethrombosis to Enhance Acute Reperfusion in Myocardial Infarction; EXPIRA, Thrombectomy With Export Catheter in Infarct-Related Artery During Primary Percutaneous Coronaiy Intervention; EXPORT, Prospective, Multicentre, Randomized Study of the Export Aspiration Catheter; INFUSE-AMI, Intracoronary Abciximab and Aspiration Thrombectomy in Patients With Large Anterior Myocardial Infarction; IS, infarct size; JETSTENT, Comparison of AngioJet Rheolytic Thrombectomy Before Direct Infarct Artery Stenting With Direct Stenting Alone in Patients With Acute Myocardial Infarction; MACCE, major adverse cardiac and cerebral events; NR, no-reflow; N/A, not applicable; OCT, Optical Coherence Tomography; PIHRATE, Polish-Italian-Hungarian Randomized Thrombectomy Trial; REMEDIA, Randomized Evaluation of the Effect of Mechanical Reduction of Distal Embolization by Thrombus Aspiration in Primary and Rescue Angioplasty; SR, slow-reflow; STR, ST-segment resolution; TAP AS, Thrombus Aspiration During Percutaneous Coronary Intervention in Acute Myocardial Infarction Study; TASTE, Thrombus Aspiration in ST-Elevation myocardial infarction in Scandinavia; tMPG, TIMI myocardial perfusion grade; TOTAL, A Trial of Routine Aspiration Thrombectomy With Percutaneous Coronary Intervention Versus PCI Alone in Patients With ST-Segment Elevation Myocardial Infarction Undergoing Primary PCI; VAMPIRE, Vacuum Aspiration Thrombus Removal; X-AMINE ST, X-sizer in AMI for Negligible Embolization and Optimal ST Resolution.

*Adapted from* Yetgin T, Magro M, van Geuns RJ, et al. Utilizing thrombectomy during PCI for STEMI. Current evidence, unresolved questions, and future trials. Cardiac Interventions Today 2012; with permission.

Aspiration and rheolytic thrombectomy devices have demonstrated a clinical benefit in patients with STEMI; however, many trials were too small and underpowered to assess clinical end points. Additionally, the variability of devices evaluated in nonuniform clinical settings imposed inherent challenges on interpreting disparate results from thrombectomy trials. To harmonize interpretation of these studies, meta-analyses have shown a trend toward a survival benefit with manual aspiration thrombectomy devices.[23,24] Mongeon and colleagues[23] identified 21 eligible trials involving 4299 patients with STEMI randomized to primary PCI with or without thrombectomy and found that thrombectomy improved early markers of reperfusion, but did not substantially effect 30-day post-MI mortality, reinfarction, and stroke. A meta-analysis done by Tamhane and colleagues[24] examined 3909 patients from 17 randomized trials of thrombectomy for STEMI, and similarly found that thrombectomy seemed to improve myocardial perfusion with a trend toward survival benefit in favor of manual aspiration thrombectomy, worsening outcomes with rheolytic thrombectomy, and no difference in overall 30-day mortality but an increased likelihood of stroke. Although no randomized controlled studies of rheolytic versus aspiration thrombectomy in STEMI have been done, the SMART-PCI[25] trial may help to answer that question in the near future.

Questions also remain as to which type of thrombectomy should be performed or if one thrombectomy catheter is superior to another. The RETAMI trial[26] was a prospective trial of 103 patients with STEMI undergoing thrombectomy with PCI using one of two different aspiration thrombectomy catheters, the Diver (Invatec, Bethlehem, PA) (n = 52) and Export (n = 51). In this small single-center study, the Export catheter seemed to remove more thrombus compared with the Diver providing greater postthrombectomy epicardial coronary flow and microvascular perfusion.

Data aside, there are technical and procedural differences to consider in evaluating which thrombectomy device to select. Rheolytic thrombectomy catheters are bulkier, have steeper learning curves, may have longer procedure times impacting door-to-balloon time, often require a temporary pacemaker to prevent associated symptomatic bradycardia,[27] and are more complex to operate than aspiration thrombectomy catheters. Despite these limitations, rheolytic devices provide superior thrombus extraction efficiency and some of the earlier limitations have been improved by using a single antegrade pass technique.[27] Aspiration thrombectomy catheters by contrast are lower in

profile, more user-friendly, and have shorter learning curves and shorter procedure times despite being less efficient in thrombus extraction. Additional unresolved issues regarding the role of thrombectomy in STEMI include whether a universal or more selective approach is superior and, if a selective approach is used, which patients should be selected and what thrombectomy device should be used.

## SUMMARY

Optimal reperfusion strategies in the management of patients with STEMI have been the subject of an iterative scientific process focusing on adjunctive pharmacotherapy and mechanical revascularization. The TAPAS trial was pivotal in demonstrating improved long-term clinical outcomes of patients with STEMI undergoing adjunctive aspiration thrombectomy. The results of the INFUSE-AMI trial have reinfused controversy into the discussion regarding the benefit of glycoprotein IIb/IIIa inhibitors in the management of patients with STEMI while also rechallenging the notion that aspiration thrombectomy provides a benefit in that setting. Furthermore, there are unresolved questions regarding whether rheolytic or aspiration thrombectomy leads to better clinical outcomes in patients with STEMI. It is hoped that the results of the TOTAL, TASTE, and SMART-PCI trials will provide further insight into how best to manage this patient population (**Figs. 1–4**; **Tables 1** and **2**).

## REFERENCES

1. Davies MJ, Woolf N, Robertson WB. Pathology of acute myocardial infarction with particular reference to occlusive coronary thrombi. Br Heart J 1976;38: 659–64.
2. Keeley EC, Boura JA, Grines CL. Primary angioplasty versus intravenous thrombolytic therapy for acute myocardial infarction: a quantitative review of 23 randomized trials. Lancet 2003;361:13–20.
3. Ito H, Tomooka T, Sakai N, et al. Lack of myocardial perfusion immediately after successful thrombolysis. A predictor of poor recovery of left ventricular function in anterior myocardial infarction. Circulation 1992;85:1699–705.
4. Rezkalla SH, Kloner RA. No-reflow phenomenon. Circulation 2002;105:656–62.
5. Ito H, Maruyama A, Iwakura K, et al. Clinical implications of the "no-reflow" phenomenon. Circulation 1996;93:223–8.
6. Kushner FG, Hand M, Smith SS, et al. 2009 focused updates: ACC/AHA guidelines for the management of patients with ST-elevation myocardial infarction (updating the 2004 guideline and 2007 focused

update) and ACC/AHA/SCAI guidelines on percutaneous coronary intervention (updating the 2005 guideline and 2007 focused update). A report of the American College of Cardiology Foundation/ American Heart Association Task Force on Practice Guidelines. J Am Coll Cardiol 2009;54:2205–41.

7. Beran G, Lang I, Schreiber W, et al. Intracoronary thrombectomy with the X-sizer catheter system improves epicardial flow and accelerates ST-segment resolution in patients with acute coronary syndrome: a prospective, randomized, controlled study. Circulation 2002;105:2355–60.

8. Lefevre T, Garcia E, Reimers B, et al. X-sizer for thrombectomy in acute myocardial improves ST-segment resolution: results of the X-sizer in AMI for negligible embolization and optimal ST resolution (X AMINE ST) trial. J Am Coll Cardiol 2005;46:246–52.

9. Ali A, Cox D, Dib N, et al. Rheolyticthrombectomy with percutaneous coronary intervention for infarct size reduction in acute myocardial infarction: 30 day results from a multi-center randomized study. J Am Coll Cardiol 2006;48:244–52.

10. Migliorini A, Stabile A, Rodriguez A, et al. Comparison of AngioJet rheolytic thrombectomy before direct infarct artery stenting with direct stenting alone in patients with acute myocardial infarction. The JETSTENT trial. J Am Coll Cardiol 2010;56(16): 1298–306.

11. Dudek D, Mielecki W, Legutko J, et al. Percutaneous thrombectomy with the RESCUE system in acute myocardial infarction. Kardiol Pol 2004;61:523–33.

12. De Luca G, van't Hof AW, Ottervanger JP, et al. Unsuccessful reperfusion in patients with ST-segment elevation myocardial infarction treated by primary angioplasty. Am Heart J 2005;150(3):557–62.

13. Silva-Orrego P, Colombo P, Bigi R, et al. Thrombus aspiration before primary angioplasty improves myocardial reperfusion in acute myocardial infarction: the DEAR-MI (Dethrombosis to Enhance Acute Reperfusion in Myocardial Infarction) study. J Am Coll Cardiol 2006;48:1552–9.

14. Kaltoft A, Mottcher M, Nielsen SS, et al. Routine thrombectomy in percutaneous coronary intervention for acute ST-segment elevation myocardial infarction: a randomized, controlled trial. Circulation 2006;114:40–7.

15. Dudek D, Mielecki W, Burzotta F, et al. Thrombus aspiration followed by direct stenting: a novel strategy of primary percutaneous coronary intervention in ST-segment elevation myocardial infarction. Results of the Polish-Italian Hungarian Randomized Thrombectomy Trial (PIHRATE Trial). Am Heart J 2010;160(5):966–72.

16. Chao CL, Hung CS, Lin YH, et al. Time-dependent benefit of initial thrombosuction on myocardial reperfusion in primary percutaneous coronary intervention. Int J Clin Pract 2008;62:555–61.

17. Svilaas T, Vlaar P, van der Horst IC, et al. Thrombus aspiration during primary percutaneous coronary intervention. N Engl J Med 2008;358:557–67.

18. Vlaar PJ, Svilaas T, van der Horst IC, et al. Cardiac death and reinfarction after 1 year in the Thrombus Aspiration during Percutaneous coronary intervention in Acute myocardial infarction Study (TAPAS): a 1-year follow-up study. Lancet 2008;371(9628):1915–20.

19. Sardella G, Mancone M, Bucciarelli-Ducci C, et al. Thrombus aspiration during primary percutaneous coronary intervention improves myocardial reperfusion and reduces infarct size. The EXPIRA (thrombectomy with Export catheter in infarct-related artery during primary percutaneous coronary intervention) prospective, randomized trial. J Am Coll Cardiol 2009;53:309–15.

20. Stone G, Maehara A, Witzenbichler B, et al. Intracoronary abciximab and aspiration thrombectomy in patients with large anterior myocardial infarction. JAMA 2012;307(17):E1–10. http://dx.doi.org/10.1001/ jama.2012.421.

21. Jolly S, Dzavik V. A Trial of Routine Aspiration Thrombectomy with Percutaneous Coronary Intervention (PCI) Versus PCI Alone in Patients with ST-Segment Elevation Myocardial Infarction (STEMI) Undergoing Primary PCI (TOTAL). Available at: ClinicalTrials.gov. Accessed April 19, 2012.

22. Frobert O, Lagerqvist B, Gudnason T, et al. Thrombus Aspiration in ST-Elevation myocardial infarction in Scandinavia (TASTE trial). A multicenter, prospective, randomized, controlled clinical registry trial based on the Swedish angiography and angioplasty registry (SCAAR) platform. Study design and rationale. Am Heart J 2010;160:1042–8.

23. Mongeon FP, Belisle P, Joseph L, et al. Adjunctive thrombectomy for acute myocardial infarction: a bayesian meta-analysis. Circ Cardiovasc Interv 2010;3:6–16.

24. Tamhane U, Chetcuti S, Hameed I, et al. Safety and efficacy of thrombectomy in patients undergoing primary percutaneous coronary intervention for acute ST elevation MI: a meta-analysis of randomized controlled trials. BMC Cardiovasc Disord 2010;10:10.

25. Antoniucci D. Comparison of manual aspiration with rheolytic thrombectomy in patients undergoing primary PCI. The SMART-PCI Trial. Avaiable at: ClinicalTrials.gov. Accessed April 19, 2012.

26. Sardella G, Mancone M, Nguyen BL, et al. The effect of thrombectomy on myocardial blush in primary angioplasty: the randomized evaluation of thrombus aspiration by two thrombectomy devices in acute myocardial infarction (RETAMI) trial. Catheter Cardiovasc Interv 2008;71:84–91.

27. Kastrati A, Byrne R, Schomig A. Is it time to jettison complex mechanical thrombectomy in favor of simple manual aspiration devices? J Am Coll Cardiol 2010; 56:1307–9.

28. Napodano M, Pasquetto G, Sacca S, et al. Intracoronary thrombectomy improves myocardial reperfusion in patients undergoing direct angioplasty for acute myocardial infarction. J Am Coll Cardiol 2003;42:1395–402.

29. Antoniucci D, Valenti R, Migliorini A, et al. Comparison of rheolytic thrombectomy before direct infarct artery stenting alone in patients undergoing percutaneous coronary intervention for acute myocardial infarction. Am J Cardiol 2004;93:1033–5.

30. Burzotta F, Trani C, Romagnoli E, et al. Manual thrombus-aspiration improves myocardial reperfusion: the randomized evaluation of the effect of mechanical reduction of distal embolization by thrombus-aspiration in primary and rescue angioplasty (REMEDIA) trial. J Am Coll Cardiol 2005;46:371–6.

31. Andersen NH, Karlsen FM, Gerdes JC, et al. No beneficial effects of coronary thrombectomy on left ventricular systolic and diastolic function in patients with acute ST-segment-elevation myocardial infarction: a randomized clinical trial. J Am Soc Echocardiogr 2007;20:724–30.

32. Lipiecki J, Monzy S, Durel N, et al. Effect of thrombus aspiration on infarct size and left ventricular function in high-risk patients with acute myocardial infarction treated by percutaneous coronary intervention: results of a prospective controlled pilot study. Am Heart J 2009;157:583.e1–7.

33. Liistro F, Grotti S, Angioli P, et al. Impact of thrombus aspiration on myocardial tissue reperfusion and left ventricular functional recovery and remodeling after primary angioplasty. Circ Cardiovasc Interv 2009;2:376–83.

34. Ciszewski M, Pregowski J, Teresinska A, et al. Aspiration coronary thrombectomy for acute myocardial infarction increases myocardial salvage: single center randomized study. Catheter Cardiovasc Interv 2011;78:523–31.

35. Ikari Y, Sakurada M, Kozuma K, et al. Upfront thrombus aspiration in primary coronary intervention for patients with ST-segment elevation acute myocardial infarction: report of the VAMPIRE (Vacuum aspiration thrombus Removal) trial. JACC Cardiovasc Interv 2008;1:424–31.

36. Chevalier B, Gilard M, Lang I, et al. Systematic primary aspiration in acute myocardial percutaneous intervention: a multicenter randomized controlled trial of the Export® aspiration catheter. Eurointervention 2008;4:222–8.

# Utility of Thrombectomy in Primary Percutaneous Coronary Intervention

Carl A. Dragstedt, DO, Anthony A. Bavry, MD, MPH*

## KEYWORDS

- Thrombus • Thrombectomy • Myocardial infarction • Coronary artery disease • Aspiration
- Rheolytic • Primary percutaneous coronary intervention • Suction

## KEY POINTS

- Embolization of thrombotic debris is common during primary percutaneous coronary intervention.
- Embolism can result in coronary no reflow and is associated with poor outcomes.
- Numerous devices are available to aid in removing thrombotic debris from the coronary circulation during primary percutaneous coronary intervention.
- Clinical trial data supports the use of thrombus removal before stent implantation.

## INTRODUCTION

Despite advances in general awareness, preventative strategies, and treatment modalities, acute myocardial infarction (MI) remains the leading primary cause of mortality in the United States as well as in developed countries, with the incidence increasing in countries of the developing world. In the United States in 2012, it is estimated that 785 000 Americans will have an acute MI; of these, approximately one-third will be classified as an ST-elevation MI (STEMI).[1] The classic pathophysiologic progression (from the disruption of a thin-cap fibro-atheromatous plaque, platelet aggregation, fibrin cross-linkage, and ultimate thrombotic occlusion of the infarct-related vessel) has been well described.[2] Indeed, a high burden of residual thrombotic material within the coronary macrocirculation and microcirculation has been shown to result in adverse outcomes.[3]

Adjunctive mechanical treatments in concert with potent pharmacotherapies offer the clinician

further opportunities to minimize the thrombotic burden and allow for additional clinical benefit. The use of distal embolic protection devices to trap thromboembolic material during balloon angioplasty and stent deployment has been evaluated in several randomized controlled trials and meta-analyses. Despite their logical rationale in capturing embolized material and preventing macrovascular/microvascular flow obstruction, the use of these devices has not yielded conclusive results as to their efficacy in preventing adverse cardiovascular outcomes. Therefore, except in the setting of saphenous vein graft interventions, their routine use is not recommended.[4,5]

Thrombectomy, or the removal of intracoronary thrombus in the setting of primary percutaneous coronary intervention (PCI) during the management of STEMI, offers the interventional clinician an additional tool in the growing armamentarium of pharmacologic and mechanical treatment strategies for this clinical problem. A variety of devices, each with unique properties and mechanisms of

Disclosures: Dr Dragstedt has no disclosures to report. Dr Bavry has received research support from Novartis Pharmaceuticals and from Eli Lilly and serves as a contractor for the American College of Cardiology's Cardiosource.
Division of Cardiovascular Medicine, University of Florida, 1600 Southwest Archer Road, Gainesville, FL 32610-0277, USA
* Corresponding author.
E-mail address: bavryaa@medicine.ufl.edu

Intervent Cardiol Clin 2 (2013) 361–374
http://dx.doi.org/10.1016/j.iccl.2012.11.004
2211-7458/13/$ – see front matter © 2013 Elsevier Inc. All rights reserved.

thrombus removal, have been developed in the era of primary PCI.

## RATIONALE FOR THROMBECTOMY USE IN ACUTE MI

A large proportion of patients undergoing primary PCI for STEMI experience the *no reflow* phenomenon, despite alleviation of the acute obstruction.[6] Despite the reestablishment of normal epicardial blood flow in patients presenting with acute MI, the incidence of particulate microvascular embolization following reperfusion may be as high as 50%.[7]

Microembolic debris is predominantly derived from the necrotic core of thin fibrous cap atheromas; histopathologic assessment of the microcirculation has demonstrated the presence of cholesterol crystals, hyalin, and platelet aggregates. These particles are similar to analyzed particulate retrieved from distal embolic protection devices. Additionally, myocyte edema, hemorrhage, and resulting capillary compression with erythrocyte rouleaux bodies further impair microvascular perfusion. In patients undergoing PCI, those with unstable atherosclerotic lesions (as opposed to those with stable-appearing plaques) have a higher likelihood of microembolization and no reflow, presumably a function of the biochemical makeup of the necrotic core and its relative embolic potential.[8,9]

Epicardial flow or coronary macrocirculation is strongly correlated with clinical outcomes. Poor outcomes are observed when thrombolysis in MI (TIMI) flow grade is less than 3. However, even when there is a TIMI 3 flow, there still may be impaired perfusion at the microvascular level.[10] The assessment of myocardial blush grade (MBG), which is scored from 0 (having no myocardial contrast enhancement and clearance) to 3 (intense myocardial contrast enhancement and clearance), has additional prognostic value in determining adverse outcomes.

MBG 0 to 1, which angiographically suggests no reflow, is present in up to 50% of patients with epicardial TIMI 3 flow.[11] Analyzed in concert, the markers of TIMI flow and MBG can be used by the clinician to determine the likelihood of adverse clinical events. Additionally, failure to resolve ST-segment elevation by at least 50% at 1 hour is a surrogate marker of microvascular obstruction and it also portends an increased mortality.[12]

Noninvasive imaging has allowed for direct post-infarction and longitudinal assessments of myocardial function. Contrast echocardiography has been used to assess the potential impact of microvascular obstruction[13]; however, cardiac magnetic resonance imaging (MRI) has emerged as a superior modality for direct objective assessment of microcirculatory dysfunction with a correlative impact on left ventricular dysfunction.[14,15]

Thrombectomy offers the opportunity to mitigate microvascular obstruction and its subsequent deleterious sequelae. Cardiac MRI performed after aspiration thrombectomy has demonstrated a lower incidence of microvascular obstruction, myocardial edema, and myocardial hemorrhage, with prevention of left ventricular remodeling.[16] Preservation of myocardial viability after aspiration has also been described.[17]

The adverse effects of microvascular obstruction and no reflow on mortality cannot be overstated. Despite the reestablishment of epicardial TIMI 3 flow, the presence of no reflow portends a worse in-hospital and 6-month mortality.[18] The long-term effects of no reflow are similarly striking. In a recent observational study of more than 1400 patients with STEMI, after adjustment for infarct size, patients with no reflow experienced higher mortality at 5 years (hazard ratio [HR] 1.66, 95% confidence interval [CI] 1.17–2.36, $P = .0004$).[19] This finding underscores the clinical opportunity to improve this marker of perfusion and perhaps long-term outcomes.

## THERAPEUTIC OPTIONS

Types of thrombectomy devices

1. Manual aspiration devices (aspiration thrombectomy)
2. Mechanical devices (rheolytic thrombectomy)
3. Excimer laser
4. Ultrasonic thrombectomy

### *Manual Aspiration Devices*

Many catheters with a similar mode of action are commercially available. This review focuses on select catheters that have either gained approval from the Food and Drug Administration (FDA) or have been studied experimentally.

The Export AP Aspiration Catheter (*Medtronic, Minneapolis, Minnesota*) is a commonly used aspiration thrombectomy catheter. The 6F system is 0.014-in wire compatible with rapid exchange. The tip is soft and allows for easy trackability. The catheter features a patented Full-Wall Variable Braid Technology with a hydrophilic coating, geared at minimizing kinking and optimizing deliverability. The proximal catheter features low-density braiding to facilitate passage, whereas the distal catheter offers higher-density braiding to minimize kinking. Despite this feature, kinking can still occur with rapid advancement of the catheter. The catheter is connected to a stopcock, and the packaging includes 2 lockable syringes. The syringes are locked with negative pressure. When the catheter is advanced proximal to the coronary lesion, the stopcock is opened to a negative-pressure syringe and aspiration occurs until that syringe is filled. Once a syringe is filled, the alternative syringe can be opened and aspiration continued. A 7F system is also available.[20]

Early experience with the Export demonstrating ease of use and feasibility, which led to several randomized controlled trials comparing the adjunctive use of the Export catheter upstream of primary PCI with primary PCI alone. The largest of these trials was the landmark Thrombus Aspiration During Percutaneous Coronary Intervention in Acute Myocardial Infarction Study (TAPAS). This single-center trial randomized 1071 patients; the primary endpoint was a post-PCI MBG of 0 or 1. The primary endpoint occurred in 17.1% in the aspiration arm as opposed to 26.3% in the conventional treatment arm (relative risk [RR] 0.63, CI 0.51–0.83, $P<.001$). Additionally, ST-segment resolution (STR) occurred in 56.6% versus 44.2% of patients (RR 1.28, CI 1.13–1.45, $P<.001$).[21]

Although the 30-day clinical outcomes demonstrated a nonsignificant trend toward death, reinfarction, and major adverse cardiac events (MACE), a 12-month follow-up analysis of the *TAPAS* trial demonstrated reduced death at 12 months (3.6% vs 6.7%, HR 1.93, CI 1.11–3.37, $P = .02$) and reduced death or nonfatal MI at 12 months (5.6% vs 9.9%, HR 1.81, CI 1.16–2.84, $P = .009$), suggesting that routine use of the Export catheter before primary PCI results in improved clinical outcomes.[22]

The Thrombectomy with Export Catheter in Infarct-Related Artery During Primary Percutaneous Coronary Intervention (EXPIRA) trial similarly randomized 175 patients to Export aspiration thrombectomy with primary PCI (n = 88) to primary PCI alone (n = 87). Primary outcomes were an MBG of 2 or more and an STR of more than 70%. A cardiac MRI substudy was performed initially and at 3 months on a subset of patients with anterior MI to assess microvascular perfusion and the extent of infarct, respectively. An MBG of 2 or more was seen more in the aspiration group than in stand-alone PCI (88% vs 60%, $P = .001$). STR also occurred more in the treatment group (64% vs 39%, $P = .001$). Among patients with anterior MI, microvascular obstruction occurred less in the Export arm and infarct size was significantly limited by routine use of aspiration.[23]

Patients in the *EXPIRA* trial were followed for 24 months. MACE rates in the treatment group were lower than the control (4.5% vs 13.6%, $P = .038$) and death (0% vs 6.4%, $P = .012$), all

of which were classified as cardiac deaths. These findings offer the greatest longitudinal follow-up for the Export catheter and, similar to *TAPAS*, are suggestive of improved long-term cardiovascular outcomes.[24]

The Diver CE MAX (*Invatec, Brescia, Italy*) aspiration catheter features a shorter tip (4 mm) with lower profile (0.023 in) and a relatively larger inner diameter relative to the Export catheter. The 6F system is 0.014-in wire compatible with a rapid-exchange platform with a hydrophilic coating to allow for enhanced deliverability. A unique feature of the Diver is an option for 2 distal circumferential side holes, which are available in both the 6F and 7F versions. Similar to the Export, the Diver catheter is accompanied by a stopcock, two 30-mL syringes, and a filter basket for thrombus collection.[25]

The Randomized Evaluation of the Effect of Mechanical Reduction of Distal Embolization by Thrombus-Aspiration in Primary and Rescue Angioplasty (REMEDIA) trial randomized patients to aspiration using the Diver catheter during primary PCI (n = 50) or PCI alone (n = 49); the primary endpoints were an MBG of 2 or more and an STR of 70% or more. The Diver arm demonstrated improved MBG (68.0% vs 58.0%, odds ratio [OR] 2.6, 95% CI 1.1–5.9, $P = .02$) and STR (44.9% vs 36.7%, OR 2.4, 95% CI 1.1–5.3, $P = .034$). The combined endpoint also favored the Diver catheter (46.0% vs 24.5%, OR 2.6, 95% CI 1.1–6.2, $P =.025$). This study demonstrated the feasibility and ease of use in unselected patients with STEMI and suggested improved angiographic and electrocardiogram resolution.[26]

The *Polish-Italian-Hungarian Randomized Thrombectomy Trial* similarly enrolled patients with STEMI into treatment with Diver plus PCI (n = 100) versus balloon angioplasty followed by stenting (n = 96). The primary outcome was a STR of more than 70% at 60 minutes after PCI. Despite not achieving the primary endpoint, numerous secondary surrogate endpoints were achieved more frequently in the Diver arm, including improved STR, MBG 3, and optimal myocardial reperfusion. Despite these surrogate endpoints, there was no difference in mortality or repeat MI for 6 months.[27]

A limited number of head-to-head comparative trials have been performed to assess for relative benefit of a particular device. The Export catheter's effect on thrombus burden, TIMI flow, and post-PCI MBG has been compared with the Diver in the Randomized Evaluation of Thrombus Aspiration by two thrombectomy devices in Acute Myocardial Infarction (RETAMI) randomized study of 103 patients with STEMI. Use of the Export resulted in a greater reduction in thrombus burden, higher TIMI flow of 2 or more, and an MBG of 2 or more (P<.05 for all outcomes). There was no difference between groups in clinical events at 1 month and 1 year.[28]

In a prospective cohort study, use of the Diver did not facilitate improved aspiration success, MBG, or STR over the Export catheter. Extracted particulate matter was histopathologically analyzed; despite a difference in inner luminal area, there was no difference in particle size noted between the Diver and Export cohorts.[29]

The Xpress-Way Rx (*Atrium Medical, Hudson, New Hampshire*) is a novel aspiration catheter recently approved in 2010 by the FDA. The 6F system is 0.014-in wire compatible with a rapid-exchange platform. It functions similarly to the Export and Diver catheters, with tubing, stopcock, and two 30-mL aspiration syringes. It is marketed as an ultralow profile system designed for the removal of fresh, soft thrombus, with enhanced crossability. Unlike other contemporary aspiration catheters, the Xpress-Way Rx features an inner stylet that minimizes kinking and facilitates easier passage. Although the stylet enhances deliverability of the device to the coronary lesion, a potential downside of this feature is that the catheter may not be activated until the catheter is distal to the lesion. At least theoretically, this could result in the embolization of thrombotic material.

Outside of the United States, an identically designed catheter is marketed as the Thrombuster II catheter (*Kaneka Corporation, Osaka, Japan*); much clinical experience and data regarding the Xpress-way's performance is extrapolated from studies abroad with this catheter.[30] A retrospective analysis of patients with STEMI in Japan treated with the Thrombuster device found reduced rates of no reflow and left ventricular remodeling, particularly for infarcts involving the left anterior descending or right coronary arteries.[31]

A large retrospective cohort of 3913 Japanese patients was also performed. Of this group, approximately 25% underwent aspiration with the Thrombuster before PCI. Overall, there was no difference in 30-day mortality, other than in those with the highest TIMI risk score. Additionally, elderly patients, patients with diabetes, and patients undergoing stent implantation benefitted from aspiration thrombectomy with the Thrombuster catheter.[32]

The Pronto family of aspiration catheters (*Vascular Solutions, Minneapolis, Minnesota*) share a common design. Most clinical experience has been with the Pronto V3, which requires a 6F guide. The catheters feature a rapid exchange platform and are compatible with 0.014-in guidewires. It features a fully braided shaft, hydrophilic coating, and a large lumen for thrombus extraction. The unique Silva tip is tapered to allow improved navigation, and the lumen orifice is sloped to theoretically accommodate larger thrombus. Rather than a variable luminal area, the catheter length features the same luminal dimension to allow for maximum capacity for extraction.

The Pronto LP features a 20% smaller profile compared with the Pronto V3. The design features are otherwise the same. The device includes an inner stylet to allow for minimization of kinking and improved deliverability, particularly into tortuous and distal vessels.[33] The Pronto V4 is new for 2012 and has an embedded longitudinal wire that provides enhanced kink resistance.

The Dethrombosis to Enhance Acute Reperfusion in Myocardial Infarction (DEAR-MI) trial was a randomized controlled clinical study of the Pronto with primary PCI versus primary PCI alone. One hundred forty-eight patients were enrolled; the primary endpoints of an STR more than 70% (68% vs 50%, P<.05) and an MBG of 3 (88% vs 44%, P<.0001) were achieved more frequently in the Pronto-treated group. In addition, the aspiration arm showed similar in-hospital clinical events but improved TIMI frame count, lower creatine kinase MB fraction, and lower no reflow (3% vs 15%, P<.05).[34] See **Table 1** for comparison of aspiration thrombectomy catheters.

The TransVascular Aspiration Catheter (TVAC) (*Nipro Corporation, Osaka, Japan*) is not currently FDA approved for use in the United States. Aspiration is performed through a 7F compatible catheter by continuous vacuum suction via an external pump. Continuous pressure of 0.9 atm is maintained during aspiration, which provides for 20 to 40 mL of aspirate with each pass. The catheter features a beak-shaped distal tip and a flexible 4.5F catheter with a monorail platform. Aspiration can also be performed by standard syringe suction if desired. Safety and feasibility have been demonstrated.[35] See **Fig. 1** for an image of TVAC.

The VAcuuM AsPIration Thrombus REmoval (VAMPIRE) trial is the only randomized study to evaluate adjunctive use of the TVAC to standalone primary PCI. In this trial, 355 patients were assigned to primary PCI with (n = 180) or without (n = 175) the use of the TVAC catheter. There was a nonstatistical trend (P = .07) toward improved no reflow (MBG <3) with TVAC among patients who presently relatively late (>6 hours). No clinical endpoints were assessed in this study.[36]

## Mechanical Devices

### X-sizer

The X-sizer Catheter System (*eV3, Inc, White Bear Lake, Minnesota*) is comprised of a rotating helical cutting device housed within the soft, atraumatic

**Table 1**
**Comparison of aspiration catheters**

| | Export AP (Medtronic) | Diver CE (Invatec) | Expressway (Atrium Medical) | Pronto V3 (Vascular Solutions) | Pronto LP (Vascular Solutions) |
|---|---|---|---|---|---|
| Tip | | | | | |
| Cross-sectional | | | | | |
| Guide compatibility | 0.070 in | 0.068 in | 0.070 in | 0.070 in | 0.070 in |
| Distal lumen | 0.043 in | 0.033 in | 0.039 in | 0.047 in | 0.031 in |
| Shaft lumen | 0.043 in | 0.039 in | 0.042 in | 0.049 in | 0.039 in |
| Wire lumen | 0.015 in | 0.016 in | 0.016 in | 0.017 in | 0.018 in |
| Catheter length | 140 cm | 145 cm | 140 cm | 140 cm | 137 cm |
| Coating | Hydrophilic | Hydrophilic | Hydrophilic | Hydrophilic | Hydrophilic |
| Braiding | Hub to tip (variable) | None | None | Hub to tip (not variable) | Proximal only |
| Tip Design | Beveled, short tip | Beveled, long tip (side holes optional) | Beveled, short tip | Rounded tip, slot cut at distal end | Rounded tip, slot cut at distal end |
| Syringe | (2) 30 mL | (1) 30 mL | (2) 30 mL | (2) 30 mL | (2) 30 mL |

catheter tip. When the vacuum is activated, the cutting device liberates and captures thrombus that is then removed from the catheter. A battery pack is attached to the externalized end of the device. The systems are based on an over-the-wire platform and require a 300-cm, 0.014-in guidewire. The cutting devices are 1.5 or 2.0 mm, requiring 7F or 8F systems, respectively. The device is powered by an enclosed battery source within the handle of the device. It achieved FDA approval for use in native coronary arteries in 2002; however, it currently is not marketed or commercially available.[37] See **Fig. 2** for an image of the X-sizer device.

The X-Sizer in AMI for Negligible Embolization and Optimal ST Resolution (X AMINE ST) trial is the largest randomized study to date evaluating the X-sizer. Patients were randomized to X-sizer thrombectomy plus primary PCI (n = 100) versus primary PCI alone (n = 101). The X-sizer group had a higher frequency of STR of more than 50% (68% vs 53%, $P = .037$), less distal embolization (2% vs 10%, $P = .033$), with similar TIMI 3 flow and MBG ($P$ = not significant). There was no difference in clinical outcomes at 6 months.[38]

The *TREAT-MI* study compared Export with the X-sizer before PCI, enrolling 201 patients. The Export exhibited a trend toward a better STR (56.6% vs 44.0%, $P = .06$). The primary endpoint was combined MACE at 3 years. The occurrence was 22.2% in the Export group and 18.6% in the X-sizer group (HR 1.20, 95% CI

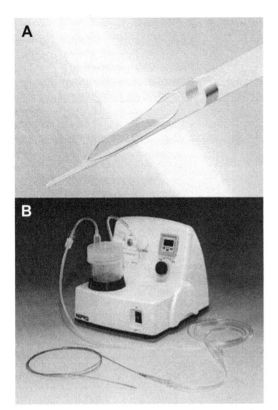

**Fig. 1.** TransVascular aspiration catheter. *Panel A* shows the detail of the catheter tip. *Panel B* shows the catheter and vacuum motor drive assembly. (*From* Sakurada M, Ikari Y, and Isshiki T. Improved performance of a new thrombus aspiration catheter: outcomes from in vitro experiments and a case presentation. Catheter Cardiovasc Interv 2004;63(3):299–306; with permission.)

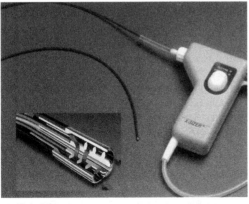

**Fig. 2.** X-sizer catheter. (*From* Constantinides S, Lo TS, Been M, et al. Early experience with a helical coronary thrombectomy device in patients with acute coronary thrombosis. Heart 2002;87(5):455–60; with permission.)

0.65–2.22, $P = .35$). Although no difference was seen in clinical outcomes, this study demonstrated that the use of the Export catheter was associated with shorter procedure times, ease in lesion crossing, and fewer complications relative to the X-sizer.[39]

### AngioJet

The AngioJet (*Medrad, Warrendale, Pennsylvania*) is a rheolytic thrombectomy system. Rheolysis, or thrombus fragmentation, is induced by negative pressure generated by directional infused saline flow dynamics via the Bernoulli-Venturi effect.[40] A variety of catheter sizes have been developed for various clinical uses, including use in the coronary arteries, saphenous vein grafts, pulmonary arteries, peripheral arteries, and arteriovenous fistulae. The manufacturer reports more than 500 000 cases have been performed using the AngioJet.[41] See **Fig. 3** for images of AngioJet and Rheolysis.

The catheters consist of 2 inner lumina and are available in both rapid-exchange and over-the-wire platforms. Saline is infused under high pressure via a dispensing ring distally, with the infusate directed retrograde toward the more proximally positioned and larger extraction lumen. Activation is by a foot pedal controlled by the operator. Typical use in the coronary circulation is with the 4F XMI or Spiroflex Rapid Exchange catheters (Medrad, Warrendale, Pennsylvania), which are 0.014-in guidewire compatible and require a 6F guide, although larger-sized catheters are available. See **Table 2** for types and specifications of AngioJet catheters.

In the prospective *Strategic Transcatheter Evaluation of New Therapies* (STENT) registry study from 2003 to 2005, more than 9000 patients with STEMI were evaluated in which AngioJet was used 3% to 4% of the time. Similar 9-month mortality outcomes were seen between the AngioJet and primary PCI cohorts, although higher thrombus burden and cardiogenic shock was evident in the AngioJet arm.[42] This registry experience established a framework for 2 pivotal randomized clinical trials evaluating the AngioJet, the AngioJet Rheolytic Thrombectomy In Patients Undergoing Primary Angioplasty for Acute Myocardial Infarction (AIMI) and AngioJET Thrombectomy and STENTing for Treatment of Acute Myocardial Infarction (JETSTENT) trials, which yielded conflicting results with regards to outcomes.

The *AIMI* study randomized 480 consecutive patients with STEMI in a 1:1 fashion to AngioJet plus PCI versus PCI alone. Thrombus visualization was not required for enrollment. Infarct lesion location and characteristics were similar between

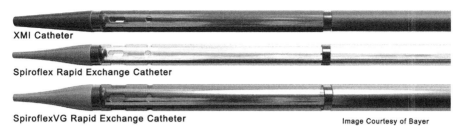

XMI Catheter

Spiroflex Rapid Exchange Catheter

SpiroflexVG Rapid Exchange Catheter

Image Courtesy of Bayer

**Fig. 3.** Diagram of available AngioJet catheters. (*Courtesy of* Bayer HealthCare LLC, Wayne, NJ; with permission.)

groups. Infarct size as determined by nuclear imaging was similar at 2 to 4 weeks in the AngioJet-treated group (12.5% ± 12.1% vs 9.8% ± 10.9%, $P$ = .03). TIMI flow grade, MBG, STR, and 30-day MACE were not improved with the use of the AngioJet. In fact, MACE events at 30 days were higher in the AngioJet group (6.7% vs 7.0%, $P$ = .01), largely driven by low event rates in the PCI-only group. Procedural times were longer with AngioJet, because of the thrombectomy plus the need for temporary pacing.[43]

The *JETSTENT* trial randomized 501 patients in a similar fashion to the *AIMI* study. Unlike the *AIMI* study, whereby only 21% had angiographically moderate or large thrombus, the presence of visible thrombus was a requisite for enrollment. Although no difference was found in TIMI 3 flow, MBG, or TIMI frame count between the groups, STR was improved in the AngioJet group (85.5% vs 78.8%, $P$ = .043). More significantly, the JETSTENT trial found that 12-month event-free survival was higher in the AngioJet group, with survival 85.2% versus 75.0% in the direct stent arm ($P$ = .009).[44]

Contrasting the conclusions from the *AIMI* study, the *JETSTENT* study has refocused the discussion on the potential role of rheolytic thrombectomy in a higher-risk patient population, namely, those with large thrombus burden.

## Excimer Laser

The Spectranetics CVX-300 Excimer Laser System (ECLA) (*Spectranetics Corporation, Colorado Springs, Colorado*) has been studied adjunctively in acute MI; however, no current FDA indication exists. Catheters are available in a range of sizes and guide compatibilities (6F to 8F), both with rapid-exchange and over-the-wire platforms. Tissue ablation is achieved by pulsed ultraviolet laser light of 308 nm, which results in dissolution of intermolecular and intramolecular bonds within thrombus. Saline is continuously infused at 2 to 3 mL/s during laser activation. Activation for periods of 5 seconds with 10-second delays is recommended by the manufacturer, with catheter advancement of 0.2 to 0.5 mm/s. Operators and those in the room are required to wear protective eyewear during laser operation.[45]

The Cohort of Acute Revascularization in Myocardial Infarction with Excimer Laser (CARMEL) multicenter trial was designed to assess the safety and efficacy of the ECLA in patients with STEMI. One hundred fifty-one patients underwent laser thrombectomy. Those patients with extensive thrombus burden achieved higher procedural success, marked by improved TIMI 3 flow and increase in minimal luminal diameter. Procedural complications included perforation (0.6%), dissection (5% major, 3% minor), acute vessel closure (0.6%), distal embolization (0.2%), and bleeding (3%).[46]

The Laser angioplasty in AMI (LaserAMI) study randomized 27 consecutive patients with STEMI to ECLA with primary PCI (n = 14) versus primary PCI alone (n = 13). ECLA was safe and feasible in all cases with no procedural complications. There was no difference in quantitative coronary angiography, TIMI flow, or MBG.[47] See **Fig. 4** for an image of the excimer laser device.

## Ultrasonic Thrombectomy

Ultrasonic vibration can potentiate microfragment thrombus into tiny particles and improve flow within a thrombus-occluded artery. The Acolysis System (*Rayfield Technology, Houston, Texas*) delivers ultrasonic energy (41.9 kHz, 18 W) causing longitudinal vibration along the catheter with delivery of ultrasonic energy into the surrounding thrombus, resulting in ultrafragmentation. The catheter requires a 7F guide and is 0.014-in guidewire compatible.[48]

Percutaneous transluminal coronary ultrasound thrombolysis was studied in a multicenter registry study of 126 patients using the Acolysis system. Sonolytic therapy was administered to patients with unstable coronary syndromes, a subset of which included patients with STEMI. Eighty-four percent of patients had occluded arteries at presentation. Recanalization, defined as TIMI flow 2 to 3 occurred in 89% of patients.[49]

Currently, FDA-approved for use in thrombotic dialysis shunts, the OmniWave Endovascular

**Table 2**
**Specifications of AngioJet catheters**

| Catheter Model | Minimum Vessel Diameter | Length | Diameter | Guidewire | Guide Catheter |
|---|---|---|---|---|---|
| XMI Catheter | 2 mm | 135 cm | 4F | 0.014 in | 6F >0.068 in |
| Spiroflex Rapid Exchange Catheter | 2 mm | 135 cm | 4F | 0.014 in | 6F >0.070 in |
| SpiroflexVG Rapid Exchange Catheter | 3 mm | 135 cm | 5F | 0.014 in | 7F >0.076 in |

Image Courtesy of Bayer

*Courtesy* of Bayer HealthCare LLC, Wayne, NJ; with permission.

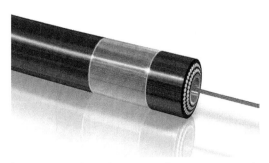

**Fig. 4.** Excimer laser. (*Courtesy of* Spectranetics, Colorado Springs, Colorado; with permission.)

System (*OmniSonics Medical Technologies, Wilmington, Massachusetts*) is a novel system that emits low-energy (20 kHz) ultrasonic waves from the distal 10 cm of a 0.018-in wire, resulting in cavitation of thrombus with no disruption of underlying endothelium.[50]

This technology may warrant further investigation in certain patient subsets, such as those with high thrombus burden during acute MI, and may one day serve a role adjunctively in acute MI.

## PROCEDURAL CONSIDERATIONS
### Predictors of Failed Thrombectomy

Aspiration thrombectomy can safely and easily be performed in most cases. Failure to cross the lesion is the most common reason for device failure and occurs in approximately 10% of cases. Several predictors of failed thrombus aspiration have been identified. Marked proximal vessel tortuosity, the presence of a calcified lesion, and bifurcation lesions have all been associated with an inability to cross the lesion and are independent predictors of failed aspiration. Additionally, patient age greater than 60 years and the circumflex as the infarct-related artery are associated with an inability to extract thrombus.[51]

A single-center experience in 200 cases using the X-sizer device identified device failure in 24% of real-world cases. The presence of an ostial lesion was the sole independent predictor of device failure, defined as failure to reach target segment, reach final TIMI 3 flow, slow or no reflow, distal embolization, or coronary perforation. Clinically, such failure portended a worse 30-day clinical event rate.[52]

Rheolytic thrombectomy confers an electrically stabilizing effect on ischemic myocardium by reducing QT dispersion[53]; however, there is a high incidence of bradyarrhythmias commonly encountered with use of the AngioJet. This occurrence is more pronounced with use in right or dominant circumflex arteries. Sinus bradycardia, junctional bradycardia, heart block, and asystole have been reported, often precipitating hypotension, with an incidence of 20% to 79%. In the AIMI trial, 58% of patients required temporary pacemaker with rheolytic thrombectomy. Although mechanistically unresolved, several theories have been postulated. These theories include distal embolization resulting in increased ischemia-mediated arrhythmia, rheolysis-associated hemolysis with adenosine liberation, and infusate activation of stretch-sensitive endothelial channels. The stimulation of vagally mediated pathways may explain the higher incidence (12%–20%) of bradyarrhythmia observed during rheolytic treatment of the pulmonary arteries or great thoracic veins.[54]

The *JETSTENT* investigators used a single-pass anterograde technique, with catheter activation 1 cm proximal to thrombus, slow advancement 1 to 3 mm/s through the thrombus, and continuous activation of catheter on pullback. Additional passes may be necessary, depending on follow-up angiography.[44] By protocol design, a temporary pacemaker was left to operator discretion. In practice, less than 1% of patients required the placement of a temporary pacemaker.

The administration of intracoronary aminophylline prior to thrombectomy (each dose 10–20 mg) may obviate pacing.[55] Preliminary experience with glycopyrrolate, a synthetic anticholinergic agent, has shown promise in reducing hemodynamically significant bradyarrhythmias.[56]

Despite the low use of temporary pacemakers in the JETSTENT trial, AngioJet's manufacturer still recommends temporary transvenous pacing in patients with STEMI undergoing rheolytic thrombectomy.[41] Because of the potential delays to primary revascularization, many clinicians may be reluctant to use the AngioJet because of the increased time needed for venous access and temporary pacing. Alternatively, guidewire pacing has been demonstrated to be an effective alternative in managing bradyarrhythmias with AngioJet use.[57]

### Complications During Thrombectomy

All thrombectomy devices carry the risk of complication. Fortunately, the rates of such events are very low, particularly with use of aspiration devices; the potential benefits outweigh the slight risk associated with their use. Dissection has been systematically evaluated in recent comparative effectiveness analysis. No comparative data exist on the rates of complications between various aspiration devices, despite industry claims of such or user intuition based on device characteristics. Rates of coronary perforation are not consistently reported, but their rate is historically low.

Aspiration thrombectomy may result in the withdrawal of thrombus from the infarct-related artery into the arterial circulation, resulting in cerebrovascular events.[5] Left main coronary artery thrombosis has also been reported following circumflex aspiration.[58]

The X-sizer device has been associated with numerous procedural complications, including coronary perforation,[59,60] coronary arteriovenous (AV) fistulization,[61] and guidewire fracture.[62,63] These complications help to explain why this device did not garner widespread clinical use.

## CLINICAL OUTCOMES

Several meta-analyses have assessed a myriad of surrogate endpoints (STR, MBG, restoration of TIMI 3 flow) and angiographic endpoints (no reflow and distal embolization), in addition to clinical outcome (mortality).

DeLuca and colleagues[64] found that aspiration thrombectomy devices (including 1 study using the TVAC) resulted in improved MBG, post-PCI TIMI 3 flow, and reduced distal embolization. Thirty-day mortality was lower in the aspiration group (1.7% vs 3.1%, $P = .04$).

Bavry and colleagues[5] demonstrated improved surrogate endpoints of MBG and STR with aspiration devices but no such difference with the use of mechanical devices (AngioJet or X-sizer). Mortality was improved at a mean follow-up of 5 months with use of aspiration but not mechanical thrombectomy (see **Fig. 5**).

The *JETSTENT* trial, which demonstrated improvement in surrogate endpoints, was not included in the Bavry analysis, whereas the largely negative *AIMI* trial was included, which accounted for most of the overall negative results for mechanical devices on both surrogate endpoints and mortality. In addition, a meta-analysis of AngioJet by Grines and colleagues[65] involving 11 studies and 1018 patients was performed before *JETSTENT's* outcome data could be included.

Burzotta and colleagues[66] reported an improvement in mortality; however, further subgroup analysis found this association only in patients treated with glycoprotein IIb/IIIa inhibitors and only in patients treated with aspiration devices.

Mongeon and colleagues[67] demonstrated an improvement in surrogate endpoints, including MBG, no reflow, post-PCI TIMI 3 flow, STR, and less distal embolization, but no improvement in 30-day mortality or 30-day combined MACE.

These meta-analyses suggest that aspiration thrombectomy consistently results in improved

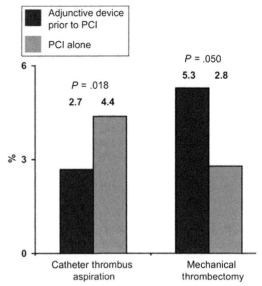

**Fig. 5.** Effect of adjunctive thrombectomy devices on mortality. Catheter thrombus aspiration includes thrombus removal by syringe suction devices and thrombus removal by continuous suction device. Mechanical thrombectomy includes the Angiojet and X-sizer devices. (*Reprinted from* Bavry AA, Kumbhani DJ, Bhatt DL. Role of adjunctive thrombectomy and embolic protection devices in acute myocardial infarction: a comprehensive meta-analysis of randomized trials. Eur Heart J 2008;29(24):2989–3001; with permission.)

surrogate endpoints that may translate into improved mortality. Mechanical thrombectomy has not demonstrated any long-term clinical benefit; however, results of the *JETSTENT* trial are encouraging in this regard.

The 2 × 2 Factorial, Randomized, Multicenter, Single-Blind Evaluation of Intracoronary Abciximab Infusion and Aspiration Thrombectomy in Patients Undergoing Percutaneous Coronary Intervention for Anterior ST-Segment Elevation Myocardial Infarction (INFUSE-AMI) trial tested 2 strategies to reduce embolization during large anterior MI.[68] By factorial design, patients were randomized to aspiration thrombectomy (Export catheter) versus no aspiration thrombectomy and also randomized to intracoronary abciximab (infused with the ClearWay catheter [Atrium Medical, Hudson, New Hampshire]) versus no intracoronary abciximab. The smallest infarct size was seen in the intracoronary abciximab group. Further studies are needed to determine the optimal use of this unique drug delivery catheter.

## GUIDELINES AND RECOMMENDATIONS

The American College of Cardiology, the American Heart Association, and the European Society of

Cardiology have issued recommendations for the use of aspiration thrombectomy in the management of patients with STEMI. A class IIa recommendation (level of evidence: B), was made with the 2009 focused update, indicating it is reasonable to perform aspiration thrombectomy. This recent update was largely attributed to improved clinical outcomes shown in the *TAPAS* and *EXPIRA* trials and meta-analysis by Bavry and colleagues.[5] Interestingly, these trials evaluated up-front use of aspiration thrombectomy regardless of thrombus burden. Questions regarding a selective or provisional use of aspiration devices remain unanswered, thus studies are still needed.[1]

## SUMMARY

A case series report from New York in 1993 described mechanical manipulation of thrombus:

> *Three techniques were used: transcatheter aspiration, clot displacement, and thrombectomy. Five patients in shock had the thrombus aspirated from the left main and right coronary arteries. Eight patients had the clot pushed by the balloon from the mid-LAD to the apical LAD to reduce the area of ischemic myocardium, and 13 patients underwent of thrombectomy of the right coronary artery. These procedures enjoyed a high rate of success in re-establishing patency and a favorable long-term clinical and angiographic follow-up. Although the applicability and role of these interventions in acute myocardial infarction are not yet defined, we conclude that they are feasible and have an acceptable success and complication rate.[69]*

Significant advancements have occurred over the past 20 years regarding the management of thrombus in the setting of STEMI, both from pharmacologic and mechanical strategies. Despite significant data supporting their use, contemporary adjunctive use of thrombectomy devices during STEMI approaches only 20% of cases.[70]

Overall, aspiration thrombectomy is safe with favorable procedural, surrogate marker, and clinical benefit. Rheolytic thrombectomy, particularly with large thrombus burden, seems to have similar benefit. The use of alternative forms of thrombectomy is not yet established during primary PCI.

## REFERENCES

1. Roger VL, Go AS, Lloyd-Jones DM, et al. Heart disease and stroke statistics—2012 update: a report from the American Heart Association. Circulation 2012;125:e2–220.

2. Fishbein MC. The vulnerable and unstable atherosclerotic plaque. Cardiovasc Pathol 2010;19(1):6–11.

3. Gibson CM, Murphy S, Menown IB, et al. Determinants of coronary blood flow after thrombolytic administration. TIMI Study Group. Thrombolysis in myocardial infarction. J Am Coll Cardiol 1999;34(5):1403–12.

4. Kunadian B, Dunning J, Vijayalakshmi K, et al. Meta-analysis of randomized trials comparing anti-embolic devices with standard PCI for improving myocardial reperfusion in patients with acute myocardial infarction. Catheter Cardiovasc Interv 2007;69(4):488–96.

5. Bavry AA, Kumbani DJ, Bhatt DL. Role of adjunctive thrombectomy and embolic protection devices in acute myocardial infarction: a comprehensive meta-analysis of randomized trials. Eur Heart J 2008;29(24):2989–3001.

6. Sobieraj DM, White CM, Kluger J, et al. Systematic review: comparative effectiveness of adjunctive devices in patients with ST-segment elevation myocardial infarction undergoing percutaneous coronary intervention of native vessels. BMC Cardiovasc Disord 2011;11:74.

7. Niccoli G, Burzotta F, Galiuto L, et al. Myocardial no-reflow in humans. J Am Coll Cardiol 2009;54(4):281–92.

8. Heusch G, Kleinbongard P, Böse D, et al. Coronary microembolization: from bedside to bench and back to bedside. Circulation 2009;120(18):1822–36.

9. Kloner RA. No-reflow phenomenon: maintaining vascular integrity. J Cardiovasc Pharmacol Ther 2011;16(3–4):244–50.

10. The Thrombolysis in Myocardial Infarction (TIMI) trial. Phase I findings. TIMI Study Group. N Engl J Med 1985;312(14):932–6.

11. van't Hof AW, Liem A, Suryapranata H, et al. Angiographic assessment of myocardial perfusion in patients treated with primary angioplasty for acute myocardial infarction: myocardial blush grade. Circulation 1998;97(23):2302–6.

12. Schröder R. Prognostic impact of early ST-segment resolution in acute ST-elevation myocardial infarction. Circulation 2004;110(21):e506–10.

13. Wu KC, Kim RJ, Bluemke DA, et al. Quantification and time course of microvascular obstruction by contrast-enhanced echocardiography and magnetic resonance imaging following acute myocardial infarction and reperfusion. J Am Coll Cardiol 1998;32(6):1756–64.

14. Wong DT, Leung MC, Richardson JD, et al. Cardiac magnetic resonance derived late microvascular obstruction assessment post ST-segment elevation myocardial infarction is the best predictor of left ventricular function: a comparison of angiographic and cardiac magnetic resonance derived measurements. Int J Cardiovasc Imaging 2012;28(8):1971–81. http://dx.doi.org/10.1007/s10554-012-0021-9.

15. Tarantini G, Razzolini R, Cacciavillani L, et al. Influence of transmurality, infarct size, and severe microvascular obstruction on left ventricular remodeling and function after primary angioplasty. Am J Cardiol 2006;98(8):1033–40.

16. Zia MI, Ghugre NR, Connelly KA, et al. Thrombus aspiration during primary percutaneous coronary intervention is associated with reduced myocardial edema, hemorrhage, microvascular obstruction, and left ventricular remodeling. J Cardiovasc Magn Reson 2012;14:19.

17. An Y, Kaji S, Kim K, et al. Successful thrombus aspiration during primary percutaneous coronary intervention reduces infarct size and preserves myocardial viability: a cardiac magnetic resonance imaging study. J Invasive Cardiol 2011;23(5):172–6.

18. Mehta RH, Harjai JK, Boura J, et al. Prognostic significance of transient no-reflow during primary percutaneous coronary intervention for ST-elevation myocardial infarction. Am J Cardiol 2003;92(12):1445–7.

19. Ndrepepa G, Tiroch K, Fusaro M, et al. 5-year prognostic value of no-reflow phenomenon after percutaneous coronary intervention in patients with acute myocardial infarction. J Am Coll Cardiol 2010;55(21):2383–9.

20. Heading: healthcare professionals, cardiovascular, catheters, aspiration catheter. Available at: www.medtronic.com. Accessed January 02, 2013.

21. Svilaas T, Vlaar PJ, van der Horst IC, et al. Thrombus aspiration during primary percutaneous coronary intervention. N Engl J Med 2008;358(6):557–67.

22. Vlaar PJ, Svilaas T, van der Horst IC, et al. Cardiac death and reinfarction after 1 year in the Thrombus Aspiration during Percutaneous coronary intervention in Acute myocardial infarction study (TAPAS): a 1-year follow-up study. Lancet 2008;371(9628):1915–20.

23. Sardella G, Mancone M, Bucciarelli-Ducci C, et al. Thrombus aspiration during primary percutaneous coronary intervention improves myocardial reperfusion and reduces infarct size: the EXPIRA (thrombectomy with export catheter in infarct-related artery during primary percutaneous coronary intervention) prospective, randomized trial. J Am Coll Cardiol 2009;53(4):309–15.

24. Sardella G, Mancone M, Canali E, et al. Impact of thrombectomy with EXPort Catheter in Infarct-Related Artery during Primary Percutaneous Coronary Intervention (EXPIRA Trial) on cardiac death. Am J Cardiol 2010;106(5):624–9.

25. Heading: products, coronary. Available at: www.invatec.com. Accessed January 2, 2013.

26. Burzotta F, Trani C, Romagnoli E, et al. Manual thrombus-aspiration improves myocardial reperfusion: the randomized evaluation of the effect of mechanical reduction of distal embolization by thrombus-aspiration and rescue angioplasty (REMEDIA) trial. J Am Coll Cardiol 2005;46(2):371–6.

27. Dudek D, Mielecki W, Burzotta F, et al. Thrombus aspiration followed by direct stenting: a novel strategy of primary percutaneous coronary intervention in ST-segment elevation myocardial infarction. Results of the Polish-Italian-Hungarian RAndomized ThrombEctomy Trial (PIHRATE Trial). Am Heart J 2010;160(5):966–72.

28. Sardella G, Mancone M, Nguyen BL, et al. The effect of thrombectomy on myocardial blush in primary angioplasty: the Randomized Evaluation of Thrombus Aspiration by two thrombectomy devices in acute Myocardial Infarction (RETAMI) trial. Catheter Cardiovasc Interv 2008;71(1):84–91.

29. Vlaar PJ, Svilaas T, Vogelzang M, et al. A comparison of 2 thrombus aspiration devices with histopathological analysis of retrieved material in patients presenting with ST-segment myocardial infarction. JACC Cardiovasc Interv 2008;1(3):258–64.

30. Heading: interventional cardiology. Available at: www.atriummed.com. Accessed January 2, 2013.

31. Kishi T, Yamada A, Okamatsu S, et al. Percutaneous coronary arterial thrombectomy for acute myocardial infarction reduces no-reflow phenomenon and protects against left ventricular remodeling related to the proximal left anterior descending and right coronary artery. Int Heart J 2007;48(3):287–302.

32. Nakatani D, Sato H, Sakata Y, et al. Effect of intracoronary thrombectomy on 30-day mortality in patients with acute myocardial infarction. Am J Cardiol 2007;100(8):1212–7.

33. Heading: our products. Available at: www.vasc.com. Accessed January 2, 2013.

34. Silva-Orrego P, Colombo P, Bigi R, et al. Thrombus aspiration before primary angioplasty improves myocardial reperfusion in acute myocardial infarction: the DEAR-MI (Dethrombosis to Enhance Acute Reperfusion in Myocardial Infarction) study. J Am Coll Cardiol 2006;48(8):1552–9.

35. Yokoyama Y, Kushibiki M, Fujiwara T, et al. Feasibility and safety of thrombectomy with TVAC aspiration catheter system for patients with acute myocardial infarction. Heart Vessels 2006;21(1):1–7.

36. Ikari Y, Sakurada M, Kozuma K, et al. Upfront thrombus aspiration in primary coronary intervention for patients with ST-segment elevation acute myocardial infarction: report of the VAMPIRE (VAcuuM asPIration thrombus REmoval) trial. JACC Cardiovasc Interv 2008;1(4):424–31.

37. Heading: U.S. product catalog. Available at: www.ev3.net. Accessed January 02, 2013.

38. Lefèvre T, Garcia E, Reimers B, et al. X-sizer for thrombectomy in acute myocardial infarction improves ST-segment resolution: results of the X-sizer in AMI for negligible embolization and optimal ST resolution (X AMINE ST) trial. J Am Coll Cardiol 2005;46(2):246–52.

39. Vink MA, Patterson MS, van Etten J, et al. A randomized comparison of manual versus mechanical thrombus removal in primary percutaneous coronary intervention in the treatment of ST-segment elevation myocardial infarction (TREAT-MI). Catheter Cardiovasc Interv 2011;78(1):14–9.

40. Nakagawa Y, Matsuo S, Kimura T, et al. Thrombectomy with AngioJet catheter in native coronary arteries for patients with acute or recent myocardial infarction. Am J Cardiol 1999;83(7):994–9.

41. Heading: products. Available at: www.medrad.com. Accessed January 2, 2013.

42. Simonton CA 3rd, Brodie BR, Wilson H, et al. Angio-Jet experience from the multi-center STENT registry. J Invasive Cardiol 2006;18(Suppl C):C22–3.

43. Ali A, Cox D, Dib N, et al, AIMI Investigators. Rheolytic thrombectomy with percutaneous coronary intervention for infarct size reduction in acute myocardial infarction: 30-day results from a multicenter randomized study. J Am Coll Cardiol 2006; 48(2):244–52.

44. Migliorini A, Stabile A, Rodriguez AE, et al, JETSTENT Trial Investigators. Comparison of AngioJet rheolytic thrombectomy before direct infarct artery stenting with direct stenting along in patients with acute myocardial infarction. The JETSTENT trial. J Am Coll Cardiol 2010;56(16):1298–306.

45. Heading: coronary vascular intervention. Available at: www.spectranetics.com. Accessed January 2, 2013.

46. Topaz O, Ebersole D, Das T, et al. Excimer laser angioplasty in acute myocardial infarction (the CARMEL multicenter trial). Am J Cardiol 2004;93(6):694–701.

47. Dörr M, Vogelgesang D, Hummel A, et al. Excimer laser thrombus elimination for prevention of distal embolization and no-reflow in patients with acute ST elevation myocardial infarction: results from the randomized LaserAMI study. Int J Cardiol 2007; 116(1):20–6.

48. Heading: Acolysis System. Available at: www. rayglobe.com. Accessed January 2, 2013.

49. Brosh D, Bartorelli AL, Cribier A, et al. Percutaneous transluminal therapeutic ultrasound for high-risk thrombus-containing lesions in native coronary arteries. Catheter Cardiovasc Interv 2002;55(1):43–9.

50. Lang EV, Kulis AM, Villani M, et al. Hemolysis comparison between the OmniSonics OmniWave Endovascular System and the Possis AngioJet in a porcine model. J Vasc Interv Radiol 2008;19(8): 1215–21.

51. Vink MA, Kramer MC, Li X, et al. Clinical and angiographic predictors and prognostic value of failed thrombus aspiration in primary percutaneous coronary intervention. JACC Cardiovasc Interv 2011; 4(6):634–42.

52. Lee CH, Tan HC, Wong HB, et al. Incidence, predictors, and outcomes of device failure of X-sizer thrombectomy: real-world experience of 200 cases in 5 years. Am Heart J 2007;153(1):14.e13–9.

53. Ali A, Malik FS, Dinshaw H, et al. Reduction in QT dispersion with rheolytic thrombectomy in acute myocardial infarction: evidence of electrical stability with reperfusion therapy. Catheter Cardiovasc Interv 2001;52(1):56–8.

54. Zhu DW. The potential mechanisms of bradyarrhythmias associated with AngioJet thrombectomy. J Invasive Cardiol 2008;20(8 Suppl A):2A–4A.

55. Murad B. Intracoronary aminophylline for management of bradyarrhythmias during thrombectomy with the AngioJet catheter. J Invasive Cardiol 2008; 20(8 Suppl A):12A–18A.

56. Syed T, Tamis-Holland J, Coven D, et al. Can glycopyrrolate replace temporary pacemaker and atropine in patients at high risk for symptomatic bradycardia undergoing AngioJet mechanical thrombectomy? J Invasive Cardiol 2008;20(8 Suppl A):19A–21A.

57. Mixon TA, Dehmer GJ, Santos RA, et al. Guidewire pacing safely and effectively treats bradyarrhythmia induced by rheolytic thrombectomy and precludes the need for transvenous pacing: the Scott & White experience. J Invasive Cardiol 2008;20(8 Suppl A):5A–8A.

58. Alazzoni A, Velianou J, Jolly SS. Left main thrombus as a complication of thrombectomy during primary percutaneous coronary intervention. J Invasive Cardiol 2011;23(2):E9–11.

59. Sanmartín M, Goicolea J, Ruis-Salmerón R, et al. Coronary perforation as a potential complication derived from coronary thrombectomy with the X-sizer device. Catheter Cardiovasc Interv 2002;56(3):378–82.

60. Lee CH, Wong PS, Tan HC, et al. Free coronary perforation after X-sizer thrombectomy: experience of two cases and review of the literature. J Invasive Cardiol 2005;17(8):445–8.

61. Porto I, Greco F, Buffon A. Coronary arteriovenous fistula following X-sizer thrombectomy. J Cardiovasc Med (Hagerstown) 2007;8(11):973–4.

62. Cafri C, Rosenstein G, Ilia R. Fracture of a coronary guidewire during graft thrombectomy with an X-sizer device. J Invasive Cardiol 2004;16(5):263–5.

63. López-Mínguez JR, Dávila E, Doblado M, et al. Rupture and intracoronary entrapment of an angioplasty guidewire with the X-sizer thromboatherectomy catheter during rescue angioplasty. Rev Esp Cardiol 2004;57(2):180–3 [in Spanish].

64. De Luca G, Dudek D, Sardella G, et al. Adjunctive manual thrombectomy improves myocardial perfusion and mortality in patients undergoing primary percutaneous coronary intervention for ST-elevation myocardial infarction: a meta-analysis of randomized trials. Eur Heart J 2008;29(24):3002–10.

65. Grines CL, Nelson TR, Safian RD, et al. A Bayesian meta-analysis comparing AngioJet thrombectomy to percutaneous coronary intervention alone in acute myocardial infarction. J Interv Cardiol 2008;21(6):459–82.

66. Burzotta F, De Vita M, Gu YL, et al. Clinical impact of thrombectomy in acute ST-elevation myocardial infarction: an individual patient-data pooled analysis of 11 trials. Eur Heart J 2009;30(18):2193–203.

67. Mongeon FP, Bélisle P, Joseph L, et al. Adjunctive thrombectomy for acute myocardial infarction: a Bayesian meta-analysis. Circ Cardiovasc Interv 2010;3(1):6–16.

68. Stone GW, Maehara A, Witzenbichler B, et al. Intracoronary abciximab and aspiration thrombectomy in patients with large anterior myocardial infarction. The INFUSE-AMI randomized trial. JAMA 2012; 307(17):1817–26.

69. Shani J, Abittan M, Gallarello F, et al. Mechanical manipulation of thrombus: coronary thrombectomy, intracoronary clot displacement, and transcatheter aspiration. Am J Cardiol 1993;72(19):116G–8G.

70. Owan TE, Roe MT, Messenger JC, et al. Contemporary use of adjunctive thrombectomy during primary percutaneous coronary intervention for ST-elevation myocardial infarction in the United States. Catheter Cardiovasc Interv 2012;80(7):1173–80.

# Adjunctive Pharmacotherapy for Thrombotic Coronary Lesions

Pei-Hsiu Huang, MD[a], Deepak L. Bhatt, MD, MPH[a,b],*

## KEYWORDS

- Intracoronary thrombus • Percutaneous coronary intervention • Thrombolytic therapy
- Glycoprotein IIb/IIIa inhibitors

## KEY POINTS

- Angiographically evident intracoronary thrombus is associated with higher rates of angioplasty failure and worse clinical outcomes.
- Thrombolytic therapy and glycoprotein IIb/IIIa inhibitors may decrease ischemic complications in percutaneous coronary intervention of thrombus-containing native coronary artery lesions.
- Embolic protection devices may be more effective than thrombolytics or glycoprotein IIb/IIIa inhibitors in the treatment of saphenous vein grafts.

## INTRODUCTION

Contemporary treatment of coronary artery disease commonly involves percutaneous coronary intervention (PCI) as a method of coronary revascularization. Advancements in technique and equipment have dramatically improved the outcomes for patients undergoing PCI in a variety of acute and elective settings. In some cases, intracoronary (IC) thrombus is discovered as part of the initial lesion presentation or is newly formed during the procedure. In either case, the presence of IC thrombus threatens the success of revascularization. Several studies clearly demonstrate the association with higher rates of angioplasty failure, abrupt closure, distal embolization, slow-flow or no-reflow phenomenon, restenosis, and worse clinical outcomes.[1–7] The prevalence of IC thrombus in patients with symptomatic ischemic heart disease is likely underestimated on angiography alone,[8] an important consideration during an era in which angiography and PCI play a large role in the management of acute coronary syndromes (ACS) as well as in the treatment of more complex coronary disease. The optimal strategy for managing IC thrombus remains uncertain, and thus continues to challenge interventional cardiologists faced with this situation. This article discusses the various pharmacologic agents to consider when treating thrombotic coronary lesions. Technical and mechanical aspects of the interventional procedure are reviewed in "Utility of Thrombectomy in Primary Percutaneous Coronary Intervention" by Carl A. Dragstedt and Anthony

Disclosures: P.H. has no relevant disclosures. D.L.B.: Advisory Board: Medscape Cardiology; Board of Directors: Boston VA Research Institute, Society of Chest Pain Centers; Chair: American Heart Association Get With The Guidelines Science Subcommittee; Honoraria: American College of Cardiology (Editor, Clinical Trials, Cardiosource), Duke Clinical Research Institute (clinical trial steering committees), Slack Publications (Chief Medical Editor, Cardiology Today Intervention), WebMD (CME steering committees); Other: Senior Associate Editor, Journal of Invasive Cardiology; Research Grants: Amarin, AstraZeneca, Bristol-Myers Squibb, Eisai, Ethicon, Medtronic, Sanofi Aventis, The Medicines Company; Unfunded Research: FlowCo, PLx Pharma, Takeda.
a Division of Cardiovascular Medicine, Brigham and Women's Hospital and Harvard Medical School, 75 Francis Street, Boston, MA 02115, USA; b Integrated Interventional Cardiovascular Program, Cardiovascular Division, VA Boston Healthcare System, 1400 VFW Parkway, Boston, MA 02132, USA
* Corresponding author. VA Boston Healthcare System, 1400 VFW Parkway, Boston, MA 02132.
E-mail address: dlbhattmd@post.harvard.edu

A. Bavry and "Thrombectomy Devices in Coronary Intervention" by Aaron Horne Jr and Matthews Chacko elsewhere in this issue.

## THROMBUS FORMATION

The hemostatic system produces thrombus as the end product of a series of events designed to preserve the integrity of the circulatory system after injury. The system quickly forms a temporary seal to protect against excessive blood loss while healing of the vessel wall occurs. The process of thrombus formation involves activation of 2 major coagulation pathways, the intrinsic and extrinsic pathways, that coalesce into a common final pathway to generate fibrin. The fibrin framework supports the aggregation of platelets and other circulating cells that organize to further stabilize the hemostatic plug.

Thrombus formation as a result of endovascular injury forms the pathologic basis of ACSs. The significance of these hemostatic mechanisms in the process of atherothrombosis plays out in the following manner. Typically, a fibrous cap isolates the lipid-laden portions of atherosclerotic plaques from the coronary artery lumen. Fissure or rupture of this fibrous cap exposes the extracellular matrix collagen and macrophage-associated tissue factor to the bloodstream, and initiates the thrombotic cascade. The contact of tissue factor and collagen with blood sets off "initiation" with the extrinsic coagulation cascade to produce thrombin. This process is somewhat inefficient and generates a small amount of thrombin, which in turn promotes activation of factors VIII and V leading to a burst of thrombin production via the intrinsic coagulation pathway.[9] During this "amplification" stage, the more efficient production of thrombin enhances the clot structure by strengthening the fibrin framework.

The composition of a coronary thrombus includes fibrin, platelets, erythrocytes, and various inflammatory cells. Platelets account for about 25% of the initial thrombus in acute myocardial infarction (MI),[10] making the mechanisms for platelet aggregation a prime pharmacologic target. Similar to fibrin formation, platelet aggregation occurs through two distinct pathways, one resulting from collagen interaction with various platelet glycoproteins and the other from generation of thrombin by the coagulation cascades after exposure to tissue factor that is independent of platelet glycoproteins and von Willebrand factor. Thrombin activates platelets by cleaving platelet surface protease-activated receptor 1 (PAR1), causing the release of adenosine diphosphate, serotonin, and thromboxane $A_2$. These substances then propagate the platelet thrombus through activation of additional platelets. As the clot ages, its composition changes to include a higher fibrin content, with the initial 25% platelet portion decreasing to around 10% in clots older than 6 hours.[10] This characteristic may impact the effectiveness of pharmacologic or mechanical therapies for coronary reperfusion in ACS.

## CONSEQUENCES OF INTRACORONARY THROMBUS

Many patients with unstable coronary syndromes undergoing angiography have evidence of IC thrombus. The Thrombolysis in Myocardial Infarction (TIMI) thrombus score is a useful method of quantitatively assessing the burden of angiographically evident thrombus (**Table 1**).[11,12] In the Coronary Angioplasty versus Excisional Atherectomy Trial (CAVEAT), around 20% of patients with symptomatic ischemic heart disease had visible thrombus on initial angiography, perhaps an underestimate, as 36% of patients had thrombus identified in atherectomy aspirates.[8] Angioscopic evidence of thrombus was found in 47% of patients undergoing angioplasty for unstable angina.[13] In patients presenting with ST-segment elevation MI, the majority have complete thrombotic occlusion of an epicardial coronary artery. The finding of thrombus on angiography has many implications and may prompt a change in the therapeutic approach. Presence of IC thrombus has been associated with an increased incidence of abrupt closure, restenosis, MI, death, and coronary artery bypass grafting (CABG) (**Table 2**).[1,3,5,6,14,15]

| Table 1 TIMI thrombus score | |
|---|---|
| Grade 0 | No angiographic evidence of thrombus |
| Grade 1 | Possible thrombus as suggested by: Reduced contrast density Haziness Irregular lesion contour Smooth convex "meniscus" at the site of total occlusion |
| Grade 2 | Definite thrombus, largest dimension ≤½ the vessel diameter |
| Grade 3 | Definite thrombus, largest dimension >½ but <2 vessel diameters |
| Grade 4 | Definite thrombus, largest dimension ≥2 vessel diameters |
| Grade 5 | Total occlusion |

**Table 2**
**Outcomes associated with angiographically evident thrombus**

|  | Odds Ratio[Ref.] |
|---|---|
| In-Hospital | |
| Death | 2.06[6] |
| MI | 1.33–3.78[6,7] |
| Death or MI | 1.30[7] |
| 30-Day | |
| Death | 2.36[15] |
| MI | 2.00[15] |
| Death or MI | 2.04[15] |
| 30-Day repeat revascularization | |
| By PCI | 1.54[15] |
| By CABG | 1.63[15] |
| Any revascularization | 2.23[15] |
| Acute closure | 2.43[1] |
| Angioplasty failure | 1.96–7.07[2] |

All odds ratios were statistically significant after multivariate adjustment within their respective studies.

*Abbreviations:* CABG, coronary artery bypass grafting; MI, myocardial infarction; PCI, percutaneous coronary intervention.

Studies from the balloon angioplasty era repeatedly demonstrated the association of IC thrombus with acute closure. In a series of 238 consecutive patients treated with balloon angioplasty between 1979 and 1983, complete vessel occlusion after angioplasty occurred in 73% of patients found to have IC thrombus and in only 8% of those without IC thrombus.[16] The incidence of acute occlusions after PCI of thrombus-containing lesions decreased to 24% in a subsequent report from the same institution on procedures performed between 1983 and 1985.[17] With the introduction of bare-metal stents, the rate of acute closure decreased further to 4%,[6] but the presence of IC thrombus remained an independent predictor of acute closure despite pharmacologic and procedural advancememts. A greater thrombus burden (≥2 mm on angiography) increased the odds of acute closure by nearly 4-fold.[3]

Whether IC thrombus affects short- and long-term mortality has been inconsistent among studies. In the Hirulog Angioplasty Study, the rate of in-hospital death after PCI among 4098 patients did not differ in those who had thrombus-containing lesions in comparison with the rest.[18] Similarly, a retrospective single-center analysis of 7184 patients did not show a significant difference in the rate of in-hospital death among patients undergoing PCI of a thrombus-containing lesion.[6] In long-term follow-up extending to 3 years, the composite end point of death or MI did not differ between patients with and without IC thrombus. A pooled analysis of data from 6 randomized trials representing 7917 patients again demonstrated no difference in the incidence of in-hospital and 6-month mortality between patients with and without thrombus identified on angiography.[7] The same finding was demonstrated on an analysis from the Evaluation of IIb/IIIa Platelet Receptor Antagonist 7E3 in Preventing Ischemic Complications (EPIC) trial, which showed that the presence of thrombus did not influence the 30-day or 6-month mortality.[19] To the contrary, an analysis of the Platelet Receptor Inhibition for Ischemic Syndrome Management in Patients Limited by Unstable Signs and Symptoms (PRISM-PLUS) trial showed that presence of thrombus increased the odds of 30-day death by greater than 2-fold.[15] IC thrombus increases the odds of MI up to 3.8-fold for both in-hospital events and at 6 months. The relationship with MI remained significant even after adjustment for additional factors and exclusion of vein-graft lesions.[7]

## ADJUNCTIVE PHARMACOLOGIC THERAPY

Proposed strategies for treating thrombus-containing lesions have largely been based on anecdotal experience and observational trials rather than on data from large-scale randomized clinical trials. We will discuss on a few frequently encountered scenarios involving ST-segment elevation MI, high thrombus burden, and saphenous vein grafts, and attempt to review the evidence on the commonly used antithrombotic and antiplatelet agents.

### Unfractionated Heparin

The routine use of unfractionated heparin (UFH) in PCI was born out of convention rather than clinical trial data, as it was the only anticoagulant available for PCI for many years.[20] Initial observations associated inadequate anticoagulation with formation of IC thrombus and complications.[21–23] Subsequent studies demonstrated that the level of anticoagulation during PCI as measured by activated clotting time (ACT) had an inverse relationship with the risk of ischemic complications, although higher levels of anticoagulation increased the risk of bleeding complications.[24–26]

In the setting of IC thrombus, some have reported that a prolonged preprocedural heparin infusion and delivery of IC heparin were effective at reducing the burden of thrombus.[21,27] However, thrombotic complications still occur despite aggressive anticoagulation with heparin, explained at least in part by the lack of adequate suppression of thrombin activity in some patients with heparin anticoagulation alone.[28] The results of 2 meta-analyses further support to the need for additional agents rather than augmenting anticoagulation with heparin alone during PCI by increasing the heparin dose only. Using data from 6 randomized clinical trials representing 5216 patients, Chew and colleagues[29] demonstrated a correlation between reduction in ischemic events with higher ACTs, a relationship not seen in the subgroup of patients receiving abciximab, representing about 66% of the total population. This subgroup of patients receiving abciximab had a lower rate of ischemic events compared with the overall population, irrespective of ACT level. The second meta-analysis used data from a more contemporary set of 4 randomized trials representing 9974 patients, and demonstrated the lack of correlation between ACT and ischemic events.[30] The important differences between these studies include the higher frequency of glycoprotein (GP) IIb/IIIa inhibitor (89% vs 66%) and coronary stent use (93% vs 15%) in the more contemporary analysis, perhaps accounting for the lower absolute overall event rates.

## Low Molecular Weight Heparin

Trials have studied low molecular weight heparin (LMWH) as an alternative to UFH for antithrombotic therapy in PCI for both elective and ACS settings.[31–33] Experience with LMWH in STEMI was initially obtained from trials of fibrinolytic therapy in which the combination of LMWH with fibrinolytics reduced the thrombus burden on angiography.[34,35] LMWH in primary PCI has been reported in observational studies and has shown a reduction in ischemic events without a significant increase in bleeding complications.[36–39] This finding was confirmed in the Acute Myocardial Infarction Treated with Primary Angioplasty and Intravenous Enoxaparin or Unfractionated Heparin to Lower Ischemic and Bleeding Events at Short- and Long-term Follow-up (ATOLL) study, which randomized 910 patients with STEMI undergoing primary PCI to anticoagulation with UFH or enoxaparin.[40] Patients treated with enoxaparin had a lower rate of ischemic events without an increase in bleeding or procedural success. Of note, radial access was used in 67% of procedures, GP IIb/IIIa inhibitors were given in 80% of patients, and 63% of patients received a clopidogrel loading dose of 600 mg or greater, reflecting the use of contemporary strategies in STEMI treatment. Some reports have found that catheter and guide-wire thrombosis may occur with the use of

LMWH as an alternative to UFH in PCI of thrombotic lesions.[41–43] Although similar complications may have occurred in ATOLL, an additional enoxaparin dose was administered when stronger anticoagulation was desired or if the procedure lasted longer than 2 hours. We suggest consideration of this strategy when LMWH is used for anticoagulation in PCI of thrombus-containing lesions.

## Bivalirudin

The results of the Randomized Evaluation in PCI Linking Angiomax to Reduced Clinical Events (REPLACE)-2,[44] the Acute Catheterization and Urgent Intervention Triage Strategy (ACUITY),[45] and the Harmonizing Outcomes with Revascularization and Stents in Acute Myocardial Infarction (HORIZONS-AMI)[46] studies provided the basis for using bivalirudin as an alternative antithrombotic agent in PCI. Its use in the treatment of thrombus-containing lesions was first examined in a subset of 567 patients from the 4098 patient Hirulog Angioplasty Study, in which bivalirudin monotherapy was not found to be more effective than heparin alone in reducing the incidence of death, MI, emergent CABG, or abrupt vessel closure at 6 months.[18] However, this trial was strictly an angioplasty study, and also did not use the higher bivalirudin dosing that is standard today or bailout GP IIb/IIIa inhibitors. The 3 contemporary randomized trials use GP IIb/IIIa inhibitors on a provisional basis, with 7% to 9% of patients in the bivalirudin treatment groups receiving these agents for various indications. In these cases, 6.5% of bivalirudin patients in ACUITY received GP IIb/IIIa for procedural complications, most commonly for the presence of new or suspected thrombus, slow flow, or no reflow. Similarly, in HORIZONS-AMI, 2.8% of bivalirudin patients received GP IIb/IIIa inhibitors for no reflow after PCI and 1.9% received GP IIb/IIIa inhibitors for development of a giant thrombus after PCI.

Adequate antiplatelet therapy before PCI seems to mitigate some of the risk of acute ischemic events while using bivalirudin for PCI. In a post hoc analysis of the ACUITY data, patients with ACSs treated with bivalirudin during PCI who received clopidogrel before or within 30 minutes of the procedure had similar rates of ischemic events compared with those treated with heparin and a GP IIb/IIIa inhibitor.[47] Patients who did not receive clopidogrel or received clopidogrel more than 30 minutes after the PCI had a higher incidence of ischemic events. Inadequate platelet inhibition may also explain the higher rate of acute stent thrombosis among bivalirudin-treated patients in HORIZONS-AMI despite administration of antiplatelet therapy immediately before PCI. The use of the newer antiplatelet agents prasugrel and ticagrelor in ACS patients undergoing PCI may improve outcomes further, as these agents achieve higher levels of platelet inhibition more rapidly than clopidogrel.[48,49]

Some investigators have proposed using a prolonged bivalirudin infusion after PCI as another strategy to reduce the risk of acute ischemic events. In a few observational reports, this strategy appeared to reduce myocardial damage as measured by levels of creatine kinase MB,[50] and led to faster ST-segment resolution[51] as well as reduced rates of acute stent thrombosis[52] in the STEMI setting.

## Thrombolytics

In the treatment of STEMI, both primary PCI and intravenous thrombolytic therapy can effectively restore flow in the culprit coronary artery. Use of thrombolytic therapy in acute MI was first described in the 1950s, but did not gain widespread use until studies implicated thrombotic coronary artery occlusion as the pathologic event in acute MI. Many of the early studies of thrombolysis in acute MI delivered various agents locally by way of invasive cardiac catheterization, and showed that a high rate of reperfusion could be achieved.[53–55] Intravenous thrombolysis was similarly effective in achieving vessel patency. However, with the advancement of PCI technology and techniques the use of IC thrombolysis decreased, taking on more of a supportive role to mechanical interventions and newer pharmacologic agents.

Studies examining the use of IC thrombolytics as a prophylactic measure against acute closure after angioplasty have not suggested a significant benefit in outcomes. Treatment with adjunctive urokinase during angioplasty appeared to lower rates of abrupt closure, MI, and emergency bypass surgery in one small study.[56] No benefit was seen in a second small study examining the use of adjunctive IC urokinase during angioplasty.[57] The larger randomized Thrombolysis and Angioplasty in Unstable Angina (TAUSA) trial studied the routine administration of IC urokinase versus placebo during PCI in 469 patients and showed that despite a mild, nonsignificant reduction in thrombus after angioplasty, patients treated with urokinase had higher incidences of acute closure, recurrent ischemia, infarction, or need for emergency CABG.[58] A similar trend was evident in the subgroup of patients with complex lesions, in whom the incidence of recurrent ischemia and acute closure, mostly thrombotic in nature, was higher among those treated with urokinase.[59] The introduction of coronary stents and the general advancement of PCI have dramatically lowered the rate of acute closure with PCI. The use of IC thrombolytics as an adjunct to contemporary PCI methods was revisited in a recent small pilot study showing that whereas measures of microvascular function improved with administration of IC streptokinase after primary PCI, left ventricular size and function did not differ from that of the placebo group at 6 months.[60]

Some investigators have advocated pharmacoinvasive therapy, describing the combined strategy of fibrinolytics and PCI, as the optimal approach to the management of thrombotic lesions. Compared with IC thrombolysis alone, additional treatment with angioplasty resulted in a lower rate of ischemic events and greater improvement in left ventricular function.[61–63] In the setting of STEMI, a recent meta-analysis of 17 trials using the combination of fibrinolytics with or without GP IIb/IIIa inhibitors resulted in an increased risk of death, reinfarction, and urgent revascularization as well as major bleeding and total and hemorrhagic stroke, compared with primary PCI.[64]

Four recent major randomized trials have also addressed this issue, and form the basis of the current American College of Cardiology/American Heart Association guidelines on pharmacoinvasive therapy.[65] The Assessment of the Safety and Efficacy of a New Treatment Strategy with Percutaneous Coronary Intervention (ASSENT-4 PCI) trial[66] compared full-dose tenecteplase followed by immediate PCI and standard primary PCI in 1667 patients with STEMI. The Facilitated Intervention with Enhanced Reperfusion to Stop Events (FINESSE) trial[67] compared PCI with upstream abciximab or full-dose reteplase and abciximab with standard primary PCI in 2452 patients with STEMI. Neither study found a benefit of the pharmacoinvasive strategy over primary PCI in clinical outcomes. However, the pharmacoinvasive groups had higher rates of adverse events including bleeding, strokes, and ischemic cardiac complications.

The 2 other trials, Combined Abciximab REteplase Stent Study in Acute Myocardial Infarction (CARESS-in-AMI)[68] and Trial of Routine Angioplasty and Stenting after Fibrinolysis to Enhance Reperfusion in Acute Myocardial Infarction (TRANSFER-AMI),[69] were designed to assess the optimal timing of PCI after fibrinolytic therapy. In both studies, patients with STEMI and high-risk features presenting to hospitals without primary PCI capabilities were given thrombolytic therapy and then randomized to early transfer to a PCI center for angiography and revascularization or standard therapy. Compared with standard therapy, early PCI after thrombolysis resulted in a lower rate of ischemic complications without a significant increase in major bleeding in these high-risk patients.

Despite the lack of benefit in routine use of adjunctive thrombolytics in the treatment of STEMI, the pharmacoinvasive approach may play a more important role in lesions with a large thrombus burden. Of note, Gurbel and colleagues[70] treated 45 patients found to have IC thrombus on angiography with the combination of IC heparin and 20 mg alteplase administered as 2-mg bolus injections every 2 minutes, and found such a strategy to be effective in reducing the thrombus size, particularly in those with large thrombi. Subsequent PCI was successful in 89% of patients. Local thrombolytic delivery using perfusion wires, catheters, and special balloon catheters have also been reported.[71–74] Two recent case reports highlight the pharmacoinvasive management of large IC thrombus in contemporary practice. Kim and colleagues[75] described a case of massive IC thrombus involving a dominant right coronary artery. After failure of aspiration thrombectomy to remove the thrombus, IC thrombolysis was performed with a 10-mg bolus injection of alteplase followed by a 1-mg/min infusion for 90 minutes. Repeat angiography showed near complete dissolution of the thrombus, allowing for an uncomplicated PCI of a proximal lesion of the right coronary artery. Agarwal[76] reported the case of a patient presenting with chest pain who was found to have thrombotic occlusion of the proximal left anterior descending artery (LAD) as well as a large thrombus in the left circumflex artery (LCx). Alteplase (20 mg) was infused through the guiding catheter followed by an additional 10 mg, resulting in dissolution of the LCx and restoration of flow in the LAD. Aspiration thrombectomy retrieved the remaining fragments of thrombus from the LAD, and the underlying lesion was treated with stenting.

When thrombotic complications occur during PCI, local administration of thrombolytics may be used to improve coronary flow. Unfortunately, this treatment strategy lacks validation in large clinical trials, so experience is derived from small observational studies using streptokinase,[14,77] urokinase,[78–81] and recombinant tissue-type plasminogen activators,[81,82] reporting success rates between 47% and 91%. In general, successful results were achieved with repeat angioplasty performed immediately after thrombolytic administration, and the incidence of reinfarction and emergency coronary bypass were reduced.

However, Lincoff and colleagues[81] found that IC thrombolytic therapy was equally ineffective for the treatment of acute occlusions caused by thrombus compared with those attributable to other mechanisms. The only study to examine the use of IC thrombolytic therapy in this setting during the current era of PCI was reported by Kelly and colleagues.[82] In the 34 patients who developed an IC thrombotic complication during PCI, IC tenecteplase led to an angiographic dissolution of thrombus and improvement in coronary flow in 91% of patients. There were 3 minor access-site bleeds and 1 major gastrointestinal bleed. GP IIb/IIIa inhibitors were used in 76% of patients.

## Glycoprotein IIb/IIIa Inhibitors

The GP IIb/IIIa inhibitors play a central role in the armamentarium for treating thrombus-containing lesions. Several randomized trials, mostly using abciximab, have studied the addition of GP IIb/IIIa inhibitors to the standard antithrombotic regimen in primary PCI for STEMI. A meta-analysis of 11 abciximab trials showed that adjunctive IIb/IIIa use in primary PCI reduced mortality and reinfarction without increasing major bleeding complications.[83] The mortality benefit from GP IIb/IIIa inhibitors appears to be related to the risk profile of patients, with a more notable impact among higher-risk patients[84,85] and in diabetic patients.[86] Pooled analyses of randomized trials suggest equivalence among the abciximab and the small-molecule inhibitors eptifibatide and tirofiban in STEMI.[87,88]

IC and intravenous delivery routes have also been compared in several studies, with mixed results. Four recent meta-analyses have uniformly concluded that IC administration of GP IIb/IIIa reduced coronary flow, reinfarction, and mortality without an increase in bleeding.[89–92] However, none of these meta-analyses included the larger randomized trials Abciximab Intracoronary versus intravenous Drug Application in ST-Elevation Myocardial Infarction (AIDA STEMI)[93] and INFUSE-AMI.[94] AIDA STEMI randomized 2065 patients undergoing primary PCI to IC or intravenous abciximab. All patients were treated with UFH and antiplatelet therapy with aspirin plus clopidogrel or prasugrel. The abciximab infusion was continued in all patients for 12 hours after the PCI. At 90 days, there was no difference in the incidence of death or reinfarction in the IC and intravenous abciximab groups. Despite a lower rate of new congestive heart failure in patients receiving IC abciximab, no difference in infarct size, ST-segment resolution, or left ventricular ejection fraction was seen between the 2 treatment groups.

In INFUSE-AMI, 452 patients with anterior STE-MI presenting within 4 hours of symptom onset were randomized in a 2 × 2 factorial fashion to IC abciximab or no abciximab, and to aspiration thrombectomy or no thrombectomy. All patients were pretreated with aspirin and either clopidogrel or prasugrel, and underwent PCI using bivalirudin as the antithrombotic agent. Infarct size at 30 days assessed by cardiac magnetic resonance imaging was reduced with IC abciximab but not by aspiration thrombectomy. The incidence of bleeding did not increase with the use of IC abciximab, suggesting that this route of administration may afford the potential benefits of GP IIb/IIIa without affecting the bleeding benefits from bivalirudin use. Whether routine aspiration thrombectomy improves outcomes in STEMI remains uncertain.

The benefit of GP IIb/IIIa inhibitors in other thrombus-containing lesions is less clear. Prior reports have shown the effectiveness of abciximab administered as a rescue treatment for acute ischemic complications during PCI to reduce thrombus burden and restore TIMI-3 flow.[95,96] The c7E3 Fab Anti Platelet Therapy in Unstable REfractory angina (CAPTURE) trial, in which patients were pretreated for 18 to 24 hours with heparin alone or heparin plus abciximab before angioplasty, showed that complete thrombus dissolution occurred more frequently in those receiving abciximab (43% vs 22%).[97] The Thrombolysis in Myocardial Infarction (TIMI) 14 trial demonstrated that abciximab added to thrombolytic therapy reduced thrombus burden more than thrombolytic therapy alone.[12] However, when clinical outcomes were examined the benefit was not as robust. A pooled analysis of randomized trials did not show any benefit for in-hospital mortality or 6-month death and MI when GP IIb/IIIa inhibitors were used during PCI of thrombus-containing lesions.[7] In the PRISM-PLUS trial, treatment with tirofiban and heparin reduced thrombus burden compared with heparin alone, although 45% of patients had persistent IC thrombus and continued to have a greater than 2-fold increase in the risk of death or MI.[15]

## Oral Antiplatelet Therapy

All patients should receive antiplatelet therapy according to the guideline recommendations for PCI.[20] This therapy is particularly important in those undergoing PCI of thrombus-containing lesions, although none of these agents have been studied in this specific situation. Patients should receive aspirin, 325 mg, before the procedure followed by daily maintenance afterward. The use of clopidogrel in STEMI is supported by the ClOpidogrel and Metoprolol in Myocardial Infarction Trial (COMMIT)[98] and CLARITY-TIMI 28[99] trial, which showed a reduction in clinical outcomes including death and recurrent MI. A loading dose of 600 mg appears to improve both procedural and clinical outcomes.[100,101] The newer and more potent antiplatelet agents prasugrel and ticagrelor have also shown benefit in primary PCI. Among STEMI patients in the Therapeutic Outcomes by Optimizing Platelet Inhibition with Prasugrel—Thrombolysis in Myocardial Infarction (TRITON-TIMI) 38 trial that compared prasugrel with clopidogrel, the risk of ischemic events including stent thrombosis was reduced with the use of prasugrel. Of note, a 300-mg loading dose of clopidogrel was used in this study. In the subset of patients with STEMI in the Platelet Inhibition and Patient Outcomes (PLATO) trial, ticagrelor similarly improved ischemic events, including stent thrombosis, in comparison with clopidogrel.[102] There was also a significant all-cause and cardiac mortality benefit in this study. No significant increase in major bleeding was seen with prasugrel or ticagrelor compared with clopidogrel among the STEMI patients in either of these trials. Post-PCI antiplatelet therapy should be given in accordance with the current guideline recommendations.

## SAPHENOUS VEIN GRAFTS

After 5 years up to 45% of venous bypass grafts have occluded, leaving a large percentage of these patients requiring PCI or a repeat CABG in the first 10 years after the original surgery.[103] PCI for vein-graft disease is commonly preferred, but outcomes are worse than for intervention on the native coronary circulation with respect to distal embolization, no reflow, and a higher rate of periprocedural MI.[4] These large bypass conduits tend to develop a high burden of atherosclerosis that may contribute to the worse outcomes during intervention, particularly in older grafts with thrombus.[104–107] Embolic protection devices have been the mainstay in the prevention of ischemic complications during vein-graft PCI.[107] In addition to the standard antithrombotic regimen used for native coronary PCI, thrombolytics and GP IIb/IIIa inhibitors have been the main adjunctive agents.

In cases involving vein grafts with large intraluminal thrombus, several reports demonstrate the utility of thrombolytics in reducing the thrombus burden. Completely occluded vein grafts have been successfully recanalized using a combination of short or long-duration thrombolytic infusions and angioplasty.[71,80,108–110] Prolonged thrombolytic infusions have often been delivered through a perfusion wire. However, the effectiveness of IC thrombolytics may be limited in comparison with mechanical thrombectomy, as suggested by the Vein Graft AngioJet Study (VeGAS 2) in which use of rheolytic thrombectomy achieved a higher procedural success rate with fewer bleeding complications than when using IC urokinase.[111]

GP IIb/IIIa inhibitors have been more extensively studied in this setting. As in native coronary arteries, evidence suggests that administration of GP IIb/IIIa inhibitors can significantly reduce the thrombus burden before mechanical treatment of the graft.[112–114] Despite the angiographic improvement, GP IIb/IIIa inhibitors may not have the same clinical benefit as seen in the treatment of native coronary arteries. A pooled analysis of 5 randomized trials showed that vein-graft PCI resulted in an approximately 2-fold increase in the incidence of death and MI at 30 days and 6 months.[115] Use of GP IIb/IIIa inhibitors in these cases did not reduce mortality or reinfarction out to 6 months. Trials of systemic versus local administration of GP IIb/IIIa inhibitors in vein-graft intervention have not been performed.

## SUMMARY

Thrombotic coronary lesions are associated with a greater risk of adverse periprocedural and long-term outcomes. Treatment of these lesions remains a challenge for the interventional cardiologist because of the lack of consensus regarding the optimal approach. Adjunctive pharmacotherapy may reduce the risk of ischemic complications in high-risk situations such as STEMI with high thrombus burden. In these cases, administration of IC thrombolytics or GP IIb/IIIa inhibitors may reduce the thrombus burden and improve outcomes, although no large randomized trials yet support this practice. In the case of saphenous vein grafts, use of distal embolic protection, when feasible, may be more effective than use of GP IIb/IIIa inhibitors or thrombolytics.

## REFERENCES

1. Detre KM, Holmes DR, Holubkov R, et al. Incidence and consequences of periprocedural occlusion. The 1985-1986 National Heart, Lung, and Blood Institute Percutaneous Transluminal Coronary Angioplasty Registry. Circulation 1990;82:739–50.
2. Reeder GS, Bryant SC, Suman VJ, et al. Intracoronary thrombus: still a risk factor for PTCA failure? Cathet Cardiovasc Diagn 1995;34:191–5.
3. Ellis SG, Roubin GS, King SB, et al. Angiographic and clinical predictors of acute closure after native vessel coronary angioplasty. Circulation 1988;77:372–9.
4. Piana RN, Paik GY, Moscucci M, et al. Incidence and treatment of 'no-reflow' after percutaneous coronary intervention. Circulation 1994;89:2514–8.
5. Violaris AG, Melkert R, Herrman JP, et al. Role of angiographically identifiable thrombus on long-term luminal renarrowing after coronary angioplasty: a quantitative angiographic analysis. Circulation 1996;93:889–97.
6. Singh M, Berger PB, Ting HH, et al. Influence of coronary thrombus on outcome of percutaneous coronary angioplasty in the current era (the Mayo Clinic experience). Am J Cardiol 2001;88:1091–6.
7. Singh M, Reeder GS, Ohman EM, et al. Does the presence of thrombus seen on a coronary angiogram affect the outcome after percutaneous coronary angioplasty? An Angiographic Trials Pool data experience. J Am Coll Cardiol 2001;38:624.
8. Topol EJ, Leya F, Pinkerton CA, et al. A comparison of directional atherectomy with coronary angioplasty in patients with coronary artery disease. The CAVEAT Study Group. N Engl J Med 1993;329:221–7.
9. Furie B, Furie BC. Mechanisms of thrombus formation. N Engl J Med 2008;359:938–49.
10. Silvain J, Collet JP, Nagaswami C, et al. Composition of coronary thrombus in acute myocardial infarction. J Am Coll Cardiol 2011;57:1359–67.
11. The TIMI IIIA Investigators. Early effects of tissue-type plasminogen activator added to conventional therapy on the culprit coronary lesion in patients presenting with ischemic cardiac pain at rest. Results of the Thrombolysis in Myocardial Ischemia (TIMI IIIA) Trial. Circulation 1993;87:38–52.
12. Gibson CM, de Lemos JA, Murphy SA, et al. Combination therapy with abciximab reduces angiographically evident thrombus in acute myocardial infarction: a TIMI 14 substudy. Circulation 2001;103:2550–4.
13. Larrazet FS, Dupouy PJ, Rande JL, et al. Angioscopy after laser and balloon coronary angioplasty. J Am Coll Cardiol 1994;23:1321–6.
14. de Feyter PJ, van den Brand M, Laarman GJ, et al. Acute coronary artery occlusion during and after percutaneous transluminal coronary angioplasty. Frequency, prediction, clinical course, management, and follow-up. Circulation 1991;83:927–36.
15. Zhao XQ, Theroux P, Snapinn SM, et al. Intracoronary thrombus and platelet glycoprotein IIb/IIIa receptor blockade with tirofiban in unstable angina or non-Q-wave myocardial infarction: angiographic results from the PRISM-PLUS trial (platelet receptor inhibition for ischemic syndrome management in patients limited by unstable signs and symptoms). Circulation 1999;100:1609–15.
16. Mabin TA, Holmes DR, Smith HC, et al. Intracoronary thrombus: role in coronary occlusion complicating percutaneous transluminal coronary angioplasty. J Am Coll Cardiol 1985;5:198–202.

17. Sugrue DD, Holmes DR, Smith HC, et al. Coronary artery thrombus as a risk factor for acute vessel occlusion during percutaneous transluminal coronary angioplasty: improving results. Br Heart J 1986;56:62–6.

18. Shah PB, Ahmed WH, Ganz P, et al. Bivalirudin compared with heparin during coronary angioplasty for thrombus-containing lesions. J Am Coll Cardiol 1997;30:1264–9.

19. Khan MM, Ellis SG, Aguirre FV, et al. Does intracoronary thrombus influence the outcome of high risk percutaneous transluminal coronary angioplasty? Clinical and angiographic outcomes in a large multicenter trial. EPIC Investigators. Evaluation of IIb/IIIa Platelet Receptor Antagonist 7E3 in Preventing Ischemic Complications. J Am Coll Cardiol 1998;31:31–6.

20. Levine GN, Bates ER, Blankenship JC, et al. 2011 ACCF/AHA/SCAI guideline for percutaneous coronary intervention: a report of the American College of Cardiology Foundation/American Heart Association Task Force on Practice Guidelines and the Society for Cardiovascular Angiography and Interventions. Circulation 2011;124:e574–651.

21. Laskey MA, Deutsch E, Hirshfeld JW, et al. Influence of heparin therapy on percutaneous transluminal coronary angioplasty outcome in patients with coronary arterial thrombus. Am J Cardiol 1990;65:179–82.

22. Grayburn PA, Willard JE, Brickner ME, et al. In vivo thrombus formation on a guidewire during intravascular ultrasound imaging: evidence for inadequate heparinization. Cathet Cardiovasc Diagn 1991;23:141–3.

23. Vaitkus PT, Herrmann HC, Laskey WK. Management and immediate outcome of patients with intracoronary thrombus during percutaneous transluminal coronary angioplasty. Am Heart J 1992;124:1–8.

24. Ferguson JJ, Dougherty KG, Gaos CM, et al. Relation between procedural activated coagulation time and outcome after percutaneous transluminal coronary angioplasty. J Am Coll Cardiol 1994;23:1061–5.

25. McGarry TF, Gottlieb RS, Morganroth J, et al. The relationship of anticoagulation level and complications after successful percutaneous transluminal coronary angioplasty. Am Heart J 1992;123:1445–51.

26. Narins CR, Hillegass WB, Nelson CL, et al. Relation between activated clotting time during angioplasty and abrupt closure. Circulation 1996;93:667–71.

27. Mooney MR, Mooney JF, Goldenberg IF, et al. Percutaneous transluminal coronary angioplasty in the setting of large intracoronary thrombi. Am J Cardiol 1990;65:427–31.

28. Oltrona L, Eisenberg PR, Lasala JM, et al. Association of heparin-resistant thrombin activity with acute ischemic complications of coronary interventions. Circulation 1996;94:2064–71.

29. Chew DP, Bhatt DL, Lincoff AM, et al. Defining the optimal activated clotting time during percutaneous coronary intervention: aggregate results from 6 randomized, controlled trials. Circulation 2001;103:961–6.

30. Brener SJ, Moliterno DJ, Lincoff AM, et al. Relationship between activated clotting time and ischemic or hemorrhagic complications: analysis of 4 recent randomized clinical trials of percutaneous coronary intervention. Circulation 2004;110:994–8.

31. Montalescot G, White HD, Gallo R, et al. Enoxaparin versus unfractionated heparin in elective percutaneous coronary intervention. N Engl J Med 2006;355:1006–17.

32. SYNERGY Trial Investigators. Enoxaparin vs unfractionated heparin in high-risk patients with non-ST-segment elevation acute coronary syndromes managed with an intended early invasive strategy: primary results of the SYNERGY randomized trial. JAMA 2004;292:45–54.

33. Bhatt DL, Lee BI, Casterella PJ, et al. Safety of concomitant therapy with eptifibatide and enoxaparin in patients undergoing percutaneous coronary intervention: results of the Coronary Revascularization Using Integrilin and Single bolus Enoxaparin Study. J Am Coll Cardiol 2003;41:20–5.

34. Wallentin L, Bergstrand L, Dellborg M, et al. Low molecular weight heparin (dalteparin) compared to unfractionated heparin as an adjunct to rt-PA (alteplase) for improvement of coronary artery patency in acute myocardial infarction-the ASSENT Plus study. Eur Heart J 2003;24:897–908.

35. Sabatine MS, Cannon CP, Gibson CM, et al. Effect of clopidogrel pretreatment before percutaneous coronary intervention in patients with ST-elevation myocardial infarction treated with fibrinolytics: the PCI-CLARITY study. JAMA 2005;294:1224–32.

36. Zeymer U, Gitt A, Jünger C, et al. Efficacy and safety of enoxaparin in unselected patients with ST-segment elevation myocardial infarction. Thromb Haemost 2008;99:150–4.

37. Zeymer U, Gitt A, Zahn R, et al. Efficacy and safety of enoxaparin in combination with and without GP IIb/IIIa inhibitors in unselected patients with ST segment elevation myocardial infarction treated with primary percutaneous coronary intervention. EuroIntervention 2009;4:524–8.

38. Li YJ, Rha SW, Chen KY, et al. Low-molecular-weight heparin versus unfractionated heparin in acute ST-segment elevation myocardial infarction patients undergoing primary percutaneous coronary intervention with drug-eluting stents. Am Heart J 2010;159:684–690.e1.

39. Brieger D, Collet JP, Silvain J, et al. Heparin or enoxaparin anticoagulation for primary percutaneous

coronary intervention. Catheter Cardiovasc Interv 2011;77:182–90.

40. Montalescot G, Zeymer U, Silvain J, et al. Intravenous enoxaparin or unfractionated heparin in primary percutaneous coronary intervention for ST-elevation myocardial infarction: the international randomised open-label ATOLL trial. Lancet 2011; 378:693–703.

41. Buller CE, Pate GE, Armstrong PW, et al. Catheter thrombosis during primary percutaneous coronary intervention for acute ST elevation myocardial infarction despite subcutaneous low-molecular-weight heparin, acetylsalicylic acid, clopidogrel and abciximab pretreatment. Can J Cardiol 2006;22:511–5.

42. Madan M, Radhakrishnan S, Reis M, et al. Comparison of enoxaparin versus heparin during elective percutaneous coronary intervention performed with either eptifibatide or tirofiban (the ACTION Trial). Am J Cardiol 2005;95:1295–301.

43. Dana A, Nguyen CM, Cloutier S, et al. Macroscopic thrombus formation on angioplasty equipment following antithrombin therapy with enoxaparin. Catheter Cardiovasc Interv 2007;70:847–53.

44. Lincoff AM, Bittl JA, Harrington RA, et al. Bivalirudin and provisional glycoprotein IIb/IIIa blockade compared with heparin and planned glycoprotein IIb/IIIa blockade during percutaneous coronary intervention: REPLACE-2 randomized trial. JAMA 2003;289:853–63.

45. Stone GW, McLaurin BT, Cox DA, et al. Bivalirudin for patients with acute coronary syndromes. N Engl J Med 2006;355:2203–16.

46. Stone GW, Witzenbichler B, Guagliumi G, et al. Bivalirudin during primary PCI in acute myocardial infarction. N Engl J Med 2008;358:2218–30.

47. Lincoff AM, Steinhubl SR, Manoukian SV, et al. Influence of timing of clopidogrel treatment on the efficacy and safety of bivalirudin in patients with non-ST-segment elevation acute coronary syndromes undergoing percutaneous coronary intervention: an analysis of the ACUITY (Acute Catheterization and Urgent Intervention Triage strategY) trial. JACC Cardiovasc Interv 2008;1:639–48.

48. Brandt JT, Payne CD, Wiviott SD, et al. A comparison of prasugrel and clopidogrel loading doses on platelet function: magnitude of platelet inhibition is related to active metabolite formation. Am Heart J 2007;153:66.e9–66.e16.

49. Gurbel PA, Bliden KP, Butler K, et al. Randomized double-blind assessment of the ONSET and OFFSET of the antiplatelet effects of ticagrelor versus clopidogrel in patients with stable coronary artery disease: the ONSET/OFFSET study. Circulation 2009;120:2577–85.

50. Cortese B, Picchi A, Micheli A, et al. Comparison of prolonged bivalirudin infusion versus intraprocedural in preventing myocardial damage after percutaneous coronary intervention in patients with angina pectoris. Am J Cardiol 2009;104: 1063–8.

51. Cortese B, Limbruno U, Severi S, et al. Effect of prolonged bivalirudin infusion on ST-segment resolution following primary percutaneous coronary intervention (from the PROBI VIRI 2 study). Am J Cardiol 2011;108:1220–4.

52. Anderson PR, Gogo PB, Ahmed B, et al. Two hour bivalirudin infusion after PCI for ST elevation myocardial infarction. J Thromb Thrombolysis 2011;31:401–6.

53. Rentrop P, Blanke H, Karsch KR, et al. Selective intracoronary thrombolysis in acute myocardial infarction and unstable angina pectoris. Circulation 1981;63:307–17.

54. Van de Werf F, Ludbrook PA, Bergmann SR, et al. Coronary thrombolysis with tissue-type plasminogen activator in patients with evolving myocardial infarction. N Engl J Med 1984;310:609–13.

55. Ganz W, Buchbinder N, Marcus H, et al. Intracoronary thrombolysis in evolving myocardial infarction. Am Heart J 1981;101:4–13.

56. Pavlides GS, Schreiber TL, Gangadharan V, et al. Safety and efficacy of urokinase during elective coronary angioplasty. Am Heart J 1991;121:731–7.

57. Zeiher AM, Kasper W, Gaissmaier C, et al. Concomitant intracoronary treatment with urokinase during PTCA does not reduce acute complications during PTCA: a double-blind randomized study (abstract). Circulation 1990;82(III):189.

58. Ambrose JA, Almeida OD, Sharma SK, et al. Adjunctive thrombolytic therapy during angioplasty for ischemic rest angina. Results of the TAUSA trial. TAUSA Investigators. Thrombolysis and Angioplasty in Unstable Angina trial. Circulation 1994; 90:69–77.

59. Mehran R, Ambrose JA, Bongu RM, et al. Angioplasty of complex lesions in ischemic rest angina: results of the Thrombolysis and Angioplasty in Unstable Angina (TAUSA) trial. J Am Coll Cardiol 1995;26:961–6.

60. Sezer M, Oflaz H, Gören T, et al. Intracoronary streptokinase after primary percutaneous coronary intervention. N Engl J Med 2007;356:1823–34.

61. Erbel R, Pop T, Henrichs KJ, et al. Percutaneous transluminal coronary angioplasty after thrombolytic therapy: a prospective controlled randomized trial. J Am Coll Cardiol 1986;8:485–95.

62. Suryapranata H, Serruys PW, de Feyter PJ, et al. Coronary angioplasty immediately after thrombolysis in 115 consecutive patients with acute myocardial infarction. Am Heart J 1988;115:519–29.

63. Vermeer F, Simoons ML, de Feyter PJ, et al. Immediate PTCA after successful thrombolysis with intracoronary streptokinase, three years follow-up. A matched pair analysis of the effect of PTCA in the

randomized multicentre trial of intracoronary strep-tokinase, conducted by the Interuniversity Cardiology Institute of The Netherlands. Eur Heart J 1988;9:346–53.

64. Keeley EC, Boura JA, Grines CL. Comparison of primary and facilitated percutaneous coronary interventions for ST-elevation myocardial infarction: quantitative review of randomised trials. Lancet 2006;367:579–88.

65. Kushner FG, Hand M, Smith SC, et al. 2009 focused updates: ACC/AHA guidelines for the management of patients with ST-elevation myocardial infarction (updating the 2004 guideline and 2007 focused update) and ACC/AHA/SCAI guidelines on percutaneous coronary intervention (updating the 2005 guideline and 2007 focused update) a report of the American College of Cardiology Foundation/American Heart Association Task Force on Practice Guidelines. J Am Coll Cardiol 2009;54:2205–41.

66. Assessment of the Safety and Efficacy of a New Treatment Strategy with Percutaneous Coronary Intervention (ASSENT-4 PCI) investigators. Primary versus tenecteplase-facilitated percutaneous coronary intervention in patients with ST-segment elevation acute myocardial infarction (ASSENT-4 PCI): randomised trial. Lancet 2006;367:569–78.

67. Ellis SG, Tendera M, de Belder MA, et al. Facilitated PCI in patients with ST-elevation myocardial infarction. N Engl J Med 2008;358:2205–17.

68. Di Mario C, Dudek D, Piscione F, et al. Immediate angioplasty versus standard therapy with rescue angioplasty after thrombolysis in the Combined Abciximab REteplase Stent Study in Acute Myocardial Infarction (CARESS-in-AMI): an open, prospective, randomised, multicentre trial. Lancet 2008;371:559–68.

69. Cantor WJ, Fitchett D, Borgundvaag B, et al. Routine early angioplasty after fibrinolysis for acute myocardial infarction. N Engl J Med 2009;360:2705–18.

70. Gurbel PA, Navetta FI, Bates ER, et al. Lesion-directed administration of alteplase with intracoronary heparin in patients with unstable angina and coronary thrombus undergoing angioplasty. Cathet Cardiovasc Diagn 1996;37:382–91.

71. Chapekis AT, George BS, Candela RJ. Rapid thrombus dissolution by continuous infusion of urokinase through an intracoronary perfusion wire prior to and following PTCA: results in native coronaries and patent saphenous vein grafts. Cathet Cardiovasc Diagn 1991;23:89–92.

72. McKay RG, Fram DB, Hirst JA, et al. Treatment of intracoronary thrombus with local urokinase infusion using a new, site-specific drug delivery system: the dispatch catheter. Cathet Cardiovasc Diagn 1994;33:181–8.

73. Mitchel JF, Barry JJ, Bow L, et al. Local urokinase delivery with the Channel balloon: device safety, pharmacokinetics of intracoronary drug delivery, and efficacy of thrombolysis. Cathet Cardiovasc Diagn 1997;41:254–60.

74. Saito T, Hokimoto S, Ishibashi F, et al. Pulse infusion thrombolysis (PIT) for large intracoronary thrombus: preventive effect against the 'no flow' phenomenon in revascularization therapy for acute myocardial infarction. Jpn Circ J 2001;65:94–8.

75. Kim JS, Kim JH, Jang HH, et al. Successful revascularization of coronary artery occluded by massive intracoronary thrombi with alteplase and percutaneous coronary intervention. J Atheroscler Thromb 2010;17:768–70.

76. Agarwal SK. Pharmacoinvasive therapy for acute myocardial infarction. Cathet Cardiovasc Diagn 2011;78:72–5.

77. Suryapranata H, de Feyter PJ, Serruys PW. Coronary angioplasty in patients with unstable angina pectoris: is there a role for thrombolysis? J Am Coll Cardiol 1988;12:69A–77A.

78. Verna E, Repetto S, Boscarini M, et al. Management of complicated coronary angioplasty by intracoronary urokinase and immediate re-angioplasty. Cathet Cardiovasc Diagn 1990;19:116–22.

79. Schieman G, Cohen BM, Kozina J, et al. Intracoronary urokinase for intracoronary thrombus accumulation complicating percutaneous transluminal coronary angioplasty in acute ischemic syndromes. Circulation 1990;82:2052–60.

80. Goudreau E, DiSciascio G, Vetrovec GW, et al. Intracoronary urokinase as an adjunct to percutaneous transluminal coronary angioplasty in patients with complex coronary narrowings or angioplasty-induced complications. Am J Cardiol 1992;69:57–62.

81. Lincoff AM, Popma JJ, Ellis SG, et al. Abrupt vessel closure complicating coronary angioplasty: clinical, angiographic and therapeutic profile. J Am Coll Cardiol 1992;19:926–35.

82. Kelly RV, Crouch E, Krumnacher H, et al. Safety of adjunctive intracoronary thrombolytic therapy during complex percutaneous coronary intervention: initial experience with intracoronary tenecteplase. Catheter Cardiovasc Interv 2005;66:327–32.

83. De Luca G, Suryapranata H, Stone GW, et al. Abciximab as adjunctive therapy to reperfusion in acute ST-segment elevation myocardial infarction: a meta-analysis of randomized trials. JAMA 2005;293:1759–65.

84. De Luca G, Suryapranata H, Stone GW, et al. Relationship between patient's risk profile and benefits in mortality from adjunctive abciximab to mechanical revascularization for ST-segment elevation myocardial infarction: a meta-regression analysis of randomized trials. J Am Coll Cardiol 2006;47:685–6.

85. De Luca G, Navarese E, Marino P. Risk profile and benefits from Gp IIb-IIIa inhibitors among patients with ST-segment elevation myocardial infarction treated with primary angioplasty: a meta-regression analysis of randomized trials. Eur Heart J 2009;30:2705–13.

86. Montalescot G, Antoniucci D, Kastrati A, et al. Abciximab in primary coronary stenting of ST-elevation myocardial infarction: a European meta-analysis on individual patients' data with long-term follow-up. Eur Heart J 2007;28:443–9.

87. Gurm HS, Tamhane U, Meier P, et al. A comparison of abciximab and small-molecule glycoprotein IIb/IIIa inhibitors in patients undergoing primary percutaneous coronary intervention: a meta-analysis of contemporary randomized controlled trials. Circ Cardiovasc Interv 2009;2:230–6.

88. De Luca G, Ucci G, Cassetti E, et al. Benefits from small molecule administration as compared with abciximab among patients with ST-segment elevation myocardial infarction treated with primary angioplasty: a meta-analysis. J Am Coll Cardiol 2009;53:1668–73.

89. Hansen PR, Iversen A, Abdulla J. Improved clinical outcomes with intracoronary compared to intravenous abciximab in patients with acute coronary syndromes undergoing percutaneous coronary intervention: a systematic review and meta-analysis. J Invasive Cardiol 2010;22:278–82.

90. Friedland S, Eisenberg MJ, Shimony A. Meta-analysis of randomized controlled trials of intracoronary versus intravenous administration of glycoprotein IIb/IIIa inhibitors during percutaneous coronary intervention for acute coronary syndrome. Am J Cardiol 2011;108:1244–51.

91. Shimada YJ, Nakra NC, Fox JT, et al. Meta-analysis of prospective randomized controlled trials comparing intracoronary versus intravenous abciximab in patients with ST-elevation myocardial infarction undergoing primary percutaneous coronary intervention. Am J Cardiol 2012;109:624–8.

92. Wang Y, Wu B, Shu X. Meta-analysis of randomized controlled trials comparing intracoronary and intravenous administration of glycoprotein IIb/IIIa inhibitors in patients with ST-elevation myocardial infarction. Am J Cardiol 2012;109:1124–30.

93. Thiele H, Wohrle J, Hambrecht R, et al. Intracoronary versus intravenous bolus abciximab during primary percutaneous coronary intervention in patients with acute ST-elevation myocardial infarction: a randomised trial. Lancet 2012;379:923–31.

94. Stone GW, Maehara A, Witzenbichler B, et al. Intracoronary abciximab and aspiration thrombectomy in patients with large anterior myocardial infarction: the INFUSE-AMI randomized trial. JAMA 2012. http://dx.doi.org/10.1001/jama.2012.421.

95. Muhlestein JB, Karagounis LA, Treehan S, et al. 'Rescue' utilization of abciximab for the dissolution of coronary thrombus developing as a complication of coronary angioplasty. J Am Coll Cardiol 1997;30:1729–34.

96. Garbarz E, Farah B, Vuillemenot A, et al. 'Rescue' abciximab for complicated percutaneous transluminal coronary angioplasty. Am J Cardiol 1998;82:800–3 A9.

97. van den Brand M, Laarman GJ, Steg PG, et al. Assessment of coronary angiograms prior to and after treatment with abciximab, and the outcome of angioplasty in refractory unstable angina patients. Angiographic results from the CAPTURE trial. Eur Heart J 1999;20:1572–8.

98. Chen ZM, Jiang LX, Chen YP, et al. Addition of clopidogrel to aspirin in 45,852 patients with acute myocardial infarction: randomised placebo-controlled trial. Lancet 2005;366:1607–21.

99. Sabatine MS, Cannon CP, Gibson CM, et al. Addition of clopidogrel to aspirin and fibrinolytic therapy for myocardial infarction with ST-segment elevation. N Engl J Med 2005;352:1179–89.

100. Dangas G, Mehran R, Guagliumi G, et al. Role of clopidogrel loading dose in patients with ST-segment elevation myocardial infarction undergoing primary angioplasty: results from the HORIZONS-AMI (harmonizing outcomes with revascularization and stents in acute myocardial infarction) trial. J Am Coll Cardiol 2009;54:1438–46.

101. Mangiacapra F, Muller O, Ntalianis A, et al. Comparison of 600 versus 300-mg clopidogrel loading dose in patients with ST-segment elevation myocardial infarction undergoing primary coronary angioplasty. Am J Cardiol 2010;106:1208–11.

102. Steg PG, James S, Harrington RA, et al. Ticagrelor versus clopidogrel in patients with ST-elevation acute coronary syndromes intended for reperfusion with primary percutaneous coronary intervention: a Platelet Inhibition and Patient Outcomes (PLATO) trial subgroup analysis. Circulation 2010;122:2131–41.

103. Seides SF, Borer JS, Kent KM, et al. Long-term anatomic fate of coronary-artery bypass grafts and functional status of patients five years after operation. N Engl J Med 1978;298:1213–7.

104. Reeves F, Bonan R, Côté G, et al. Long-term angiographic follow-up after angioplasty of venous coronary bypass grafts. Am Heart J 1991;122:620–7.

105. Frimerman A, Rechavia E, Eigler N, et al. Long-term follow-up of a high risk cohort after stent implantation in saphenous vein grafts. J Am Coll Cardiol 1997;30:1277–83.

106. de Feyter PJ, van Suylen RJ, de Jaegere PP, et al. Balloon angioplasty for the treatment of lesions in saphenous vein bypass grafts. J Am Coll Cardiol 1993;21:1539–49.

107. Coolong A, Baim DS, Kuntz RE, et al. Saphenous vein graft stenting and major adverse cardiac events: a predictive model derived from a pooled analysis of 3958 patients. Circulation 2008;117:790–7.

108. Marx M, Armstrong WT, Brent BN, et al. Transcatheter recanalization of a chronically occluded saphenous aortocoronary bypass graft. AJR Am J Roentgenol 1987;148:375–7.

109. Hartmann J, McKeever L, Teran J, et al. Prolonged infusion of urokinase for recanalization of chronically occluded aortocoronary bypass grafts. Am J Cardiol 1988;61:189–91.

110. Marx M, Armstrong WP, Wack JP, et al. Short-duration, high-dose urokinase infusion for recanalization of occluded saphenous aortocoronary bypass grafts. AJR Am J Roentgenol 1989;153:167–71.

111. Kuntz RE, Baim DS, Cohen DJ, et al. A trial comparing rheolytic thrombectomy with intracoronary urokinase for coronary and vein graft thrombus (the Vein Graft AngioJet Study [VeGAS 2]). Am J Cardiol 2002;89:326–30.

112. Robinson N, Barakat K, Dymond D. Platelet IIb/IIIa antagonists followed by delayed stent implantation. A new treatment for vein graft lesions containing massive thrombus. Heart 1999;81:434–7.

113. Barsness GW, Buller C, Ohman EM, et al. Reduced thrombus burden with abciximab delivered locally before percutaneous intervention in saphenous vein grafts. Am Heart J 2000;139:824–9.

114. Gruberg L, Amikam S. Prolonged systemic delivery of tirofiban in a thrombus-laden saphenous vein graft. Int J Cardiovasc Intervent 2003;5:92–4.

115. Roffi M, Mukherjee D, Chew DP, et al. Lack of benefit from intravenous platelet glycoprotein IIb/IIIa receptor inhibition as adjunctive treatment for percutaneous interventions of aortocoronary bypass grafts a pooled analysis of five randomized clinical trials. Circulation 2002;106:3063–7.

# Index

Intervent Cardiol Clin 2 (2013) 389–395
http://dx.doi.org/10.1016/S2211-7458(13)00010-2
2211-7458/13/$ – see front matter © 2013 Elsevier Inc. All rights reserved.

Printed and bound by CPI Group (UK) Ltd, Croydon, CR0 4YY

12/10/2024

01773417-0001